THE ELK HUNT

THE ELK HUNT

ALAN E. NOURSE, M.D.

MACMILLAN PUBLISHING COMPANY
New York

Macmillan Publishing Company
866 Third Avenue, New York, N.Y. 10022
Collier Macmillan Canada, Inc.

Library of Congress Cataloging-in-Publication Data
Nourse, Alan Edward.
The elk hunt.
Includes index.
1. Coronary heart disease—Popular works.   I. Title.
RC685.C6N66   1986   616.1'23   86-8332
ISBN 0-02-590700-X

Macmillan books are available at special discounts for bulk purchases
for sales promotions, premiums, fund-raising, or educational use.
For details, contact:

Special Sales Director
Macmillan Publishing Company
866 Third Avenue
New York, N.Y. 10022

10 9 8 7 6 5 4 3 2 1

Printed in the United States of America

For Ann, who was there, with love

and for

Fred E. Cleveland, Jr., M.D.,
Robin R. Johnston, M.D., and
Richard P. Anderson, M.D.,
with gratitude

— CONTENTS —

INTRODUCTION

ix

I

CATASTROPHE

1

II

INVESTIGATIONS

93

III

BENCHMARKS

151

IV

THE CUTTING EDGE

211

CONTENTS

AFTERWORD
293

INDEX
295

─ INTRODUCTION ─

This book has a great deal to say about coronary artery disease—where it comes from, what it can do to you, and how you can prevent it from happening.

When my oldest son, Ben, age twenty-seven, read the first draft of the manuscript he said, "It's a good book—but nobody's going to read it until they've already had a heart attack."

I profoundly hope that he is wrong.

Six years ago, on the night of October 24, 1980, at the age of fifty-two, and without any warning, I suffered a severe and massive heart attack—an acute myocardial infarction, to use the medical term. That night changed my life—and it changed my children's lives as well. In the course of that night I presented Ben, as well as my two other sons and my daughter, with a most unkind and involuntary burden: an active family history of coronary artery disease, a major risk factor for a disease that had never existed before in our family.

Ben and the others must now live and deal with this risk factor for the rest of their lives. Twenty or thirty years from now any one of them may follow in their father's footsteps—but they don't have to. Explicit in this book is a body of basic knowledge about the ways that they, and multitudes of others like them, can escape.

In spite of its title, this is not a book about hunting elk. But in a very real sense it is a book about an elk hunt—a continuing search for an elusive quarry: a search for solutions to a dreadful disease. Parts of the book are very much about *me* and my individual experience, but far more important, it is a sourcebook for *you* to use, ideally before catastrophe strikes.

The best of all possible solutions to coronary artery disease is prevention, and in that sense knowledge is power. No one can use basic knowledge about this disease to protect you better than you yourself can, and the earlier you start, the better—but you are the one who must do it. Thirty years ago nobody knew too much about how you could protect yourself; today we know a great deal, and we know that prevention *works*. I hope this book will open a door.

—Alan E. Nourse, M.D.
Thorp, Washington
June 1986

THE ELK HUNT

I

CATASTROPHE

— 1 —

It was almost two o'clock on a brilliant late October afternoon when I finally saw the bull elk that Ann and I had been searching for since dawn.

From daybreak on we had been working our way through brush and forest in one of our favorite hunting spots—down below Cedar Meadows, down over the edge of the mountain on the steep north slope of Cle Elum Ridge in the eastern foothills of the Washington Cascades near our home. At first light that day we had driven down a mile or so of steep logging road and parked the Bronco on a small landing; from there we proceeded on foot. At this point the forested hillside was interrupted by a broad, sloping bench of land some three miles wide and a mile across. To the north the land fell gently to a broad saddle and then rose again to a major promontory before plunging steeply down to the valley floor far below. It was the kind of country the elk loved—dense and protected, with a steep escapeway nearby—and we had spotted elk in this area many times in previous years—always, it seemed, at the wrong time or in the wrong season. On this particular day the opening of the coming elk season was still a week away, and we were pretending we were hunting deer, but the truth was we were scouting for elk, hoping the great animals would be there again this year when the season finally began.

We knew from the start it would be a hard and exhausting day's hunting. The country was steep up-and-down, filled with dense brush and thickets. I was fifty-two years old at the time, six feet tall, a flabby 220 pounds, and not exactly an Olympic athlete. Although I was apparently healthy enough, I didn't believe in exercise except during hunting season, and I smoked two packs of cigarettes a day. My wife, Ann, at age forty-eight, was a little more spry, but

3

not a great deal; at least she had never smoked. But we were accustomed to hard hunting days during elk season. As we moved
away from the car, we fell into a hunting pattern we had used here
many times before. We separated, with Ann moving off to the right,
following an old cat road along the top of the bench to the head of
a large gully, then cutting downhill in a broad curve to the saddle
three-quarters of a mile below. I turned to the left, following a well-
used game trail along the bench, keeping to the upper side of a
number of small ridges, and then gradually dropping down and down
into a densely wooded pocket. At the bottom of the pocket, some
two miles from Ann's saddle, an ancient lake had dried up into a
small swamp surrounded by dense vine maple and Douglas fir thickets. A broad game trail circumnavigated that swamp and then passed
through a large open forest of fir and pine, a major crossing point
and meeting place for elk passing through. It was our plan that I
would hunt the swamp and thickets slowly and quietly while Ann
circled down from the saddle to meet me at the lower edge of the
forest two or three hours later.

The day was bright and crisply cold, a perfect Cascades autumn
day. My route down into the pocket passed through beautiful elk
country: old fir and pine forest, dense but open, with areas free from
underbrush; scattered clusters of aspen trees turning golden green,
and scarlet vine maples. The floor of the forest was crisscrossed with
windfalls but open enough for easy travel. I made my way along
slowly and silently, stopping now and then to sit on a log, motionless
for five or ten minutes, listening and watching. Like all game trails
in the area, this one was constantly forking, frequently joined by
side trails, sometimes disappearing completely and then reappearing
a little farther on, but generally this was a major elk path. It had
rained the night before, but dozens of tracks remained in the damp
earth and pine duff, some obviously old, some so recent that the
hoof marks were sharp, the ground freshly scuffed. One could fairly
sense the imminent presence of the animals in these woods, yet all
the way down into the pocket the only animal I actually saw was a
big old porcupine waddling off the trail into the woods when he saw
me coming.

Once down in the bottom of the pocket, I rested awhile, watching
and listening. Then I moved around the swamp as silently as possible,
checking out side trails into the thickets. Presently I found the broad
game trail through the thick woods beyond the swamp, reached a
huge log where Ann and I usually met, and sat down to post. It was
a lonely place, beautiful and silent, and once again I had the strong
sense of déjà vu I often felt here. I knew I sometimes dreamed about

this place, and now an eerie sixth sense told me that elk had been through here very recently.

The elk that frequented these wooded mountain slopes were the native Roosevelt elk, or *wapiti*, from the Shawnee Indian term meaning "white rump"—canniest and most elusive of the great forest deer. They are startlingly *big* animals. A cow elk, encountered in the woods, will appear absolutely enormous, with her gray-brown body; her blackish head, neck and legs; and her beige-colored rump. When startled she will bolt away with an enormous crashing of brush and snapping of tree limbs, sounding like a freight train going through the woods, and then—abruptly—vanish so swiftly and suddenly that you just can't believe that anything that big could possibly disappear that fast. A bull elk may stand as high as a horse, with antlers rising up another four feet and spreading out three feet or more—a majestic creature. Sometimes bulls will run with the cows during the hunting season, but more often they tend to be solitary, bursting out of their cover with a speed and agility that defy description. We had seen such bulls at close quarters, now and then, over the years and knew that a single glimpse of one in the woods is worth all the hard work of a whole hunting season.

Ann and I had hunted elk faithfully every season since we had first come to the Cascade foothills decades before. Those two autumn weeks in the woods were, for us, the high point of every year. We would spend the winter trading hunting tales with our friends, spring and summer poring over maps of our favorite hunting areas, eager for the fall. We were no serious menace to the wildlife; in more than two decades of hunting, neither Ann nor I had actually taken a bull elk, and sometimes we would pause to ask ourselves why we kept doing this—but every autumn we were back exploring the logging roads and game trails as the excitement and anticipation grew. Someday, who could tell, we might just be at the right place at the right time. . . .

Now, sitting and waiting, I heard a twig snap off to my right, and then saw Ann in her red hat coming down through the woods toward me. While she rested, we debated where to go next. There was another area we could explore from this point—a long, hard hunt seldom tried by other hunters. Beyond the swamp was a major game trail disappearing into dense forest, a veritable "elk highway" that traversed the steep slope of the ridge for a mile or more. There the trail worked its way up a wooded side hill onto a beautiful promontory, a flat benchlike area covered with long grass dappled with sunlight coming down through the pines. The first time we had come upon that rise of land we had named it the Elk Tuileries, a stately

5

Enchanted Forest of a place—"Exactly the spot I'd go to if I were an elk," as Ann had put it.

We started off a little before noon on the slow, difficult trip. Though the trail was well beaten, it was by no means wide or commodious—no more than six inches across, frequently disappearing into patches of brush and then reappearing farther on. The slope it traversed was extremely steep, in some places so sheer that if one lost his footing he might slide down two hundred feet or more before he could stop himself. We made our way along slowly and unsteadily, rifles slung on our shoulders, climbing up over windfalls and down into two or three dry gullies. The tall trees here obscured the sun, creating an odd midday twilight. Gradually the trail worked its way downward around the shoulder of the hill and into a deep, swampy ravine with running water in it, an area literally torn up with fresh elk tracks.

We stopped to rest in the ravine before starting up the trail that curved around the side of the next steep hill. I was feeling surprisingly tired by them, and the climb up that hill looked formidable, but that was all right, I thought—it would slow us down. I took the lead, with Ann a few feet behind me, taking two or three steps, then stopping to watch and listen, then taking two or three more steps. It was one in the afternoon by then, but we had plenty of time.

Quiet and cautious as we were, we weren't cautious enough. As I approached the top of the rise, the trail leveled out just below the crown of the hill, and it was just at that point that I saw the bull elk rise up from his bed fifty yards above me.

He was a magnificent creature, with a great rack of horns thrown back on his shoulders, his chin raised high in the air. Whether it was scent or sound that had warned him I could only guess, but he didn't pause or look back. He rose from the ground at a dead run and dropped straight down over the steep side of the hill. I saw his full body for less than a second; then his tawny haunches and white rump were disappearing down the slope through the trees, gone within another two seconds. The cracking and snapping of branches and underbrush in his path seemed to go on forever.

I knew there was no point going down the hill after him—we were scouting, not hunting. We knew that elk might very well go five miles before stopping, with no perceptible trail to follow. We climbed on up into the Elk Tuileries and found a dozen new-looking beds—a whole herd of elk had been frequenting the place. By then it was almost two o'clock. We sat down to munch our lunchtime sandwiches and prepare for the long trip back. As it happened, a piano tuner was due at our house at four, and we had to be there to meet him.

We started back along the trail, slipping and misstepping as we tried to hurry. Suddenly I found that I was very tired—far more tired than I had any reason to be. I began stopping to catch my breath, repeatedly slowing us down, and I thought we would never get back to the pocket. Once there, we then had the long climb up to the car. I panted and puffed, pausing frequently to rest and sweating profusely, although clouds were coming in and the air had turned cold. At one point I told Ann to go on ahead, I just couldn't keep up with her, so we stopped for a ten-minute break. Finally, and it seemed like forever, we got back to the car and were heading for home a little before four.

The piano tuner was waiting when we got there. He tinkled and twanged for an hour and a half while I showered and changed, still totally exhausted. Ann started a fireplace fire and made martinis; the piano tuner joined us for a Mexican beer before he left. Ann had popped a beef heart into the oven on slow-bake before we'd left that morning, so she finished preparing supper and we ate like starving hounds. By eight in the evening we had our clothing laid out for a quick departure in the morning and were both in bed, anticipating the next day's hunting. My mind was still filled with the bull elk I'd seen that afternoon; I had never before so badly wanted an elk hunt to begin.

I went to sleep, exhausted. Then, a little before midnight, I woke up with an agonizing, crushing pain in my chest, a choking pain that would not go away, and I knew that there wasn't going to be any elk hunt for me that year.

— 2 —

One of the problems of being a doctor faced with a personal medical calamity is knowing too much about what's going on—and doing all the wrong things just the same.

As a doctor, I knew perfectly well what was happening to me when I woke up with that pain in my chest. There was never any question in my mind, yet I could not believe or accept it, so I did a long series of stupid things instead of what I should have done.

First, I sat up in bed motionless for almost five minutes waiting for the pain to go away. Of course, it didn't, but during that time the pain *changed*, and it was a very singular kind of pain. At first it seemed like a vast, crushing pressure in my chest, just to the left of the breastbone. Moment by moment it grew more heavy and severe; at one point there almost seemed to be a sound to it. At the same time I began perspiring and felt cold and slightly short of breath. I tried taking my pulse: It was racing, but very weak and thready, so I could barely feel it—a characteristic, I knew, of heart attacks. Within a few minutes the pain, while still centered in my chest, seemed to spread down my entire left arm—a deep, aching pain, down the shoulder, the elbow, the wrist, until my thumb and one or two of my fingers were throbbing. Then, in addition, I felt it in my neck and up into my jaw on the left side, almost up to the ear. I remember that the teeth in my lower jaw began aching fiercely on the left side, but the pain stopped abruptly at the midline—the teeth on the right side felt just fine.

Within five minutes I couldn't sit still any longer—the pain was too intense—so I got up from bed, went out into the kitchen and mixed a little bicarbonate of soda in some water and drank it, telling myself maybe this was just indigestion from eating too much rich dinner. For a while I paced the floor back and forth, waiting for the bicarbonate to help, but, of course, it didn't. I even lit a cigarette and smoked it, my invariable habit anytime I awakened at night for any reason, even though I knew at that moment that this was perhaps the least sane action I could have taken. Finally I went back and sat on the edge of the bed, hoping against hope that the pain would simply subside.

I must have delayed a full half-hour from the beginning of that chest pain before I finally reached over and shook Ann awake. "I think you'd better get up and get dressed," I told her. "I'm having a heart attack, and I'm afraid we're going to have to do something about it."

The question was what to do, and it was a good question. We were living in a house at the edge of a remote wilderness area, on a creek up a narrow canyon, with the nearest neighbor a quarter-mile away. The place was located sixteen miles from the small town of Cle Elum to the west, fifteen miles from the larger town of Ellensburg to the east.

We were new to the area. Although we had had this vacation home there for years, we had only come to live there full-time a few months earlier, and we knew very little about local medical facilities. We knew there was a small community hospital in Ellensburg but had met none of the doctors there. In Cle Elum there was a family practice clinic with an emergency room, and Ann, a physical therapist, had met Dr. John Anderson, a general practitioner there, through her physical therapy work. It struck me at the time that I would rather contact a doctor one of us had met than take off blind to an institution where we knew nobody, so Ann called the Cle Elum clinic number. She talked to a nurse on duty and told her what was happening. The nurse said she would contact the doctor right away and to hang up so that he could call back. I moved over to sit near the phone while Ann hastily got dressed. In less than five minutes Dr. Anderson was on the phone. I told him as briefly as possible what was happening, answered a question or two. When I finished, he said, "Don't come here, you'll lose too much time. Have your wife take you directly to the hospital in Ellensburg. They have facilities for coronary care there that I don't have here, and it sounds as though you may need them. Call the hospital before you leave so they can be contacting whichever doctor is on call down there while you're on your way."

I reported this to Ann. At first she was annoyed that Dr. Anderson didn't want to see me himself, but after a moment's reflection we realized he had given me absolutely the best advice possible. I knew enough to know that if this really was a heart attack, there were quite a number of serious things to worry about, and they were not things any doctor could hope to deal with effectively anywhere other than in a well-equipped hospital. Of course I couldn't be certain it was a heart attack, but there was no question that something malign was going on inside my chest. Rather than easing or subsiding, the pain was steadily deepening and thickening, not so much a sharp pain now as a grinding, crushing ache, continuous and unremitting, involving my chest, shoulder, left arm, and jaw. I was also aware of a deepening, deadening exhaustion; I was having trouble breathing and could hardly muster strength even to talk. I just sat there next to the phone while Ann placed a call to the hospital to tell them what was happening and that we were coming. Then she ran outside to start the car.

When she came back, she was sopping wet—it was pouring rain outside. She brought me my bathrobe and slippers and helped me struggle into them; I knew there was no way I could get fully dressed. It seemed to take forever, getting my arms into the sleeves. I clearly remember thinking, maybe this is it, buster, maybe you're just going out right here and now, and it puzzled me that I wasn't feeling scared when I should have been terrified. All I felt was the pain and wanting it to stop at any cost. Maybe I wasn't thinking clearly enough to be scared. Once the robe was on, Ann had to half support me as I staggered to the door and down the steps to the car. By the time I got into the passenger seat I was pretty much out of it. All I could do was sit hunched over, clutching the armrest and hoping that we

9

could get somewhere soon. From that point on Ann's account, re-corded later, tells the story far more clearly than anything I can remember:*

When I ran out to start the car, I had taken the dog and put her in the backseat because I had no idea how long we might be. Once Alan had his robe on, we started out the door. He was obviously very uncomfortable, but was able to get out of the house and down the steps by hanging on to me and the railing. Finally he was in the car. We left there with all the doors of the house wide open and all the lights still on, and I drove as fast as I could toward the highway, which was not easy because it was raining so hard. I didn't know if this was really a heart attack or not, but I knew that something terrible had happened, and I remember telling Alan that I loved him because I was afraid he was about to die; I don't know if he even heard me. He didn't talk to me at all, but he was breathing and was not unconscious. I tried to drive as carefully as I could and still keep an eye on him to be sure he didn't slump over or lose consciousness, because I knew that might mean cardiac arrest, and then it would be important to do cardiopulmonary resuscitation. (I had reviewed CPR techniques every six months for probably the last ten years while I was working at University Hospital and later at Providence Hospital in Seattle, so at least I had some basic idea how to do it.) Fortunately, he did not stop breathing or go into cardiac arrest, two of the terrible things that I knew could happen during a heart attack. I drove down the back road alongside the freeway to the first interchange, then took the freeway from there to Ellensburg.

When we got to the hospital door I parked the car right there and rang the emergency bell. A young man came out with a wheelchair, and we got Alan into it, even though he protested that he could walk, and hurried him down the hall. A nurse appeared and took him into a room that was used as this small hospital's Coronary Care Unit or CCU. I told the nurse that Alan was a physician and thought he was having a heart attack and I was pretty sure he was. We helped him get onto the bed, taking off the robe and slippers. The clock on the wall said just five minutes to one in the morning, so we hadn't lost as much time as I thought we had.

Other nurses came into the room, including a middle-aged woman with blond hair who immediately started putting an IV line into Alan's left wrist. (They *always* start an intravenous infusion into any patient's vein the minute they get him into bed, in case they have to get emergency medications into him *immediately*. It's routine—it doesn't even take a doctor's order.) She had a lot of difficulty getting the IV in, and Alan was

---

* Ann says she is not a writer and never will be, but when it became clear that I was going to write The Elk Hunt, she agreed to write out her impressions of things that happened during the critical period, to record details that I might not recall or couldn't have been aware of.

extremely uncomfortable. Another nurse, who had already been in contact with a doctor on call, asked Alan if he'd ever had any allergic trouble with Demerol, then gave him a 100-milligram injection. She said it would help relieve the chest pain, and after five or ten minutes Alan indicated that the pain was easing up a little—but, then, five minutes later, he suddenly became very nauseated and said he had to throw up. I remember helping the nurse hold him up and get an emesis basin to him just in time, and this happened a couple more times in the next ten minutes. Whether this was a reaction to the medicine or just part of the illness I didn't know, but I think the pain medication was later changed to morphine. (I suppose Alan's two martinis and rich dinner a few hours earlier didn't help much, either.)

While this was going on, another young woman came in and took an electrocardiogram. One of the nurses told me that the doctor on call for the Valley Clinic, a Dr. Homer Coppock, was on his way. He arrived within fifteen minutes: an older man with gray hair, dressed in an open-necked shirt, trousers, and a brown sweater. He was a quiet-looking person, slightly sleepy, but aware of what was going on and obviously at ease with this situation. He looked at the EKG tracing and then showed it to me, pointing out some things I didn't understand having to do with T-waves and ST segments. He said that the cardiogram showed that Alan had had, or was having, a heart attack involving the lateral or inferior (underneath) area of the heart, rather than the anterior part. He said that this kind of heart attack wasn't as likely as some others to cause instant death, but it often caused problems with arhythmia that made it just as potentially dangerous. Dr. Coppock said that he would need to see the results of some blood enzyme tests that already has been started before he could be absolutely sure of the diagnosis, but he didn't think there was very much doubt about what it was. As for prognosis, he just shook his head and said that Alan was in very critical condition, and that the next three days would probably be the most critical of all.

Later on, I could remember Dr. Coppock's first visit only very vaguely. I had a fuzzy impression of a small, gray, gentle man who looked very tired and behaved exactly as though this kind of illness was an old, old story to him. I had heard what he told Ann about the electrocardiogram but I didn't really follow him or comprehend much that he said. I was far too groggy from the medicine by then, and wanted nothing more than to put my head back and go to sleep undisturbed. After he left, I was aware of the nurses taping telemetry leads to my chest to start continuous heart monitoring, an endless, ongoing EKG tracing that registered as a jagged green line crawling across the face of an oscilloscope planted near the side of the bed. It registered simultaneously on a similar scope in the nurses' station.

I remember having new IVs hooked up and some other amount of fiddle-faddle having to do with my body, but I guess I dozed off in the middle of it and simply slept.

When I saw Dr. Coppock next it was daylight, and I woke up with a start when he came in the room. The medication must have worn off because I was quite alert and the chest pain was back, although only about half as severe as the night before.

I asked him if the enzyme tests were back yet. He nodded. "We'll run repeats today just to assess progress," he said, "but the first ones confirm the EKG findings."

"Then I really have had a heart attack," I said.

He nodded again and hesitated for a moment. Then, perhaps, he was more candid than usual, knowing I was a doctor, because he told me precisely how things stood in clear medical terms. "You've had an acute posterior MI, and it looks like a major one. It's knocked out a good deal of your right ventricle. You're still with us, so far, but we're going to have to walk on eggs for a while."

The words brought a shock of reality: It hadn't seriously occurred to me that, once I got to the hospital, I might just turn up my toes and die at any moment, but I knew what the medical terms meant. I realized then—with a jolt—that the events of that awful night had irrevocably and permanently altered my life. Whatever else might happen, things were never going to be the same again.

— 3 —

Most often, you will hear it called a *heart attack* or *cardiac attack*. Doctors are more likely to call it a *myocardial infarction*, an MI. Sometimes they will speak of it as a *coronary thrombosis*, a *coronary occlusion*, or just a *coronary*.

All these terms refer, in general, to roughly the same catastrophe, but each term has its own specific meaning. Heart attack, or cardiac attack, for example, are somewhat vague laymen's terms that can refer to almost any sudden, usually painful physical event involving malfunction or damage to the heart, without indicating just what that malfunction might be. When people say, "Jones is a cardiac case," they simply mean that Jones has some (usually unspecified) kind of heart trouble.

The medical term myocardial infarction is much more specific: It refers to the infarction or death of cells or tissues in some portion of the myocardium—the heart muscle itself. The terms coronary, coronary occlusion or coronary thrombosis refer specifically to trouble involving the *coronary arteries,* the small but utterly vital blood vessels that carry oxygenated blood directly into the heart muscle itself and thus keep the heart functioning. When something such as a blood clot or *thrombus* blocks or *occludes* a branch of a coronary artery such that fresh blood cannot get through to a portion of myocardium, the heart muscle cells there begin to starve and die very quickly—in a matter of hours. Those cells become *infarcted* or destroyed, and once this has happened, they will never recover or regenerate. It may not be too bad if only a small section of heart muscle is damaged in this way, but if too much is involved, the injury and shock can cause the heart to lose so much pumping power that the victim dies. Since the layman's term "heart attack" usually refers to this sequence of events, it is generally considered synonymous with a coronary or MI.

A myocardial infarction most often begins as a sudden, catastrophic event—but this does not mean that it takes place instantly and then is all over. Rather, it is a dynamic, progressive sequence of events that starts abruptly but then follows a changing course over a period of minutes, hours, days, even months. We can't really consider it an end point of anything unless the initial damage to the heart is so severe that the patient dies during the first few hours. But underlying the acute onset of a myocardial infarction—leading up to it and bringing it about—is a much more prolonged and continuing disease process known medically as *atherosclerotic heart disease* or ASHD, more commonly called *coronary artery disease* or CAD—still the number-one killer disease in our society today.

This may seem like a great deal of medical jargon packed into a few paragraphs, but these medical terms are loaded with real, down-to-earth meaning for every reader of this book, once we come to understand them. Since the very real hopes we now have of halting the murderous onslaught of this terrible disease depends upon what one can do *before* an acute myocardial infarction occurs as well as what can be done *after* it occurs, it is extremely important for every potential victim of this killer-in-waiting to know some basic facts, as they are understood today, about coronary artery disease from the very beginning.

Who are these potential victims? Every year some 500,000 people in the United States alone suffer acute myocardial infarctions. About 40 percent of those people die within the first few hours after the attack begins. Those who survive will have to live the rest of their lives with the heart damage that ultimately results from the acute attack. Sooner or later almost every family is going to be touched in *some* way, with some member afflicted by coronary artery disease to some degree or another.

These are plain facts. As little as twenty-five years ago, knowing all this wasn't very useful. When a heart attack struck it came out of the blue, as a sort of act of God, and once it had occurred, there wasn't a great deal that even the best of doctors could do but make the patient as comfortable as possible, and hope that he might survive the acute attack and limp along for a while with whatever heart damage had occurred. Sometimes, in those days, it seemed that the less the patient knew about what was actually going on, the better— knowing a lot wasn't going to be any help, to speak of.

Today all this has changed dramatically. In the past twenty-five years we have seen almost incredible advances in our understanding of how and why coronary artery disease comes about in the first place, and what modern medicine and surgery can do about it when it strikes. We are no longer helpless in the face of this disease. Today we are on the cutting edge of remarkable medical and technological progress in dealing with this killer when it appears—progress that is saving thousands of lives that might have been lost just a few years ago. Most important of all, today the notion that the catastrophes of coronary artery disease *can in large part be prevented before they occur* is finally coming into focus. We know that the potential victim can take active, practical, matter-of-fact steps to protect him- or herself from disaster—given enough solid knowledge to put those steps into action.

How much can or should the average layman know about coronary artery disease? I am convinced that the more any person knows about this enemy, the more effectively he can guard against catastrophe or cope with it when it strikes. As a doctor, I already knew a good deal more about heart disease than most people do long before that night in October when my number came up. That knowledge didn't help me prevent my catastrophe—I had been doing too many things wrong for too many years, and like so many others, was too heedless to try to change. But, as we will see, that knowledge was an enormous help to me in dealing with what subsequently happened. Surely it affected the course and outcome of my treatment. It helped me protect myself, and it affected my ability to communicate with my doctors and them with me.

That knowledge worked strongly for me. What was more, I added to it constantly—after all, I had a box seat from which to witness everything that happened, to ask the questions that my doctors had to answer to clarify confusing points in my mind. I believe that knowledge can work strongly for others, too. It is my goal in writing this book to pass on as much of that knowledge as possible, as accurately as possible, but in terms that are clear and simple enough for any nondoctor to understand.

Part of this book is an intensely personal chronological account of a catastrophe that happened to me, as I perceived it, and how it affected me, my wife, my family, and my future. Another part is a detailed picture of the disease itself—how it comes about, what it can do, how it can be dealt with today, and, above all, how it can be prevented. Basically, coronary artery disease is a disease of blood vessels, and the place to begin understanding it is to look more closely at these remarkable structures and consider briefly what can sometimes happen to them.

The Vital Blood Vessels

As everyone knows, the function of all of our body organs, the very maintenance of life itself, depends on the continuous circulation of blood to all the organs and tissues in the body. Blood carries the nutrients—protein, carbohydrates, and fats (or lipids)—required by the body for healthy growth and maintenance. Even more important for the continuing life of every cell, the blood must carry oxygen to all the body's tissues and pick up and cart away waste materials for disposal. To carry out these vital tasks, the blood must constantly be circulated through a series of tubes and pipes, the so-called blood vessels or *vascular system*, by the action of a great central pump—the heart—past an oxygen pickup station—the lungs—and then to nutrient pickup stations associated with the gastrointestinal tract and the liver.

In the vascular system, the blood is carried through three different kinds of tubes, or pipes, to do its work. The *arteries* carry the blood away from the heart and out to all the organs and tissues of the body. The *veins* carry blood back from the body tissues to the heart. Connecting the arteries on one side with the veins on the other are a multitude of tiny *capillaries* passing in close contact with all the cells and tissues in the body. Figure 1 (page 16) is a schematic diagram of how these three kinds of blood vessels are connected into a complete, closed circulation system.

Each of the three components of the vascular system is specially constructed for the job it has to do. Figure 2 (page 17) illustrates the differences. The arteries, for example, are a high-pressure piping system. They must be built to survive a constant pounding as the heart forces blood through them in a series of forceful rhythmic pulses, much the way a piston pump forces water through a pipe.

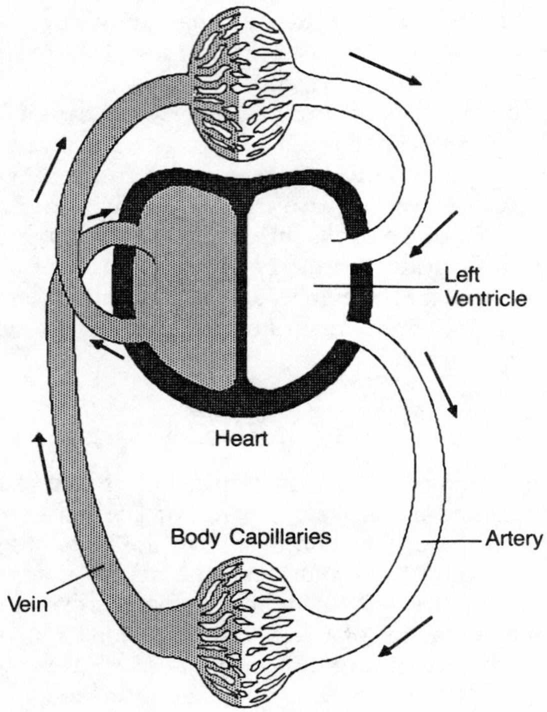

Figure 1   Arteries, capillaries, and veins form a complete, closed circulation system.

To accommodate to the rise and fall in pressure with each pulsation or heartbeat, the arteries must be thick walled, rubbery, and resilient, able to stretch a little, then spring back after each pulsation. Thus, all the arteries, from the great aorta, for example, rising out of the heart to the medium-size arteries in the wrist or the groin, down to the much smaller branch arteries or *arterioles* (literally, "little arteries") feeding into muscle tissue or skin, all are constructed in three main layers. The inside of the arterial tube is coated with a thin inner layer of smooth, slippery cells that allow the blood to pass along without clotting. This inner surface of the artery is called the *intima*. Surrounding this inner tube is a middle layer of tough muscle tissue, rubbery and resilient, called the *muscularis* or *media*. This layer of smooth muscle will stretch slightly and then spring back, just from the pressure of the blood pulsing through the tube. In addition, it is supplied with nerve fibers that can make the muscle cells relax and stretch when more blood is needed in an area, thus

16

Arteries and Arterioles

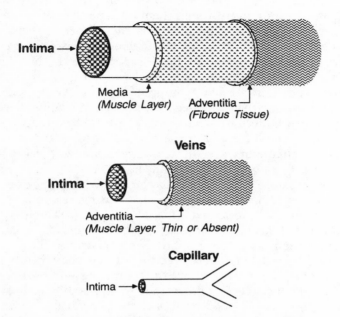

Veins

Capillary

Figure 2   Basic structure of arteries, veins, and capillaries.

widening the pipe, so to speak, to allow increased blood flow. When less blood is needed, these nerve fibers can cause the muscle layer to pinch down or contract, temporarily restricting blood flow and raising the pressure of the blood in the tube at the same time. Finally, the arteries have an outer layer composed of tough fibrous strands and rubbery connective tissue fibers, called the *adventitia*, supporting the artery in place and keeping it from bulging too much under high pressure.

The veins have much less punishment to put up with than do the arteries, and, therefore, do not need to be so thick walled and tough. The blood seeping out of the tissues into the veins for return to the heart flows under a relatively low pressure without pulsation; the veins simply act as conducting tubes, equipped in some places with interior valves to prevent back flow. Like the arteries, the interiors of the veins are lined with a thin layer of slippery cells, or intima, to allow blood to flow smoothly and without obstruction, but most of the veins lack the heavy middle layer of muscle that the arteries have, and they have a much thinner outer layer of fibrous and connective tissue.

The capillaries, connecting the smallest branch arteries entering an organ with the veins leaving the organ, are tiny blood vessels not even a hair's breadth in diameter, so very thin and narrow that red blood cells can just move through them one at a time. The main task of these capillaries is to allow nutrients and oxygen to seep out from the bloodstream into the tissue cells and allow waste materials such as carbon dioxide to seep in to be carried away. Thus, the capillaries are extremely thin walled vessels, constructed of just a single layer of cells that are not even glued together very closely, more like a meshwork than a closed vessel, leaving "holes" large enough for oxygen molecules or nutrients to pass through into the tissues but far too small for any of the blood cells to escape.

How does this circulatory system work in practice? Central to its operation is a great pumping machine—the heart. Actually, the heart consists of two separate pumps built side by side with a thick muscular partition or *septum* between them: a "right heart pump" and a "left heart pump," so to speak. This double pump is necessary because all the blood must actually pass through two separate circuits or circulatory systems, one after another, not just one. Blood returning to the heart from the far reaches of the body has been depleted of most of the oxygen it carried. It must have that oxygen replenished somehow before it moves out to the body's cells and tissues again. Thus, when blood returns to the heart it flows into a right-sided collecting chamber, the *right atrium*, and then into the corresponding right heart pumping chamber, the *right ventricle*. From there the blood is pumped out through *pulmonary arteries* to the lungs to pick up fresh oxygen at a great rate. The freshly oxygenated blood is returned by way of *pulmonary veins* to the left-sided collecting chamber of the heart, the *left atrium*, and thence into the left heart pumping chamber, the *left ventricle*. From there the blood is pumped out into the aorta to supply fresh oxygen to all parts of the body.

Among the first branch arteries to receive this freshly oxygenated blood are the two *coronary arteries*, which spring directly from the aorta and carry oxygenated blood to the heart muscle itself. These are the arteries that keep the pump running. Also early on, freshly oxygenated blood is fed into the two *carotid arteries* that supply blood to the brain, an organ so very hungry for oxygen that it consumes approximately 15 percent of all the oxygen available to the body. The diagram in Figure 3 shows how this double pump system of the heart with its double circulatory systems—the *pulmonary circulation* and the *systemic circulation*—works.

If it strikes you that this whole cardiovascular and circulatory system is extremely complicated, you are perfectly right. The truly amazing thing is that it works just incredibly well under normal,

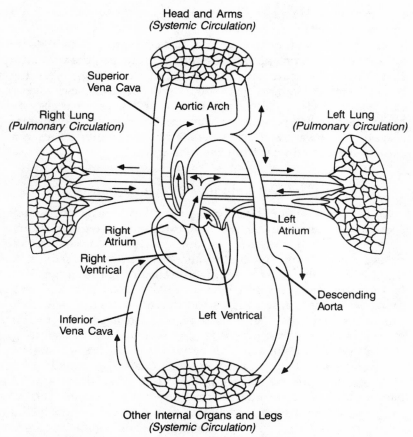

Head and Arms
(Systemic Circulation)

Superior
Vena Cava

Aortic Arch

Right Lung
(Pulmonary Circulation)

Left Lung
(Pulmonary Circulation)

Right
Atrium

Left
Atrium

Right
Ventrical

Descending
Aorta

Inferior
Vena Cava

Left Ventrical

Other Internal Organs and Legs
(Systemic Circulation)

Figure 3   The double-pump system of the heart, with its double circulatory system: the pulmonary circulation, and the systemic circulation.

healthy circumstances. The heart beats an average of 70 times a minute; 4,200 times an hour; 100,800 times a day; 36,792,000 beats a year; year in and year out, driving the blood through tens of thousands of miles of arteries, capillaries, and veins with each pulsation. A given drop of blood takes only about twenty seconds to make a complete circuit of the body, through both circulatory systems. Under normal circumstances, this cardiovascular system can sustain life in a human being for eighty, ninety or a hundred years or even more. But such performance depends upon the heart muscle itself receiving a constant, unbroken, and ample supply of both nutrients and oxygen. And to the heart muscle, it is *oxygen* that is of supreme importance. If something happens to cut off the oxygen to a person's heart muscle, that person is in immediate trouble. And if that trouble forces the heart to stop pumping, everything else comes to a stop, too.

Unfortunately, for many people, this circulatory system does not always remain in tip-top working condition. In fact, the very arteries that supply the heart with its vitally important oxygen are themselves extremely vulnerable to some subtle, progressive changes that can lead to disaster over a period of years. These changes, which bring about what we call coronary artery disease, are intimately related to the way our bodies handle nutrient materials, especially carbohydrates and fats, from the food we eat.

The Development of Atheromata

To remain alive and healthy, we must have a constant supply of protein materials from the foods we eat, in order to grow, maintain, or replace cells in our muscles, our skin, our bone, and all other tissues. In addition, for energy and heat our bodies require fuels that can be easily oxidized within our cells, using the oxygen carried in from the outside world by way of the bloodstream. Carbohydrates—various kinds of sugars and starches—are the main energy-producing fuels that our bodies require, so a certain amount of carbohydrate is necessary every day to maintain the status quo. Various fatty, or lipid, materials derived from the fats we eat provide another source of fuel. These fatty materials also provide a body-wide reservoir for the storage of extra fuel when there is more on hand at a given moment than the body actually needs. Fats taken in by our bodies are converted to a variety of compounds, including *fatty acids* and *triglycerides*. The triglycerides often link up with protein materials to form immensely complicated molecules known as *lipoproteins*. In addition, part of our bodies' fatty resources come from an oddball chemical present in many foods, known as *cholesterol*.

Cholesterol itself is not exactly a fat. Rather, it is a waxy, fat-soluble substance that contributes to the body's welfare in a number of very positive ways. Among other things, cholesterol molecules form the base for a wide variety of life-regulating hormones, including the male and female sex hormones—the androgens, estrogens and progestogens—and a number of the cortisonelike hormones manufactured by the outer layer or cortex of the adrenal glands. Indeed, the body cannot do without a certain amount of cholesterol. Ordinarily it manufactures about 70 percent of what is needed, and when the intake of cholesterol from the diet falls short, the body simply manufactures more.

Of these three groups of nutrient substances—proteins, carbohydrates, fats—the body needs a certain amount of each for maintenance and no more. When excess nutrients are taken in, the excess has to be stored somewhere. Ordinarily, excess proteins and carbohydrates are not stored as such; when an excess of either occurs, they are rearranged or bound into fatty materials and stored as fat.

Under normal circumstances fat is stored in a number of places in the body as fatty or adipose tissue—under the skin, in the abdomen, surrounding the heart or the kidneys, and, in obese or sedentary people, even in patches throughout muscle tissue.

Up to reasonable limits, the storage of fat is not necessarily an unhealthy thing. It can even be beneficial at times—as a protection against starvation, for instance. Unfortunately, however, in a great many people the normal storage of fat may be accompanied by high levels of fatty materials in the blood, and this can lead to a highly abnormal, dangerous phenomenon: the deposit of fatty material and cholesterol in the walls of the arteries throughout the body. Medically this abnormal process is known as *atherosclerosis*, from Greek words meaning "hardened mush"; the fatty deposits themselves are called *atheromata*.

Nobody knows exactly how early in life these fatty deposits begin to form in the artery walls. They may well start in early childhood in some individuals. Pathologists performing autopsies on eighteen- and nineteen-year-old American servicemen killed in the Korean War were appalled to discover that as many as 25 percent of these youthful war victims had discernible fat and cholesterol deposits in the walls of their arteries. Some, even at that age, already had atherosclerotic disease involving their coronary arteries.

Atherosclerosis doesn't happen all at once; it is a slow, silent process that grows steadily more severe over a prolonged period of time. Whenever the process begins, the first step is a microscopic deposition of fat in patchy areas under the cells lining the interior of the arteries, between the intima and the muscular tissue. In many people this small amount of deposited fat acts as an irritating foreign body, and the body responds to it by developing an inflammatory reaction. There is swelling of the tissue around the fatty deposits, and multitudes of white blood cells gather in the area in an attempt to attack the "foreign body" fat. Irritated smooth muscle cells from the muscular layer of the artery divide and pile up around the fatty deposits. This inflammatory reaction is very low grade, and again utterly silent. It produces no warning symptoms whatsoever but progresses slowly over a period of years.

During this time the body makes repeated efforts to heal these inflamed areas of artery wall. Bits of fibrous tissue and scar tissue build up in the region of the inflammation. At the same time more

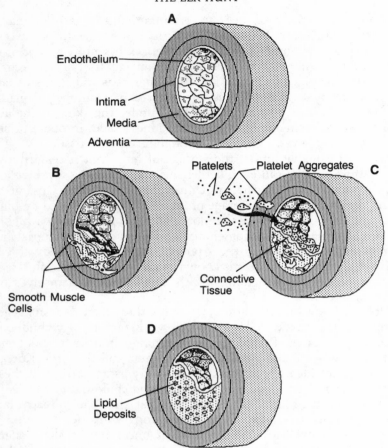

Figure 4 The stepwise development of an atheroma in an artery.

and more fatty material, especially cholesterol, is deposited in these areas. Presently, the affected arteries become studded with thick, waxy plaques composed of cholesterol, fibrous tissue, scar tissue, and dead cells lying just underneath the inner lining of the arteries. Still later, calcium is deposited in these lesions, so that they become progressively more firm and rigid, sometimes even rocklike. The result is a progressive hardening and thickening of the artery wall and a narrowing of the *lumen*, or opening, through which the blood can pass. We can see these changes diagrammed in Figure 4.

These atheromatous plaques seem to develop in certain specially vulnerable places. For example, they tend to form at arterial branch points, or places where arteries bend sharply, much like the accumulation of silt in a riverbed. But there seem to be no fixed rules as to how extensive they may become or how long it may take for the process to develop to the point of serious disease. In many people, however, the most severe atherosclerosis develops in the small to medium-size arteries, most particularly the carotid arteries that supply the brain and the coronary arteries that feed blood to the heart muscle itself. And of all the arteries in the body, it is those coronary arteries that are often the most seriously affected.

As we have seen, atherosclerosis is both slow to develop and silent as well. As the years go by and the atheromata become thicker and more extensive, there are virtually no symptoms to indicate that anything untoward is happening. There are no simple laboratory tests to demonstrate that an active, dangerous disease is in process. What does happen is that, gradually, bit by bit, the blood flow through the affected artery becomes more and more constricted as the enlarging fatty plaques block more and more of the artery's interior channel. If the affected artery is a coronary artery, this means that gradually less and less oxygenated blood can pass through that artery to supply oxygen and nutrition to the heart muscle with each heartbeat. But the blood flow through such an artery may become quite severely restricted before the heart muscle becomes hungry enough for oxygen that warning symptoms begin to appear. Because of the physics of fluid flow through a tube, up to 70 percent of the passageway of a major coronary artery may be blocked with no symptoms at all. Above 70 percent blockage, however, small decreases in diameter can produce drastic reductions in flow, and a first major symptom of coronary artery disease may appear—a type of intermittent chest pain commonly known as *angina pectoris.*

The Warning Role Of Angina

Angina pectoris plays such an extremely important part in all aspects of coronary artery disease that we will want to discuss it in much greater detail a little later in this book. Here we need to consider just one role that angina can play: as an important early warning symptom of real and dangerous trouble ahead. The word *angina* simply means pain; *angina pectoris* is chest pain. This pain can appear in many different and subtle forms in different individuals, but for many people it first appears as a deep-seated, diffuse, poorly localized, aching pain felt deep in the chest just to the left of the breastbone. Typically it tends to occur during a period of exertion, and subsides when the victim rests for a few moments. In many cases, when exertion is continued, the pain seems to spread up into the shoulder, the neck, the jaw or the arm, wrist or hand, usually on the left side. Such pain occurring in regions away from the chest is spoken of as *referred pain*.

The particular pattern of angina may differ considerably from one individual to another, but for most people who have it, the pain itself is very characteristic. People often describe it as gripping, vise-like, or crushing. Others may speak of it as a dull pain, a pressure in the chest, or merely an annoying ache. It is nothing like the acute pain of a burn, for instance, or the stabbing pain that arises from a broken bone.

Angina pectoris occurs when the oxygen supply to a portion of heart muscle suddenly becomes inadequate for the work it is doing at the moment. It is the heart's response to temporary, localized oxygen starvation, usually resulting from impairment of the arterial blood flow to a portion of heart muscle. Doctors call this kind of oxygen starvation *ischemia*, from Greek words meaning "to obstruct blood," and coronary artery disease is sometimes characterized as *ischemic heart disease*.

Again, most typically angina begins to appear only during active exertion, when a sudden demand is put on the heart to increase its rate of beating and to pump more blood. A heart that may be just barely limping along with the oxygen it is getting while the person is at rest will not produce the pain of angina, yet it may become virtually starved for oxygen if it is suddenly forced to work faster and harder during an interval of exertion. Thus angina pectoris may suddenly appear out of the blue when a person begins chopping firewood, sprinting for a bus, climbing stairs, or playing tennis. The person who feels perfectly fine at rest may abruptly find his chest hurting so much that he has to stop whatever he's doing the moment he starts some strenuous exertion. Then, as soon as the exertion is stopped, the anginal pain disappears quickly and completely; it may not recur until the next time the person starts exerting again.

Needless to say, this kind of off-and-on pain, sometimes severe enough to make the person gasp, can be disconcerting. But the person who begins experiencing it may, in fact, be extremely fortunate. Any chest pain that appears during exertion and disappears after resting may be a very clear early warning that something is seriously wrong with that person's coronary arteries.

Just a few years ago it was not possible to discover much detail about what was going on with the coronary arteries when angina pectoris appeared; even if it had been possible, the information would have been useless because there was very little in those days that a person could do but sit around waiting for disaster to strike. Today, of course, the picture has totally changed. As a first clue to the presence of coronary artery disease, angina may appear at the age of thirty or thirty-five in some people, or in the mid-fifties, even the early sixties in others. But whenever it occurs, it is today a sign that, if heeded, can lead to an orderly, nonemergency diagnostic investigation and highly successful, appropriate treatment without having to wait for a life-threatening disaster to occur.

For the person who is developing coronary artery disease, this would be the best of all possible scenarios. It doesn't always work that way, unfortunately. Sometimes events brought about by the physical changes of atherosclerosis take a different, far more dangerous direction, without benefit of any early warning.

Thrombosis and Occlusion

Obviously the development of thick atheromatous plaques in the artery walls has a serious effect on how well those arteries can do their job carrying oxygenated blood. As the artery walls become thickened and hardened, the blood-conducting channel becomes narrowed. And, as this disease slowly progresses, another kind of damage to the arteries can also occur: The layer of slippery cells lining the arterial channel can become irritated and ultimately begin to break down or ulcerate. Unfortunately, breaking the smooth integrity of that inner lining of cells can start a dangerous chain of events. One reason that the blood flows smoothly through the arteries and veins without forming clots is that the inner cell lining of those vessels normally forms an unbroken and *nonwettable* surface in contact with the flowing blood. Blood can flow past that surface without wetting it, much the same as water will run off a silicone-coated surface without wetting it. But when a blood vessel wall is damaged—by a razor nick, for example—the nonwettable interior surface is disrupted, and blood tends to wet and cling to the broken edges. One of the cellular components of the blood, the tiny blood platelets, tend to stick to the broken surface at the site of such a wound and then explode, releasing special chemicals. These chemicals then trigger a whole cascade of complex biochemical reactions that result in the formation of a sticky, gelatinous *blood clot* at the site of the injury. This clotting reaction, of course, explains why bleeding from a razor nick will ordinarily stop within a few minutes all by itself, without any need for outside measures.

When the inner surface of an artery begins to erode and ulcerate because of an atheroma in the artery wall, a similar situation can occur: The area of ulceration becomes wettable, and blood tends to "stick" to it as it sweeps by. Sticky platelets build up on the ulcerated area and trigger a clotting reaction. Presently, a layer of clotted blood can cover the ulceration—actually, this is part of the body's natural effort to heal the ulcerated surface. In a fairly large artery, such a clot may develop and build to quite some size without impeding the flow of blood through the vessel at all and may ultimately become incorporated in the process of healing the ulcerated area. But in a small to medium-size artery, such as a main coronary artery, or one of its smaller branches, fatty "sludge" from an atheroma may break through an ulcerated area and plug the artery completely. Even more likely, a blood clot may form at the area of the ulceration and then grow larger until it fills the whole artery channel, blocking off the blood flow. Very often this may happen without warning, very abruptly—and, suddenly, *no more blood is getting through that artery*.

This action of a clot or *thrombus* wedging itself tightly in an arterial channel is spoken of as *thrombosis*. In a medium- or small-size artery, it can cause complete obstruction, or *occlusion*, of blood flow through that vessel at that point. If the occlusion occurs in either one of the two main coronary arteries, or in any of the major branches of either of those arteries, the event is called a *coronary thrombosis*, leading to a *coronary occlusion*. And this is the major catastrophic event that triggers a classic coronary or heart attack.

What happens to a person when such an event occurs? First, and most important, the flow of oxygen-rich blood through that occluded artery is either blocked completely, or it is suddenly and severely impaired. Even if the flow is not completely obstructed, the injury to the artery at the point of the thrombosis may make it go into spasm and pinch down, so that whatever blood flow is left may be severely reduced. Because of the obstructed blood flow, a portion of the heart muscle that is normally supplied with blood and oxygen through that artery suddenly becomes acutely ischemic—starved for blood and therefore starved for oxygen.

This state of affairs triggers a whole succession of untoward events. The ischemia in the blood-starved heart muscle causes sudden, severe pain—the kind of crushing, pressing, breathtaking, deep-seated chest pain that I experienced the night of my heart attack. Deprived of oxygen and nutrients, the affected portion of heart muscle is immediately prevented from doing its normal job of contracting—it is so severely impaired that the pumping ability of the whole heart is impaired and diminished temporarily. As oxygen starvation in the segment of heart muscle continues, muscle cells begin to die—first a few, then more and more, then great numbers. Over a period of hours the whole area of heart muscle affected by the obstruction may die, or, as doctors would say, become *infarcted*. One of the terrible realities of this kind of catastrophe is that once those cells die they can never be revived or regenerated—they are gone forever.

Cells in the adjoining area that are merely injured or weakened—even gravely injured—may slowly recover if their blood supply is restored, or the heart is strengthened again, but the section of heart muscle cells that is dead will merely degenerate slowly into fibrous scar tissue, never to function again.

As these things happen, other events are occurring simultaneously. The normal smooth flow of electrical activity that ordinarily passes through the heart with each heartbeat is altered, because electrical impulses cannot move properly through the injured heart muscle. Thus, during an acute heart attack, the electrocardiograph tracing, or EKG, that ordinarily registers a characteristic normal-wave pattern of electrical activity with each heartbeat may show changes indicating damage to a specific section of heart muscle. One of the first things a doctor will look for when he or she suspects that a heart attack is taking place is a revealing "current of injury" showing up on the electrocardiogram. At the same time injured and dying muscle cells in the heart begin breaking down and releasing certain enzymes that ordinarily are never found outside the heart muscle cells themselves. These enzymes, over a period of several hours, may suddenly appear in greater and greater quantities in the bloodstream—another clue that a heart attack has taken place.

Other things may commonly happen during a heart attack. Since a severe blow to the heart is a severe blow to the entire body, the patient will often go into an episode of severe shock. The blood pressure will drop, the heartbeat will become very fast, the pulse weak, the patient gray and shaky, sweating, sometimes nauseated or vomiting. You can't tell anything very specific about a heart attack, either impending or occurring, from the pulse alone, but when the heart is laboring under the extreme stress of a myocardial infarction, the pulse is likely to become very rapid and so weak that you can hardly feel it. This isn't likely to happen during a "false heart attack" due to some gastrointestinal upset that seems to cause chest pain.

Another dangerous complication can occur if so much of the heart muscle is damaged that the heart as a whole cannot continue pumping blood adequately to meet the body's needs: a condition known as *heart failure*. Many of the early deaths in the midst of a heart attack result from such heart failure.

Finally, and perhaps most dangerous of all, if the area of injury is very large or involves critical parts of the heart's electrical conducting system, the pacing of the heartbeat may be thrown off, leading to an exceedingly threatening uneven or arrhythmic heartbeat known as *ventricular fibrillation*, in which the heart muscle stops contracting altogether and merely twitches, so that circulation to the whole body stops. This event, sometimes called *cardiac arrest*, can be a major cause of sudden death in the midst of a heart attack unless the fibrillation is detected and reversed very quickly.

It's important to point out here that dangerous cardiac arrhythmias such as ventricular fibrillation are not necessarily and exclusively triggered by heart attacks. Ventricular fibrillation, for example, can be triggered by heart damage from other kinds of heart disease, by too much alcohol, by an electrical shock—especially from a 110-volt AC house current—or by a dozen other possible factors. Sometimes it happens from causes that simply can't be discerned—the rare jogger who suddenly drops dead. The heart muscle injury of a myocardial infarction is just one possible trigger—but the most common one. Interestingly enough, a brief period of ventricular fibrillation, if quickly reversed, doesn't necessarily hurt the heart, in and of itself: It simply stops the heart from pumping blood to the rest of the body, or to the heart muscle, or to the brain. The heart muscle itself will only begin showing progressive damage after about thirty minutes, reaching a maximum between three and six hours—but irreversible brain damage begins within four to five *minutes* of the onset of ventricular fibrillation. Thus, if it continues for as little as four minutes without being corrected and the heartbeat restarted, either by CPR or with an emergency room shock box, death follows quickly. Immediate reversal of ventricular fibrillation is really the main reason for the existence of modern coronary care units. Undiagnosed and untreated ventricular fibrillation is one of the major causes of immediate death during an acute myocardial infarction, or during the tricky recovery period from such a catastrophe, when its occurrence is usually recorded as "sudden death syndrome" or "cardiac sudden death."

The Worst and Best Cases

How grave is the situation likely to be, then, in the event that a coronary attack occurs? Clearly the gravity in any individual case may depend upon many different factors. Which branch or branches of which coronary arteries are involved? How much total heart muscle is involved in the damage? Just where in the heart was the damage done? And what measures can be taken to treat the patient and guard against further damage? Other factors can also have an important bearing—the patient's age, for example, the body's capacity to cope with the blow, or the presence or absence of other illness. In persons with first heart attacks, which are often the first evidence that the patient has coronary artery disease at all, the gravity of the situation can hardly be exaggerated, and, even today, with all the advancements that have been made in detecting and treating coronary artery disease, there are still some 300,000 deaths among such people each year in the United States alone. For those who survive beyond the first few hours after an attack, what ultimately happens to them will depend heavily upon exactly what has happened to the heart as a result of the catastrophe and what measures can be taken to improve the chances of long survival.

Heart attacks, obviously, can vary greatly in severity. When just a tiny branch of a coronary artery is obstructed or occluded, only a small segment of heart muscle may be injured or killed. The damage may be confined to an *intramural*, "between the walls," area of the heart and not extend entirely through the heart muscle at any point. In such a case, the victim may have far milder symptoms, less risk of sudden death or dangerous complications, and far better chances of recovery, than if more damage had occurred. With such patients, doctors may have more time and greater opportunity to investigate the exact nature and extent of the coronary artery disease that is present, and be able to take measures to prevent a later, more disastrous heart attack. But not always: Even a small amount of heart damage may trigger fatal ventricular fibrillation. Claude Beck, one of the developers of the "shock box," the defibrillator, used to speak of "the hearts too good to die"—the young men with small myocardial infarctions who nevertheless died from ventricular fibrillation before the shock box had been devised to reverse it.

Whatever the nature and severity of the damage, time is of the essence when a heart attack occurs. The more quickly the catastrophe can be recognized, and the victim of a heart attack brought to a place where protective and supportive measures can be taken, the better the chances of surviving even a severe heart attack. As doctors have learned more about this disease, more and more ways have been found to *intervene* in the course of events, to protect against further damage and to preserve life—but no time must be lost getting the heart attack victim to medical help. Even a few minutes may make the difference between life and death.

There is no way that a coronary attack, whether mild or severe, proved or merely suspected, can be taken lightly. Until it has been demonstrated otherwise, anyone suspected of having a heart attack must be assumed to have one foot in the grave and the other on a banana peel. Many victims will survive, but *any* heart attack represents nothing less than a close encounter with death. Just how that encounter may evolve in any given case can depend very greatly on the victim himself.

Even as a doctor, I doubt that I was any smarter or better prepared than most other heart attack victims. I had no family history whatever of coronary artery disease; although both my parents died young (my father at forty-eight of cancer, my mother of pneumonia at age thirty-two), neither of *their* parents nor any of their brothers or sisters had ever had heart attacks. The diet I ate all my life was essentially the same diet my family had always eaten. True, I was overweight, and a heavy cigarette smoker since age thirteen, but these were easy things to ignore. The truth was that I was simply *not expecting* any such thing to happen to me. I had had regular annual physical exams with no suggestion of any impending cardiovascular disease or any other illness, and I was totally unprepared emotionally, even though intellectually, as a physician, I suppose I should have realized that I was a sitting duck, so to speak.

But one thing was absolutely clear to me the moment that chest pain began: Something terrible was happening to my body, and I knew that I was facing a close encounter with death. Exactly how my body and my mind responded to that encounter is the next part of this story.

— 4 —

I am convinced that on certain occasions, in times of desperate physical crisis, a person's body and subconscious mind may seize control of events in a most amazing fashion and save a person's life, almost in spite of himself. I had one such experience years ago, when I was caught in an undertow on the beach and nearly drowned. In the face of panic then, my subconscious mind told me *exactly* what to do *right then* to swim to safety, and later even told me what foods to eat to help my body recover from the near-exhaustion that ensued.

My body and subconscious mind took charge on the night of my heart attack, too. There are very few sudden physical events any more devastatingly traumatic to the human body than an acute coronary thrombosis and myocardial infarction. The trauma and physical injury involved are of the same order of magnitude as being hit in the head with shrapnel or run down by a truck, but the damage is all hidden inside. I don't believe there is any such thing as a "mild" heart attack or a "minor" myocardial infarction. However "mild" or "minor" as it may ultimately prove to be, any such event is a terrible blow to the body, a close encounter with death almost by definition, because life and death inevitably hang in the balance for minutes, hours, days, even longer. An arrhythmia, heart failure, or shock can kill, and any one of them can happen. And in the face of such an event, both the body and mind may take desperate measures to protect and preserve life—measures that may seem very strange indeed.

In my own case, during those first few hours and days of my heart attack, my body and mind collaborated in a way that was perfectly sensible, totally appropriate, and to the point: I was seized with a perfectly abysmal fatigue, and I went to sleep. This is not to say that I passed out or that I went into a coma or anything like that. What did happen was that I felt continuously and indescribably weary during whatever little time I was awake, and that I drifted into and out of sleep—mostly into sleep—continually for the next seven days or so.

I remember many odd bits and pieces from that period of time. Other things that I should have remembered I seemed to have forgotten completely until somebody told me about them later. I remember clearly when Dr. Coppock, the doctor who saw me on admission to the Ellensburg hospital, told me the nature of my condition, and I understood clearly what he was saying. He told me that my MI was large and located in the posterior part of the heart— the back side lying closest to the rear of the chest wall. This meant that it probably involved a good portion of the right ventricle, the half of the great pump that receives oxygen-exhausted venous blood returning from distant parts of the body and pumps it through the pulmonary artery into the lungs for fresh oxygen, and part of the left ventricle as well. This also meant that the injury probably involved a major branch of the right coronary artery.

An infarction involving this particular part of the heart can be especially bad news for several reasons. For one, a frequent complication of this kind of MI is the development of *congestive heart failure*. This can occur if so much of the right ventricle is injured that it can't carry on its pumping function adequately, so that blood and fluid back up behind the injured pump and cause congestion or swelling in the liver and other organs. It is also the kind of MI that can be complicated by dangerous heart arrhythmias or cardiac arrest that can occur quite suddenly and without warning.

I was perfectly aware of all this when Dr. Coppock described what was going on. I found it intellectually interesting, in a distant sort of way, but it didn't seem very important to *me* at the time; certainly it didn't seem particularly alarming or frightening. It was as though he were talking about somebody in a bed three rooms down the hall. What did seem important was that the crushing chest pain was gone, that suddenly absolutely nothing was expected of me but to lie there, that I felt totally exhausted and that I knew that the moment I closed my eyes I would be asleep, which was exactly the sum total of all that I wanted to do right then.

Sleep I did—long, long hours interspersed with very brief intervals of wakening and awareness. When I woke up, or was awakened by someone, I was immediately alert and refreshed for about five to ten minutes and then went to sleep again. There was a large round electric clock on the far wall directly in my field of vision, and it said all sorts of meaningless things like 2:30, or 5:12, or 9:23, but gave me no hint whether the time was A.M. or P.M., or what day it was. I was fleetingly aware of shaded daylight coming into the room at certain times and night-lighted darkness at other times, but none of this seemed to relate in any way to what the clock said.

From the first I was aware of a large dark eye up near the side of my bed with a bright green wiggly line moving across it, and a green digital number down below it blinking on and off, saying such things as "63" or "77" or "85"—the electrocardiograph monitor that was busy telling the world exactly what my heart was doing at that particular instant, seemingly far more alert and sentient than I was at the time. There was a little plastic tube affair across my face, with little tubes going up each nostril—an additional oxygen supply, I realized—but it was irritating and I kept pulling it out. A nurse kept coming around and putting it back in again. Indeed, the nurses seemed to be coming in constantly, fiddling with things on my chest, rolling me halfway on my side and propping a pillow behind me, fiddling with the oxygen, endlessly taking my blood pressure, drawing blood, taking my pulse, or shoving the dry, unnaturally warm business end of an electronic thermometer under my tongue. If I awoke at such times, more often than not I would go back to sleep before the nurse's chores were even finished.

It was some time during this period of almost continuous sleeping that I had the first odd dream—or delusion—or hallucination—about the elk hunt.

I suppose this wasn't surprising. I didn't care for this heart attack or anything that went with it, but what made me *really* unhappy was the awareness that I wasn't going to have any elk hunt that year. It was the one solid, acute, recurring disappointment that my mind kept returning to—not just that I wasn't going to get out hunting as much as I would like, but that there wasn't going to be any hunting at all. That maybe there wouldn't *ever* be another elk hunt, for me. This consciously distressed me, and it wasn't strange that I should enter into some half-dozing, half-dreaming rumination about an activity I loved so much—the elk hunt—in an area I loved so much—the beautiful mountain foothills near our home.

The dream was very simple, and very odd. In it I was walking up the series of wooded ridges or benches that rise sharply across the creek from our house, walking slowly upward, my rifle slung on my shoulder, my old beat-up English hunting hat on my head. It was just after dawn on a bright, warm day, and the brush underfoot was crackly. I was just climbing up onto the top of the second bench from the bottom when I glanced up the hill and saw movement in the trees a hundred yards above me. Then, almost magically, two bull elk appeared—a spike and a three-point—walking briefly out into the open, then crossing into a grove of trees.

It was not a good sighting at all, just the briefest of glimpses, and in my dream I froze, watching to see them again. A light breeze was coming from the east, not into them at all, and I thought that possibly they hadn't seen me. They had been moving toward a gully off to my left that I knew might hide me from sight if they went on into it. After a moment, I started slowly uphill, circling slightly to my right, my pulse pounding in my ears, trying to get up to their elevation with as little noise as possible, pausing now and then to listen for the great crash of brush that would signal that they had been spooked and were on their way.

For a few moments, I didn't see a thing, and I began getting tired from climbing. Then, quite abruptly, I saw the elk again—this time over to my right and much closer. They were standing together at the edge of the woods and they were both looking directly at me.

I knew at once that something wasn't right. Those elk should have wheeled away the moment they saw me, crashed once or twice through the woods, and vanished instantly as only bull elk can do when they have been startled by something. I tried to shrug the rifle off my shoulder without moving significantly, hoping against hope that I might get it up to my shoulder and get a shot off before they moved, but the sling hung up on my jacket somehow. Then, abruptly, they were gone. They didn't move or make a sound; they were just *gone*, and didn't reappear, although I searched the woods for movement for long moments after they vanished. At the same time I felt an odd sense of alarm as I realized that those animals must have come *downhill* directly *toward me* after I first glimpsed them, and not off into the gully to the left, where they had seemed to be heading.

I remember waking up in the hospital bed with that odd sense of alarm in my mind and seeing a nurse fiddling with an IV just out of my range of vision. It had been a strangely disturbing dream, yet

I felt a sense of perverse satisfaction about it. At least the game was afoot in my mind, I thought, even if my body couldn't play it. And then a bizarre thought: unless *this* was the *real* elk hunt. . . .

This was by no means the only peculiar experience I had during those critical hours. My mind seemed to be doing funny things as if to protect me. For example, I had no real conscious awareness of any chest pain whatever after the first injection of Demerol when I arrived at the hospital; yet my hospital record, when I checked it later,* revealed clearly that I was indeed having recurrent pain, and lots of it, reflected both in the EKG wave pattern on the heart monitor and in my own complaints that the nurses recorded but that I simply can't remember. Dr. Coppock had ordered morphine to be given by injection every three to four hours as needed to keep me free of chest pain, and apparently it *was* needed because it was recorded as having been given quite frequently during those first days. There were also those messy smears of nitroglycerin paste (an antidote for heart pain) plastered to my chest from time to time, although I didn't know what they were then.

Neither was I aware of any hunger whatever, maybe because an IV bottle of glucose water was hanging just above my head, dripping constantly—one of the things the nurses fiddled with most. I remember only one actual meal during this period: a cup of lukewarm chicken broth that I was allowed to suck up through a straw, and a dish of some indescribable red gelatin that somebody fed me with a spoon until I fell asleep on whoever it was. Of the succession of nurses I remember very little: a long series of large or small females of indefinite age, and one male nurse who seemed to be around at night, a large, moon-faced fellow I would find peering down at me over the bedside at the rare times I happened to wake up at night.

My mind began pulling other cute tricks during this period as well. At one point, during a period of alertness on the first day or so after the heart attack, I began to feel an urgent need to communicate with my agent, Carl Brandt, in New York, although I knew that Ann had already called him earlier to tell him of the catastrophe. I was worried because I was already past the deadline on a column for *Good Housekeeping*, which I had planned to write during that last week of deer season before the elk season began in order to clear the decks for hunting, and now it was clear that column was not going to be written. I was also long overdue drafting my novel *The Fourth Horseman* for Harper and Row, and felt that Buz Wyeth, my editor there, ought to be aware of a delay. But on a deeper level I was concerned that news of a serious heart attack was, perhaps,

---

* You *can* check your own hospital records, you know.

not the best thing for me to have spread abroad too widely through the publishing world, and I wanted to urge Carl to keep quiet about it as much as possible except for those who absolutely had to be informed.

Naturally, nobody at the hospital was the least bit interested in letting me get stirred up over business matters at that time. Absolutely no telephone calls could be made or received by a patient in the coronary care unit except by very special dispensation, but apparently I felt a call to Carl was imperative and became quite upset about it. Ann's journal entry described it nicely.

By Sunday afternoon (thirty-six hours after the heart attack began) Alan was getting so agitated about not being able to use the phone that Dr. Coppock finally gave permission for him to call Carl Brandt on Sunday evening, and also to walk with assistance to the bathroom to use the toilet when he had to go. I put a call through to Carl at home that evening and Alan talked with him briefly. I heard Alan saying that he was feeling much better, and that Carl shouldn't be worried, and they discussed a little bit about what to say at *Good Housekeeping* and to Buz Wyeth, but it was a very brief call. I was surprised to hear Alan saying how well he was doing because it didn't seem to me that he was doing all that well by any means.

There would be absolutely nothing remarkable about this episode, nor anything worth reporting here, except for the curious fact that the moment I finished that call to Carl and hung up the receiver, my mind blanked it out completely, just blocked it off as if it had never happened. Some three months later, when Ann made some offhand remark about my call to Carl a day or so after the heart attack, I didn't know what she was talking about. It was not until Carl himself later confirmed that I had indeed made the call and told me what I had said to him that the mental doors suddenly opened and I remembered.

In retrospect, I know that this kind of so-called *retrograde amnesia*, an action of the mind to blot out the memory of things occurring just before or during a period of terrible stress, is a very common protective device the mind uses to diminish the emotional jolt of a shock or trauma at a time when a person can't really cope with it. This told me that something deep in my mind and beyond my conscious control was aware that I was in a far more precarious state than I realized, and had simply moved in and taken over to ensure that nothing—but nothing—disturbed my necessary placidity and composure if it could possibly be helped.

Other games my mind played were more difficult to interpret. As I drifted in and out of sleep, I would be aware from time to time that people were there—people who shouldn't have been because they weren't anywhere near. It seemed that Ann was there constantly, day or night, although it didn't seem likely that she could be. (She later confirmed that she was.) Usually she would be sitting in a chair at the far side of the room, dozing when it seemed to be nighttime, perhaps reading when it seemed to be day. Then, at one awakening, sometime in the middle of the night (or so I thought), it wasn't Ann sitting in the chair but my daughter Becky, whom I had thought was busily studying over at Whitman College in Walla Walla. I spoke to her, and she answered back and it was indeed Becky. She said something ridiculous about Mom going home to turn off the lights. Then at some completely different time, again at night, my brother Bill from Spokane was in the room. He was up at the head of the bed, so that I had to look up over my right shoulder to see him. To my memory we conversed for a very short while, but I don't remember a thing that we said. I do remember thinking, "My God, he must think I'm on death's doorstep or something." How long he was there I could not say, but I didn't remember seeing him again. Later still my son Chris was there, sitting in the same chair that Becky had been sitting in.

In a way all these various visitations had a dreamlike quality, popping in and out of my awareness as I slept. They were not hallucinations; they were real enough, but merely seemed unreal to me. Above all this seems to me to illustrate the extreme self-centeredness that overtakes one during catastrophic illness of this sort. The only thing that I was really aware of during this period was *me*; the others around me were sort of shadowy stage actors who came and went without seeming to have anything precisely to do with me, so I didn't pay very much attention to them. It was only later that the obvious became clear: *I* was the one who had stopped dead center while the rest of the universe continued to revolve. The truth is that a heart attack affects others besides the victim, creating enormous problems and pressures. And in my case, of course, those problems and pressures came to rest squarely upon Ann.

How does the family close to a heart attack victim react, and what do they do? Probably nobody ever sits down and thinks about this in advance; the victim's spouse suddenly is faced with a totally different, terribly threatening situation and, abruptly, has to play it entirely by ear. This is illustrated clearly in portions of the journal that Ann later recorded of this period:

Even on the way into the hospital with Alan that night in late October, I had debated calling our kids, but realized that there was absolutely nothing that they could do, since they were all so far away, and that I might have more to tell them a little bit later. (There were four of them. Becky, our daughter, age twenty, was in Walla Walla at Whitman College; Ben, age twenty-two, was working in Santa Cruz, California; Jon, nineteen, was in classes at the Colorado School of Mines in Golden, and Chris, eighteen, was on duty aboard the Coast Guard cutter *Confidence*, docked in Portland at that time.) It seemed to me that even if Alan should die suddenly, there was no way the kids could be there at this time. I told the nurse that I wanted to be staying in the room with him, and there seemed to be no objection to this, but I asked them to wake me up about six A.M., in case I fell asleep, so that I could call the kids.

I did not sleep. I don't think I even dozed; I tried but I just couldn't. Sometime during the night I did go out, around three A.M., and walked the dog and moved the car to the parking lot away from the front door. Then at six o'clock in the morning I started calling the kids.

Becky's phone in Walla Walla (the only number I could remember off-hand) was answered, but her roommate said she had left the night before for a volleyball game in Spokane and she did not know where she was staying. She offered to check with the dean of students, who might know where Becky could be reached and get a message to her.

Next I got Ben's number in Santa Cruz, California, from Information. Fortunately, he was home, since this was a Saturday morning. I remembered always hearing that when you have bad news to tell someone over the telephone you should try to break it gradually and not just blurt it out right away, and I was thinking then of the day when my father died, when Alan had come and put his arms around me and said, "Your mother called today and I have bad news." I had known right then that it was Daddy, and Alan had said yes it was, and I asked if he was dead, and he said yes again. So I tried to think what I might say to the kids that would make it easier for them. When Ben answered the phone, I told him I was calling from the hospital in Ellensburg, and that I had some bad news, that his father had had a heart attack; that he was still alive but was seriously ill, and the doctor had indicated that the next three days would probably be the most critical. Ben's first question was, "Are you alone? Is anybody there with you?" I told him I was alone but that I'd tried to reach Becky, and also wanted to let the other boys know but didn't have their phone numbers there at the hospital. He offered to contact them for me but I said no, I thought I should talk to them myself. He found the numbers in his address book. I then suggested that he *could* save me a call if he would contact his Uncle Bill—Alan's only brother—in Spokane for me.

I really was feeling very much alone at that moment. We had just moved to Thorp two months previously, and although we had good neighbors up the road from us, I didn't feel I knew them very well, and I knew absolutely nobody else in Ellensburg or Cle Elum. Ben asked if he should come, but

I told him maybe to wait. I promised to keep him apprised of what was going on, but there was really nothing he could do at that moment. Alan was either going to make it through this crisis or he wasn't, and by the time Ben got here from Santa Cruz, we would know one way or the other, and if Alan did die there was nothing Ben could do anyway. He probably wouldn't arrive in time to be very helpful.

When I reached Jon in Colorado I told him essentially the same thing. He gave me telephone numbers of a friend or two where he could be reached if he was not at his own apartment. Chris, who had actually visited us about three weeks before on a short leave, was then in Portland, where his ship, the *Confidence*, was about ready to take off for Alaska. When I got the duty officer on the ship, I just explained that I was Chris's mother and that it was a medical emergency and I had to reach him. I held on for what seemed like forever while they dug him up and got him to the phone. His response was very emotional, and he asked if he could come, said he wanted to come, and I told him yes, if he could get permission to get away, then come along. I was feeling more lonely by the minute and wanted to have one of the kids around. I figured that Chris could probably get a bus and get to Ellensburg at least by the end of the day.

Then I went back to Alan's room and just waited. A little later in the morning, around 8:30 or so, the nurse called me out because Becky was on the phone. Somebody had reached her in Spokane and told her what had happened. She wanted to come home—it was just 170 miles—but of course in those days she didn't have a car. I mentioned that Ben was contacting her Uncle Bill there in Spokane and suggested she call him and see what he was planning. Somehow they must have gotten together, because she called back a short time later and said that Bill was driving over and would bring her with him.

I stayed in Alan's room most of the morning then, except for going down to the hospital cafeteria for a quick bite to eat at lunchtime. At about one o'clock Bill and Becky arrived and went in to see Alan for a few minutes. Earlier, when Alan had awakened for a moment or two, I had told him that they were coming, and he had said, "Why?" to which I said, "They want to." He didn't seem to understand quite what I was talking about. Alan seemed almost completely knocked out at the time they arrived, so they only stayed with him about five minutes and then I walked them out to Bill's car. Bill, five years older than Alan, asked if there was anything he could do right then, and I suggested that he go out to the house, turn off the lights and lock the doors, take the dog for a run and bring me back my address book because I wanted to let Carl Brandt know what had happened and couldn't remember his number offhand. I also asked Becky if she would bring me some clean underwear and clean clothes, since I had on the dirty jeans I'd worn hunting all the day before. And I suggested that they bring our other car back so that Becky, who said she could stay a day or so at least, would have a car available and still leave one for me at the hospital. They did these things and came back about three in the afternoon. Then Bill left to return to Spokane. There was no real point to him staying, nothing more that he could do, but I did ask him to pray a lot.

After Bill and Becky's short visit with Alan, the head nurse told me that even that brief disturbance had apparently been very stressful; Alan's blood pressure had changed a great deal during the visit, and he seemed to be having recurring runs of irregular heartbeats ever since. They were obviously concerned about this, and I fully agreed that we should confine ourselves to sitting quietly in a chair at the other side of the room and not make any effort to converse or communicate.

After Bill left, Becky spelled me sitting with Alan for a bit. I couldn't really be sure how frightening this might be for her; unlike me, who had been doing physical therapy work in hospitals for years, she had no familiarity whatever with hospitals, and even less with heart attacks.

I told her to watch the monitor and call the nurses if it suddenly changed in some way. I knew they had one going right in the nurses' station across the hall, but I was afraid they just might not be paying attention to it—not a nice thought, but I didn't know the hospital then as well as I do now.

Quite late that afternoon I went out to make a final call to Carl Brandt at his home in Rhinebeck, New York. He was obviously distressed, but I told him I couldn't think of anything he could do until we knew what was going to happen, except possibly get some word to *Good Housekeeping*, because I knew that Alan was overdue with a column he had been working on before the weekend. Finally, at 5:30, I went over to the bus station to meet Chris, who threw his arms around me and gave me a great big hug. I was really glad to see him. We went back to the hospital immediately, looking in to see Alan very briefly, maybe for twenty to thirty seconds, since I knew Bill's and Becky's visit earlier had apparently not been so good for Alan. But I felt that Chris at least ought to be able to see his father and talk with him briefly. Later the nurse showed us to a waiting room down the corridor that had a couple of comfortable chairs and a couch. Becky took the first watch with Alan for a couple of hours while I slept on the couch; then the kids slept in the waiting room while I stayed with Alan.

Quite early the next morning—Sunday—I woke up from dozing in the chair because Alan called my name. He was awake and apparently quite uneasy; he said that all of a sudden he was feeling very faint and not very good. I went across the hall to tell the nurses and they came in. Apparently he had had a sudden drop in blood pressure. There was communication by phone with Dr. Coppock, who ordered a change of medication. It was at this time that Alan complained, maybe for the second or third time since he got to the hospital, about pain in his feet and ankles, which seemed a little irrelevant to me since he wasn't using his feet and ankles, but they seemed to be bothering him more than anything that was going on in his chest.

Later that morning Dr. Coppock came in to see Alan. When he finished examining him, he motioned to me to come out into the hall, and he started walking slowly down the hall with me. He said he'd heard that two of the kids were there. I said yes, that was a relief, and I was thinking that maybe I could go home for a few hours since they were there. Dr. Coppock put his arm around my shoulders and said, "Maybe you'd better not. Maybe you'd better stick around for a while yet." That was all he said, but it was enough to make me extremely apprehensive.

I had not been aware of any apprehension, but if Ann felt apprehensive about Dr. Coppock's remark, the doctor himself was apparently apprehensive as well. According to my hospital medical record, my blood pressure had been fluctuating sharply all day Sunday and Sunday night, too high at some times, sagging off almost alarmingly low at others. In addition, I was having irregular showers, or runs, of arrhythmic heartbeat, presumably due to injury to heart muscle, that did not seem to be well controlled with the medication that Dr. Coppock was ordering. This wasn't a disastrous arrhythmia like ventricular fibrillation. The heart just kept missing beats and then following up with fast premature beats, and these irregular spells would run for three or four minutes at a time. As a general practitioner working in a small rural hospital facility, Dr. Coppock had taken care of plenty of uncomplicated heart attack patients in his time, but he was clearly becoming concerned that I was perhaps not such an uncomplicated case, or might not be going to stay uncomplicated. In any event, when he came in for rounds the following morning, Monday morning, he told Ann and me that he thought I probably ought to be transferred from this hospital to some medical center that would have better acute-care facilities, and he wondered where I would like to go.

He didn't say that anything in particular was wrong at that time, simply that he felt it would be a good thing in general for me as a patient. He mentioned facilities in both Yakima and Spokane as possibilities. I wasn't at all pleased at the prospect of going *anywhere*, but said that if I had to go somewhere, I'd prefer the Virginia Mason Hospital in Seattle, since I knew the people there so well. Dr. Coppock asked whom he should contact, and I suggested Dr. Fred Cleveland at the Mason Clinic. He said that he would plan to talk to him, and then arrange to transfer me to Seattle by ambulance on Wednesday, with a coronary care Registered Nurse in attendance as well as the ambulance driver.

One thing that we *didn't* have to worry about in the course of all this was the cost of medical care. As a member of the King County Medical Association for many years, I was covered, together with Ann, by an excellent group plan with King County Medical–Blue Shield, and it paid virtually everything necessary, with just a few minor exceptions. We had groused from time to time about the high premiums we had to pay—about $2,000 a year at the time—but when the catastrophe struck, we were very thankful that we had it.

Monday evening, Becky had to get back to school in Walla Walla. I remember thinking at the time that it seemed a pity for her to be sitting around, missing classes, and I thought it a little odd that Ann felt that one of them absolutely had to be there at all times, as if I might be going to drop dead at any minute. I didn't realize it then, but at that point even Ann had begun to notice something funny going on with my head.

Sometime Monday it began to strike me that Alan was acting decidedly strangely. He seemed to be very angry at some of the nurses, particularly when he wanted to stand up at the bedside to urinate and some of them still tried to talk him out of it even though the doctor had said that he could. He wouldn't eat very much, and took quite a dislike to one of the physicians (not his own) who came to the nurses' station right across the hall to give orders and to discuss things that Alan could overhear a little bit and didn't like the sound of.

Alan also kept complaining about the Oriental cleaning personnel. Now, Ellensburg is a town in the central part of Washington State, and although there are a number of Hispanics in the area and a couple of black families, there were very few Orientals in town other than one or two Cambodian refugee families, and there were *no* Orientals at all on the hospital staff. I began wondering if he was having some kind of toxic problem with his medications, or, even worse, if in the course of his heart attack he had suffered some lack of oxygen to his brain or had a small stroke, since it seemed to me that this odd behavior and these remarks were similar to some I had encountered in some brain-damaged physical therapy patients I had treated. He also seemed to have quite a bit of tremor in his hands, and this seemed to be getting worse as time went on.

Along about this time I was also starting to get some vibes from the nursing staff that maybe I really shouldn't be hanging around so much. I could see their point, in a way, yet I didn't feel comfortable just going home. Our house was a long way from the hospital, and it seemed to me that if Alan was in such serious condition that he needed to be transferred to a major medical center, then he really wasn't out of the woods yet, so I just ignored the nurses and continued to hang around.

It was never spelled out to me exactly what Dr. Coppock was implying by a "bigger, better-equipped medical center," but my imagination filled in for me. I knew that this little hospital had no facilities for doing coronary artery by-pass operations, whether elective or emergency, and no surgeon in town was experienced in doing them. (I had heard that somebody in Yakima was doing such things, but I suspected that it was on a sort of once-a-month basis.) This hospital didn't even have facilities for cardiac catheterization and angiograms, a procedure I knew was used for determining which coronary arteries were blocked and how much. Certainly they weren't equipped to do some of the things I'd heard some heart surgeons over in Spokane were doing, taking patients in for by-pass operations practically the minute they stepped across the threshold of the hospital—very controversial at that time. I did feel comfortable with the choice of Virginia Mason in Seattle, because of Alan's internship and long association there. I was quite sure they were not doing any radical, terribly experimental things there, and I knew that the Mason Clinic had great doctors, some of whom I knew personally and had full confidence in. Above all, I knew of Alan's long-standing admiration and respect for Dr. Fred Cleveland, a cardiologist there and sort of an old friend as well, and that alone made me feel really good about the proposed transfer. I heard from Dr. Coppock that Dr. Cleveland had said he would accept Alan; I got the impression that Dr. Cleveland was not really wild about having him transferred at that particular point in his treatment, but Dr. Coppock thought Alan was stable enough to make the trip.

On Tuesday Alan seemed a little more bright, awake a little more and talking more. He did not, however, seem to be thinking very clearly. We had been planning a trip some three weeks later to go to Denver to visit our number-two son Jon at the Colorado School of Mines, and then on to San Antonio for Alan to receive an Arthritis Foundation award for his writing. Now he was talking as though we would certainly be going. I knew we certainly wouldn't be, and I called the travel bureau and canceled our reservations.

On Wednesday morning they were busy getting Alan ready to go. The ambulance people came at ten and got him all ready on a stretcher. There was not only the driver but a special registered nurse on hand to go along. About five minutes before Alan was to be wheeled out of the room, the hospital called a Code Blue* and a moment later Dr. Coppock appeared at the door, extremely concerned that the code had been called for Alan. In this case it happened to be for a woman down the hall who had just stopped breathing, but from Dr. Coppock's concern, I got the impression that he, too, felt extremely nervous about Alan's condition.

I hated to see Alan go. I was not permitted to go in the ambulance but had to drive separately, with Chris following in tandem with the other car.

* An emergency signal that some patient has suffered some disaster such as a cardiac arrest.

I had arranged to stay some nights with friends in North Bend, just a short drive from Seattle, and stopped there briefly to park the Bronco; then Chris and I went on into the city. When we finally reached Virginia Mason, I was extremely relieved to learn that Alan had been admitted and was already in the coronary care unit. At least, I realized, that meant that he had survived the trip.

—5—

That ambulance trip to Seattle, to whatever small degree that I was aware of it, seemed to me to be much ado about nothing. There were people here, people there, people rushing around, people doing things. It was like getting a knight in armor mounted for a joust: lifting him up on cranes and pulleys, backing the horse under him, dropping him down, then easing off cautiously on the rope to see if he stayed on. All the IV bottles had to go along with me; other tubes had to be plugged up and left in place, and all the cardiograph leads had to be disconnected. They woke me up out of a dead sleep to commence all this, and I went back into a dead sleep again before we had even departed. Somebody jogged my feet, and I became aware that my ankles were swollen grotesquely and hurt like hell. I felt weak as a kitten, and my hands shook fiercely every time I moved my arms. In addition, it struck me that if I was thinking at all, I wasn't thinking very clearly. Once or twice in the course of the hundred-mile trip over the mountains from Ellensburg to Seattle, I roused enough to be aware of jouncing along the highway; at one point in the bright midday sunlight there was a stop for a seemingly interminable length of time at a place I recognized as the summit of Snoqualmie Pass, with people doing a great deal of fiddling with me, though I don't recall what they were fiddling with. Later on I woke up long enough to recognize the emergency entrance at Virginia Mason Hospital on the Terry Avenue side. The next thing I knew I was once again in a hospital bed, once again hooked up to EKG leads and IV tubes and nasal oxygen tubes in a strange, dimly lighted room, and Dr. Fred Cleveland was staring down at me owlishly through those big hornrim glasses of his.

We didn't do much talking at that point, but I was very glad to see him. I had known Fred from the very first of my intern days at

Virginia Mason twenty-five years before, and I had seen him a number of times professionally during the intervening years at the Mason Clinic for physical checkups and medical treatment. Over the years he hadn't changed very much except that his dark brown hair had gotten steadily grayer. I think we had always regarded one another with respect and a certain degree of quizzical amusement. His manner had always seemed a little pompous; when he spoke, what he had to say often came across in the nature of a pronouncement rather than conversation, but he was always precise in what he said. He always knew what he was talking about, and he moved and acted decisively. Above all, I knew he was not a person to mince words. I remember once in his office after an examination years before, when he had leaned back in his chair, looked at me disdainfully through his owly glasses and said, "Al, you're just too damned fat."

"But Fred, I like to eat," I had said.

He had given me his disgusted look number three. "We all like to eat," he said, "but we don't all carry thirty-five extra pounds of blubber around with us all the time."

At other times in clinic visits he had made an issue about my continued cigarette smoking, urging me to quit cold while I had a chance, advice I had never taken—I had made a couple of stabs at it but never stuck it out. "What are you waiting for?" he asked me on one occasion, pointing to my chest X ray on his view screen. "Are you waiting to see a spot on that film before you stop? When you see a spot there, the game's all over—you know that, don't you? When you see that spot, you don't have the chance of a snowflake in hell of lasting more than eighteen months. So why wait?" And another time he had shaken his head sadly with his "you poor sap" expression number fourteen and said, "You don't really have many aspirations for longevity, do you?"

Seeing him now, at this time, I knew two things: Fred Cleveland was not going to do anything wild, and he was probably not going to do anything wrong, either. I was in good hands.

Fred examined me briefly then, listening to my heart and lungs, feeling for my liver, checking my pulse and blood pressure, and he didn't look terribly pleased. He had reason enough not to. After all, he was seeing a patient for the first time five days after a massive MI, just at the point when the damaged or destroyed myocardium really begins to rot, when the heart wall is at its very weakest. He was seeing that patient at the end of a hundred-mile ambulance trip that the patient had hardly noticed but everybody else seemed to think must have been terribly exhausting. To top it off, this patient had to be a doctor, and doctors are bad news as patients, as anyone in medicine can testify. With a doctor for a patient, Murphy's First Law always prevails: If anything can go wrong, it will.

After Fred left, the parade that I remembered so well from my intern days began: the nurses, the attendants, the hooking me up to the monitor, and the long stream of physicians. There was the medical student, the intern, the junior resident, the senior resident, each taking the same history, asking the same questions, getting the same answers, as though not one of them ever spoke to any of the others at any time. I remember distinctly that I wanted nothing more than to go to sleep, but every time I got my eyes closed, there was another one jogging me awake. At first I was annoyed, then actively irritated, and then, I'm afraid, my sometimes-unfortunate sense of whimsy began to take over. Somewhere along there, the fourth one of these people in a row asked me how much alcohol I used.

"Not much," I said.

The young man, I think the chief resident, frowned and said, "How much is that?"

"No more than eight or ten double martinis a day," I said.

"For very long?"

"Oh, for years. I doubt if there's much of my liver left."

The resident dutifully jotted this down in his admission note—and, bless his soul, called it to Fred Cleveland's attention, too. Later Ann told me that Fred had come to her and said, "Ann, how much does Alan *really* drink?" She told him a couple of drinks before dinner in the evening was all. Then Fred showed her the resident's note in my chart. "There's a question whether this shaking of the hands and the mental confusion might not be the DTs."

Ann was taken aback, and said, "Fred, I don't think my husband is a closet drinker, and I've never known him to drink eight or ten double martinis a day anytime in his life."

When I heard this later, I, too, was taken aback. I remembered very clearly giving that spurious history to the resident, and I had thought I was being funny—perhaps an indication of just how confused I was.

From Ann's account of that admission afternoon, it was clear that Dr. Cleveland was concerned about my mental confusion too.

After the admission paperwork was done, Chris and I went up to CCU, knocked at the door of the section and asked if we could see Alan. The nurse said the doctors were with him and we would have to wait. I guess waiting rooms are not very pleasant places in any event; you either have nothing to read at all or nothing but a pile of very old magazines, and you don't feel like reading anyway. It seemed like forever before Dr. Cleveland came out. He said Alan was very tired from the trip but seemed to be relatively stable, at least for the moment, and I could go in to see him briefly. The CCU visiting regulations at Virginia Mason were far more strict than at the Ellensburg Hospital; only members of the family were allowed to visit at all, and then only for about five minutes of every hour. It was at this point that Dr. Cleveland raised the question about Alan's drinking. I did comment that Alan had seemed to have some difficulty with his reasoning in Ellensburg and that the tremor of the hands had been getting worse in the last twenty-four hours. Then Dr. Cleveland asked me in detail about the medicines that Alan had been taking before and since the heart attack: some vitamins, some aminophyllin to help clear the gunk out of his chest in the mornings, and some lithium that Dr. Melson at the Mason Clinic had been having him take for some time to help combat the spells of depression that had bothered Alan for ages and had seemed to be getting worse in recent years. Dr. Cleveland said, "That's interesting. You can get a flat-out toxic psychosis with an overdose of that stuff." He said that they'd check Alan's serum lithium level and maybe just take him off that medicine completely.

Chris and I finally got in to see Alan about two o'oclock in the afternoon, and he roused a little bit and talked with us briefly. The room was very small, actually only about half as big as the room at the Ellensburg hospital, and it all seemed very gray and gloomy. He was right across the hall from the nurses' station and had the usual monitoring hookup, the IV lines, the nasal oxygen—the works. There was a much bigger, more complicated room across the hall where they were just wheeling in a patient from coronary by-pass surgery. When the appointed five minutes were up, Chris and I went back to wait until we could go back in again, but Alan seemed to be less and less communicative, more and more torpid, with each visit. I finally decided that we should go back to North Bend and try to get some rest. At least I knew he was in good hands here, with a thoroughly experienced staff and a physician on hand twenty seconds away, even if he wasn't right in the room holding the patient's hand.

What little I can tell you about the next thirty-six-hour period— that first night in the Virginia Mason CCU, the next day and the following night—is necessarily going to be spotty, disconnected, and confused, because beyond question my conscious awareness was confused. As to what actually happened to me during that interval, I remember very little—just bits, pieces and fragments; but as to what happened *inside*, subjectively, I was clearly aware, and to this day I can remember so vividly that I could almost still be there.

In retrospect, piecing it together from remarks and comments that Fred Cleveland made later, and with the cold data from my hospital record before me, I believe that it was during this period of thirty-six hours that the total response of my body and mind to the terrible physical insult of the myocardial infarction reached its lowest point. If, indeed, any such insult to the function of the heart represents a close encounter with death, it was during this interval that the encounter occurred.

Maybe the things that I remember really were related to some minor degree of brain damage that occurred at the time of the MI, as Ann thought possible, or a toxic psychosis due to medication. But in retrospect, I think another far more basic interpretation is much closer to the truth: That during that interval my body, with the aid of my doctor's wisdom, the support of medication, and the attendance of the nursing staff, was quietly engaged in a last-ditch stand, a desperate make-or-break struggle for survival; and that my mind, in the weird, ass-backward way that a mind sometimes works, was keeping me informed of that struggle, moment by moment, on a level of unreality that would let me know what I had to know but could not hurt me. I have never understood much about the classic mental defense mechanisms that are widely accepted in the medical world, or how such mental mechanisms actually work to defend the body, but I am firmly convinced that *my* mind, at this time, began working in metaphors, trying to protect me from bald awareness of the mortal danger that I was in but still gently preparing me for whatever, good or bad, might evolve from that danger.

From the account Ann recorded later, I am quite certain that she was totally unaware of what my mind was doing. Maybe Fred Cleveland was aware of part of it as it happened, but only part. It was not until days later, when it was all over, that I was able to see a glimpse of what had really gone on.

The bits and pieces were jumbled, in no discernible chronology: At one point, something happened; at another something else; which came first, which later, I do not know. I do remember that first afternoon that it seemed irritating to me that Ann and Chris kept popping into the room time and again, each time just as I was settling back to sleep (or had been sleeping and they woke me up), and I thought of saying something about it but simultaneously felt guilty for feeling that way, and finally decided that this was one grand opportunity for me to keep my big trap shut.

At last Ann said that they were leaving for North Bend. This must have been in the late afternoon or early evening, but I realized that I had no way to tell. When they had gone and I really looked around that room for the first time, I realized that the only outside window looked out at the shadowy wall of another building. It was a tiny box of a room, almost completely filled with the bed, the monitors, IV stands, and equipment, with gray walls and a tiny dim night light, and a big round electric clock up on the wall, just like the one in Ellensburg, offering no hint of anything except that it was such-and-such o'clock *sometime*.

There were curtains on a runner around the bed, but they were practically never closed. On the corridor side of the room, however, along with the door (which remained perpetually open), there was a large picture window looking out on the corridor and across to the nurses' station. Looking out that window might have seemed pretty dull sport, except that this nurses' station didn't stay the same all the time. It kept changing, and I kept seeing new, different and mysterious things going on there every time I looked. I'm quite sure that more than once when the curtains were drawn I asked a nurse to open them so that I could see what had happened in that nurses' station since the last time I'd looked.*

At first that nurses' station looked like any other nurses' station, except that it was a very large room, being the central control room and monitoring station for all the coronary care unit rooms and the larger intensive care unit rooms used for immediately postoperative coronary by-pass surgery patients. It was really a huge box, glassed in on the corridor on my side and glassed in from the corridor on the other side, containing a whole succession of desks or writing tables as well as banks of monitoring equipment, all brilliantly lighted. It also seemed always to be full of people, at first: uniformed nurses, doctors in their long white clinical coats, and various other attendants, both male and female, wearing what seemed to be blue-green surgical scrub suits. Some time later, however, all that changed, and the things going on in that room (or those rooms) became more and more peculiar and incomprehensible.

At one point the whole station seemed to have been tipped up on its side so that then, instead of a large room, there were three or four vertical tiers of nurses' stations extending from the corridor floor up to the ceiling. Each tier, like a narrow balcony, contained three or four of the writing desks and three or four people, who seemed to be periodically appearing and disappearing in totally mysterious random fashion. At some different time I decided to try to watch these people more closely to try to figure out where they were going and what, exactly, they were doing. At first, as I watched, they stopped doing anything at all except writing diligently on their writing desks. Then I distinctly saw one of them, a young male

---

* How very odd to remember *right now* how John W. Campbell, Jr., editor of *Astounding Science Fiction* magazine, pointed out to me many, many years ago the basic, recurrent underlying theme in almost all my early science fiction stories: *Nothing is ever really what it seems to be.*

attendant, disappear under his desk. Presently he popped back up again, but then another attendant on another tier disappeared beneath his desk. This kept going on for some time in random fashion, but after a while there came a point when, suddenly, they *all* popped beneath their desks and there wasn't a soul in sight in any of the tiers. Faced with this baffling phenomenon—hallucinations seem very real to the hallucinator—I drifted off to sleep, still trying to puzzle out *what they were doing down under their desks.*

Meanwhile, as I slept and woke, slept and woke, things definitely happened to me or around me. At one point I awoke abruptly, really wide awake, to discover two nurses, one on either side of my bed. They had me half-undressed and were scratching away at my chest with their fingernails. When I objected, one of them said angrily, "You keep pulling the leads off!"

"What leads?" I said.

"The monitor leads. You keep tearing them off and the monitor doesn't work."

"I haven't touched the leads."

"You have too. This is the third time—you've got to leave them alone!"

"All I did was try to turn over."

"You're tearing the leads off, Doctor, and you've got to leave them alone."

"Well, goddamnit, if you people can't stick them on there so they stay put, I can't help it if the damn things keep falling off."

At yet another time I sensed someone nearby and looked up to see (or dream) that a very young nurse was standing at the bedside, staring at me intently in the dim night light. It seemed to me she had been taking my blood pressure or checking my pulse or something. She was Oriental—Japanese—and extremely beautiful, with that absolutely pristine, china doll–like perfection of face and carriage that one occasionally sees in Japanese women. Overriding all this, however, was the fact that she absolutely reeked of tobacco smoke, fresh on her breath, stale on her body. I remember thinking, Lord in heaven! and wanting to turn my head away from this overpowering stench, wondering if this beautiful creature had any realization that she literally stank. And then I thought, maybe it's mostly me—after all, I had suddenly discontinued a lifetime of heavy cigarette smoking, perforce, only a few nights before, and maybe my sense of smell was just beginning to rebound from years of bludgeoning.

At other times doctors were in the room, none I recognized, looking at something, fiddling with something, muttering about something, then leaving the room. At yet another time, incredibly, two absolutely immense middle-aged female nurses' aides appeared, one on either side of the bed, to give me a bed bath. The clock said 3:22, and I thought *Seriously? A bed bath at three in the morning?* Three in the morning or not, they proceeded with the job, sloshing and soaping me, while carrying on this ridiculously coy repartee, remarking upon the mole on my back, the spare tire I carried around my waist, how thin my legs were, and so forth. Finally they became even more cute and told me that now that they had washed the mentionable, I would have to wash the unmentionable, and left me with a pan of water and a soapy washcloth, and then stood outside the drapes tittering while I scrubbed my crotch. I remember thinking, my God, these two old bawds have probably had more experience with "the unmentionable" than I would ever live to witness, and here they are giggling like schoolgirls!

Still another time I entered into a long, fuguelike repetitive dream, or fantasy, that seemed to go on for hours and hours. Part of the dream involved the strange tiered nurses' station with the people bobbing up and down from behind their desks, which in some peculiar fashion I now identified with Hong Kong. Another part of the dream involved driving a car endlessly on a tortuous, winding road up an extremely steep mountainside overlooking a great city while simultaneously piecing together in my mind the many details and step-by-step cooking procedure for an enormously complex Chinese dinner. (One of my hobbies was Chinese-style cooking.) The driving was difficult, and I had no pad and paper, so I had no way to record the menu details as I worked them out; and since they were long and complicated, with everything planned in exactly the right order to get it all to come out right, details kept drifting away from me and I had to go back and start over. Presently I found that some of the earlier stages in the instructions became so firmly entrenched in my mind that I set them aside in boxes like the tiers in the nurses' station so I could just draw them out and plop them in place, but each time I did that I lost something at the other end and the whole procedure had to be started from the beginning again. I finally reached the top of the mountain with the automobile but found that the road ended there. There was no other road down, and such a tiny parking place at the top that I simply couldn't get the car turned around to go back the way I came up. One might think that this would be a good place to end such a dream and wake up, but apparently this was just the first showing, because it started all over again like a rather dull, scratchy, badly exposed television tape—I knew I'd seen it before, I had been through it all before, I knew what happened, I knew where it went, but none of that mattered. Here we were going through an instant replay, as if to make sure that I paid attention and remembered this time.

There were other such things occurring during this interval, other people coming and going, but overriding them all was a far more pervasive and sinister fantasy intermingled with all the rest, appearing again and again *in different episodes*, but all carrying the same message. These episodes were all involved with an ongoing elk hunt.

At one point I was once again walking up the series of hills and ridges rising up across the creek from our house—the exact place I had dreamed of the two elk I had seen sometime earlier. But this was a totally different day, cold and blustery, with a little snow hitting me in the face. The hill looked different than I remembered, yet I was certain those two bull elk were still up there. How I knew this, I didn't know, but there was no question in my mind. I kept climbing up and up, watching the woods above me closely. Now and then I would think I saw or heard something up in those woods—a flicker of movement or a crack of brush. I knew that some quarter of a mile ahead the woods gave way to a large expanse of rolling sagebrush hills before starting again on the far side, and I kept thinking that if the elk were moving ahead of me, tiptoeing away, they would have to break out into that open area sooner or later. If I could just move up there fast enough, there could be a clear sighting—and a close encounter with death.

I made my way down into a small gully and up the other side, trying to move quietly, but hurrying as well, tripping over windfalls as I moved, but the distance up through the forest seemed to become greater and greater, the traveling more and more difficult. Then at last I saw the edge of the forest and the open fields beyond just ahead of me. I paused to bring my rifle up to ready, placed my thumb on the safety, and made a final effort to rush up into the open, so certain was I that I would see those bulls making their way across the fields. But when I reached the forest edge, nothing was in sight, nothing but open sagebrush and a great hollow silence.

Another time and another dream: This time, I was driving the old Bronco down the rough logging road to the parking landing on the steep north face of Cle Elum ridge. It was just barely dawn on a cold wintry morning, with six inches of crusty snow on the ground. As I left the car, I realized it was still too dark to see any detail in the woods, so I found a place with a view up an open scree slope, a large tumbled slide area of small broken rocks and debris from the cliffs above, and settled down to wait for more light.

I had just found a spot when, quite suddenly, I heard an enormous crashing and scraping and rolling of rock at the top of the slope. I had heard this sound many times before and knew instantly what was happening: a group of elk were running and crashing down that scree slope, spooked by something above, and heading straight toward me. In a moment I saw them: half a dozen dark, shadowy shapes against the snow-speckled slope, coming down fast, and two of them seemed to have horns.

In the dream, I expected them to turn when they saw me or smelled me. To my amazement, they didn't. They came straight on. I could hear the crashing of brush, the thump of their hooves, and it dawned on me that they were coming right to the point where I was standing. I was out in the open, with no nearby tree to move behind; instinctively I crouched on the ground. Then two enormous cows appeared directly in front of me. One crashed past on my left, within a foot of me, a dark moving form in the dim light. The second stopped dead in her tracks twenty feet from me. She raised her head, her snout high, big ears sticking out, staring at me in stupefied surprise. Then she veered away, but three or four more came trampling straight at me as I ducked my head down. They came pounding past me and around me and over me, thumping and crashing on down the hill while I remained crouched on the ground, wondering if I had been stepped on or run over, wondering if I were hurt and if so, how badly. And then in the silence another hunter appeared and said, "There were two bulls with them! Why didn't you shoot?"

Mixed in with these dreams, at some point or another, I had a visit from Bob Dlouhy, a long-time Seattle friend who had the summer home just up the creek from us at Thorp. This was no dream, but my perception of the visit was strangely distorted. Bob had apparently brazened his way in by telling the staff that he was my best friend, and suddenly there he was, big as life, sitting in a chair at the end of the bed for a brief interval, and, it seemed to me, looking absolutely terrible. Ordinarily a big, genial, smiling fellow, Bob seemed to look shrunken and gray in the dim light, his face skeletal under the balding dome of his skull, terribly ill at ease and out of his element as he sat kneading his old cowboy hat in his hands. I guess this was a fair exchange, however, because Bob told me later that whereas *he* felt just fine, he thought that *I* looked absolutely terrible. When he left the place he was convinced that I was a goner for sure and he wished he hadn't come, I had looked so awful. Perhaps mercifully for both of us, the visit was brief. I drifted back to sleep . . .

And back to dreaming once again. This time I found myself hunting in the beautiful Elk Tuileries on the side of Cle Elum ridge, on a warm, bright day in early morning. I had just climbed up the trail to this elk haven, and I was sweating profusely, heavily overdressed for the warm day. As I walked along, I saw new signs of elk at every turn—fresh droppings, recent scuff marks in the pine needles, freshly churned tracks on the game trails, and freshly pressed bedding spots here and there with the musky odor of elk still hanging about them. But the elk themselves were not there—or at least I couldn't see them.

As I searched, however, I realized that they were very close, all around me, and it struck me that maybe I couldn't see them but *they* could see *me* perfectly. Suddenly, in the dream, I realized that I didn't have my rifle with me: I had left it down in the gully because it had seemed too heavy to carry up to this place. And then, as I walked along, I became aware of a subtle change in the place—not a change in the colors or the light or the warmness, but an odd and somehow sinister change in the air. Something about the place was wrong—and then I realized that *I* was what was wrong. This was not *my* place, my mind seemed to be saying; I had no business being there, there was nothing but danger there for me. Within moments this gathering sense of unease solidified into a totally terrifying sense of death in the air. In some bizarre fashion I suddenly recognized that I had better *leave* that place, get away *now*, not later, that there was *very little time left*. And then, in my dream, I was running for my life, stumbling down the trail into the gully again, sliding, thumping under the tangles of vine maples that lay across the trail, not stopping or looking back until I had reached the bottom and started up the other side, and then pausing to glance back, expecting something terrible to be coming after me—

Finally there came a time later, perhaps several hours later, when a nurse was shaking my shoulder, saying, "Better wake up, the doctor's here," and Fred Cleveland was in the room. I woke up this time, *really* woke up, both eyes in focus, feeling rested enough to keep my eyes open awhile. It even seemed to me that I might be a little hungry, for once. I was sure that Fred had been in several times before to check me, but always alone, or so it had seemed. This time he was accompanied by his full retinue: the chief resident, a first-year resident, the intern, a medical student, a nurse or two, all crammed into that little CCU room. I sat up in bed while Fred listened to my heart and lungs for a long, long time, shook his head, took my blood pressure, then shook his head again.

"What's wrong?" I said.

"Nothing," he said. "In fact, I think you're doing better."

"Of course I am," I said. "Look who my doctor is."

"Yes, well, be that as it may," Fred said, "I think it's about time we got you out of this cell. Someplace where there's some daylight, an honest window to look through, maybe a book to read or a TV set to watch. Something to occupy your mind. I think you're thinking too much." He looked at the charge nurse. "So let's fix that, shall we? Tomorrow morning send him up to the fourth floor. And get some X rays of those puffy ankles, too." Fred looked at the chief resident and then at me and said, "Dr. Wilske thinks he's got an attack of gout. How's that for gall, pulling something like that on us in the middle of an MI?"

After Fred left, trailing his retinue behind him, I found for the first time since arriving there that I didn't feel like going back to sleep immediately. The 5:15 I saw on the clock must have meant P.M., because when Ann came in a little later she was followed by a nurse bearing a bowl of thin gray gruel for me and a regular patient's tray for her, so we had "dinner" together. Then we talked for an hour or so, more or less coherently. After she left, I noticed that the nurses' station across the corridor seemed to be back in its proper order again. I watched the activity in the corridor for a while and then I did go to sleep—but that night, for once, I really *slept*.

— 6 —

Room 464, on a general medical floor on the fourth floor of the hospital, was a change, all right—an improvement of several orders of magnitude. The morning I was moved up there, exactly one week since the heart attack, my head was finally clear enough to recognize the significance of the change: a clear dividing line between a dim half-world of imminent death in that underground grotto of a CCU, and a sense of coming out into daylight again. I was in a private room, for which I was duly grateful—I was not yet ready to cope with somebody with liver disease in an adjacent bed—and it seemed both immensely large and immensely bright even though it was pouring rain outside the window. Like most of Seattle's large center-city hospitals, Virginia Mason was up on a high hill, with a splendid view of the downtown buildings and Elliot Bay below. My windows looked out over the rooftop of one of the older hospital buildings; off to the northwest, the Space Needle was just visible, and a high-rise downtown condominium was in the final stages of construction below me. Hospital rooms are interior-decorated these days, and somebody had had a field day with this one, all pale blues and whites, with restful abstract patterns painted on the walls. A television set was perched on a rack in the right-hand corner. Gone was the continuous monitor and the chest leads, gone the little nasal oxygen rig that had been strapped to my cheek, gone, too, most of the other paraphernalia that had crowded the little CCU room. An IV was maintained in my right arm, running glucose at a slow drip, just in case some medication had to be given fast, but aside from that I was detached from the machinery, my own person again.

It was here in room 464 that I first became aware of what was going on with my body as well as my mind and could recognize a clear pattern of day-to-day improvement.

I still slept a great deal, dozing for an hour or so after every small spurt of activity (eating a meal, having a bed bath, reading for half an hour, etc.), but the fantasies, hallucinations, dreams, and illusions were gone, even though I remembered them with perfect clarity. I realized with something of a shock that my private, subconscious-mind elk hunt was over, at least for the moment, and that both the elk and I had survived. From that first day on in room 464, my mind was looking forward, not inward—but I knew with absolute conviction that presently a book would have to be written about what had happened, and what was yet to come, and the title would be *The Elk Hunt*; nothing else could possibly do. That metaphor for a close encounter with death, still resonating in my mind, told the story far better than anything else I could imagine.

As for my body, it was no delight to behold. My ankles were grotesquely swollen, red, and intensely painful, especially when I tried to put weight on them. If I had had an attack of gout along with the heart attack (and apparently I had), it had made a real mess of my ankles. My arms were covered with purple and green splotches where IVs had been implanted and blood samples taken. My first glimpse of myself in a mirror was a revelation: I looked like walking death, sallow and cadaverous. I seemed to have no chest pain whatever, but every single thing I did was absolutely exhausting. A single trip to the bathroom and back, using a walker to take the weight off my ankles, was a full morning's hard labor. I could only read for about twenty minutes before my eyes began to cross and I would drop off to sleep. With Fred's blessing, Ann had brought in a huge pile of accumulated mail, and I wallowed in it, but only for about ten minutes at a stretch. Fred had said that that would be all right, just as long as I didn't try to do any work. I assured him solemnly that nothing was further from my mind.

I was also allowed to use the telephone, and on the second day in room 464 I called Bob Liles, the medical editor of *Good Housekeep-*

ing. He confirmed that he did have on hand enough material already submitted to piece together the February column that had been overdue when all this started. I assured him that I was coming along splendidly and would surely have the March column finished on deadline (about three weeks away), although I really had no idea whether this was going to be possible or not. Later that morning, John Mack Carter telephoned me from the magazine to cheer me on; I found myself engaged in a perfectly ridiculous conversation with him celebrating the benefits of having a heart attack as long as you didn't die from it. These calls helped bring me back in contact with the real world and set my mind at rest about one major concern: that my editors might assume I was going to be totally incapacitated and immediately start hunting up a replacement. There was no indication they had any such thing in mind, and, indeed, no such thing happened—the magazine's cheerful support throughout those critical days never once flagged. I also talked again with Carl Brandt in New York, and had calls from nephews off in Wisconsin and California. The use of the telephone was, to me, a new and totally delightful freedom.

I was allowed a broader range of visitors then, too. Ann and Chris were there every day for part of the time (Chris had taken an additional ten days' leave), and there were brief visits from old Seattle friends as well as from doctors from the Mason Clinic and elsewhere. Jennings Borgen and David Hurlbut, my doctor-partners at the North Bend Clinic years before, stopped in separately almost every day in the course of their regular hospital rounds; and I was deeply touched that Joel Baker, the chief of surgery at Virginia Mason during my intern days, now retired, stopped in one day to chat, and that Robert King, the Mason Clinic's chief of medicine and cardiology when I was an intern, also came in to say hello. Dr. King went out of his way to assure me that people nowadays bounced right back from this sort of thing; it wasn't like the old days. He said he'd had one patient who'd had twenty coronaries over the course of thirty years and had sprung back from every one of them, except the last—

At this time Dr. Ken Wilske, a Mason Clinic rheumatologist, finally decided to get moving on my ankles, which were still enormously swollen and painful. He said that the uric acid tests indicated beyond question that the trouble was gout, so he injected me with cortisone to get the acute inflammation under control and then began feeding me colchicine and allopurinol; slowly, slowly, the sore ankles began to subside.

Meanwhile, each day that Fred Cleveland came in he had something new to add about what was going on. He began talking about things to do and not to do when and if he decided to release me from the hospital. Of course the smoking had to go, he said. Carefully apportioned aliquots of rest and exercise would be in order—just slow walking, certainly no jogging, no swimming yet, and no lifting or arm-and-shoulder work whatever; he regarded that as particularly hazardous. Diet? Reduce the salt as much as possible, reduce the red meats and saturated fats to whatever limits I found tolerable. I asked him especially about cholesterol monitoring or using medicines to reduce it, and he shook his head. Yes, he knew about the work that was going on in that area, but he wasn't convinced that there was much I could do to alter anything at this stage of the game.

"Work with your diet as much as you want, that can't do any harm, but I don't want you on any medicine to mess around with your cholesterol."

I told Fred how surprised I was that I wasn't having any sign of chest pain. He gave me a long look. "Don't be impatient," he said.

"Well, I haven't even had a twinge since I got here, that I can remember."

"I assure you that you had quite enough chest pain to suit *me* the first few days you were here. Sure, you don't need morphine anymore—but then you're not doing anything but sitting in this bed like a toad on a rock. In addition, I've got you loaded up on a beta-blocker that prevents a whole lot of trouble you might otherwise be having. You'll have pain enough when the time comes, believe me, and when you do, you'd better let me know, too."

Thinking about that later, I realized that I really didn't know what medicines I was taking or what they were supposed to be doing. Neither, for that matter, did I have any idea what might be coming up in the future when I started stirring around a bit. I wasn't even sure that I wanted to know. So the next time Fred came around; I raised the subject as obliquely as possible. When Fred asked me how I was feeling, I said, "It seems to me that I'm recovering remarkably well."

"The fact is that you haven't even started recovering," he said. "All we've been doing so far is just keeping you alive, nothing more. And that's been fine, as far as I'm concerned. In some medical centers you might have been catheterized and on the operating table within six hours of the minute you walked in the door, but when you turned up here, I wasn't too sure you were going to live six hours, and neither was the surgeon, so we chose to play it very conservatively." He smiled and spread his hands. "So you're still among us," he said, "and that's an achievement. But it doesn't tell us where to go next. At this point I really don't have the slightest idea of *exactly* what happened to your heart the night you got sick, except that you plugged up a big coronary artery, and until I know *exactly* what happened, I'm not going to know which way to move next."

"Well, you certainly know I had an MI," I said.

"Oh, you had an MI all right. You had a whopper. We know that from the cardiograms, the enzyme tests, and the clinical course. We even know that the damage was posterior, on the under side of the heart, and through and through the myocardium. The trouble is, that's not enough. We don't know which coronary artery was involved—whether it was a main artery, or just one of the major branches, or whatever. We don't know *how much* of your heart may still be hanging on by a thread. We don't know how much your heart is able to do right now, or how much it's ever going to be able to do. We don't know how close to heart failure you may be right now as a result of the damage, or how likely you are to have another coronary any old minute. In other words, we know the gross pathology, all right, we just don't have any detail."

"Do we need that much detail?"

Fred hesitated. "Thirty years ago, none of this would have made any difference, because we couldn't have done anything anyway. Thirty years ago, we'd have kept you flat in bed for thirty to sixty days, and digitalized you if you went into heart failure, and then let you tiptoe around for whatever time you had left, living in mortal fear of the next coronary that would wipe you out. The kind of detail I'm talking about would have been totally academic in those days—completely useless information. Today things are different, thank God. Today we have some real options—really good, life-prolonging medical treatment on one hand, or several very promising avenues of surgical treatment on the other. In order to choose which option is right for you, we have to know everything we can know about that academic business of what happened to your heart last week and what may be about to happen sometime later."

"So let's get on with finding out," I said. "I'm here, without much else to do. Why not start now?"

"Well, for one reason, because we *don't* know very much about where you are right now. For another, the things we have to do to find out what we need to know aren't necessarily easy or comfortable, and those things themselves carry a certain risk. Right now I want you further down the road from your acute attack before we start meddling. Ideally, I'd like you to spend about three months getting out of the woods, taking things one day at a time, gradually increasing your activities, getting a little closer to the beginning of real recovery without rocking the boat before we start introducing any variables that we don't have to. With this disease, you don't like to start rocking the boat, because once that boat starts rocking, you sometimes can't get it stopped."

We left it at that for the moment. Over the next few days I edged closer and closer to the point of leaving the hospital, and Fred added a little bit each day to what I would need to know when I did so. One day he let me sit on the chair in the shower room and take the first real bath I'd had since the night of the attack, with a nurse hovering just outside the door in case something dreadful should come to pass. My hospital diet began to look more like food, although it was devoid of salt, offered little or no fried food, and nothing even vaguely resembling an egg. I spent more time reading and watching TV and less time sleeping, and found myself feeling more energetic every day.

Fred made rounds the next Monday morning, after a weekend away, and announced that Wednesday morning I could be discharged. Tuesday, November 4, was Election Day, and Ann and I were prepared for a long evening's entertainment watching the returns, only to find that the entertainment ended about 6:30 P.M. when President Carter conceded the election an hour and a half before the polls had even closed on the West Coast. And although Ann carefully didn't say anything about it, I was acutely aware that that day had also been the second day of elk season, and wondered if any of our friends had had any luck yet, and realized again that there would be no hunting for me at all this season.

The following morning on his rounds, Fred listened to my heart, and my lungs, and affirmed that I could be discharged from the hospital—but not home to Thorp just yet. For the next ten days or so he wanted me right there in Seattle, somewhere very close to the hospital where I could easily call him or see him any time of the day or night, or be hauled bodily into the emergency room if necessary. He had suggested the nearby Mason House facility, but our writer friends the Busbys had a small vacant apartment that they were renting in the building adjacent to their home on the western shoulder of Queen Anne Hill, used mostly for book and manuscript storage, and they had offered to let us use it. Fred said that sounded fine. He also outlined the medicines he wanted me to continue using when I got to the apartment, especially a beta-blocker known as propranolol (trade name Inderal). This drug, essentially, reduces the effect of adrenaline on the action of the heart muscle, slowing down the heart rate, reducing the amount of oxygen the heart muscle requires, and, in many cases, protecting against the pain of angina. He told me to continue with the allopurinol and colchicine for the gout, and provided a little bottle of nitroglycerin pills and a tube of

nitroglycerin paste to use in the event that I did get any chest pain—
"But be sure to let me know if you do," he added. "In fact, let me
know if anything at all seems out of the ordinary to you."

At ten o'clock Wednesday morning, after doctors' rounds were
over, we left the hospital in the prescribed fashion. I wasn't allowed
to walk out under my own power; Chris brought our car around to
the hospital entrance and I was wheeled down the corridor, into the
elevator, and out to the front door in a wheelchair, accompanied by
Ann and a nurse. It was the first time I had actually been outdoors
in almost two weeks, and I was greeted by typical Seattle weather
for November—gray, rainy, windy, raw. Ann had to stop to do some
grocery shopping on the way to the apartment, and Chris went in
to help her; I sat in the car in the parking lot, watching people hustle
past, cars driving around, the wind blowing people's hats off, feeling
slightly overwhelmed that I'd actually made it that far. By the time
we reached the Busbys' and I walked up the few steps to the porch
of the ground-level apartment, I was feeling totally exhausted and
chilled to the bone, despite the fact that I was wearing plenty of
clothes, a down jacket, and a wool cap. Inside, the heat had not yet
been turned on, so I immediately went to bed and pulled the blankets
up for a couple of hours before warming up enough to feel like
getting up and having a small bowl of soup for lunch.

This was the beginning of a sort of limping daily routine: getting
up, getting dressed, then lying down to rest, then getting up again,
then lying down to rest again. It was a tiny apartment: just a living
room, kitchen, bedroom, bath, without much room to move around
in. When I was "up," I was mostly sitting in a chair, but even that
seemed to require an enormous effort. There were plenty of sedentary things for me to do—piled-up mail to read and respond to, a
stack of medical journals to review for material for the next *Good
Housekeeping* column, a John D. MacDonald murder mystery to
read, and the rest of Craig Claiborne's no-salt cookbook, which I
had been reading one recipe at a time. In addition, Ann went out
and rented a television set so that I could sit and watch the Mind-
Stealer whenever I felt so inclined.

Even so, an hour or two of "being up" at a time was about all I
could manage. Just composing, typing, addressing, and sealing a two-
line response to a letter from Carl somehow seemed to evolve into
a full morning's work. I would get up early in the morning and
have breakfast with Ann—shredded wheat with milk or some such
thing—and then intermittently shuffle around and lie down while
she went out shopping for an hour at a time, the longest she dared
to be away during the first few days. Later on she would take off

for Thorp to resume seeing her patients, leaving at six in the morning and getting back around six in the evening, while I spent the day more or less vegetating. Watching Dan Rather on the evening news became one of the high spots in an otherwise stupid day; so also was the cocktail before dinner that Fred permitted me, and occasionally the Busbys would drop in to visit for half an hour in the evening. The big effort of each day went into the two daily "exercise periods" Fred had prescribed, one in the morning and one in the late afternoon. Each time, in addition to my corduroy pants, wool socks, wool shirt, and sweater, I would bundle into a scarf, down jacket, and my wool Indian hat, as though I were going out to face the Russian winter, and then I would slowly, slowly walk out onto the porch, down the steps, and take a very slow, five-minute walk up the street from the apartment and back. I must have looked to the neighbors like a walking corpse, but those were the orders, and that was what I did.

It was on the second or third day of such adventures that I made my first personal acquaintance with one of the nightmare realities of coronary artery disease: angina pectoris.

Maybe I had some angina right from the start and just didn't recognize what was going on. The first episode that I *knew* was angina, and absolutely nothing else, occurred on the second or third evening in the Busbys' apartment. It was about 5:30 P.M. and Ann was out shopping for groceries. We had invited the Busbys to come over for a drink after Elinor got home from work, but I had completely forgotten it. As it happened, I was in the bathroom at the rear of that small apartment when I heard somebody rapping on the front door. Startled, I hiked my trousers up as quickly as I could and rushed down the hall into the living room, concerned that our guests might figure we had forgotten and just leave.

I could see the Busbys through the front door glass, and they could see me, but I got just halfway across the living room and no farther. Without warning I was hit by a sudden intense groundswell of chest pain, a deep, dirty pain under the breastbone that spread in a matter of seconds into my left shoulder and down into my left wrist. I could feel my heart pounding in my ears from the simple exertion of moving that far that fast (a matter of perhaps fifty feet), but the pain continued to rise in a crescendo wave, taking my breath away until it began to crest and subside. By the time I had walked very slowly the rest of the way to the door and opened it, the pain was gone as if it had never been there at all.

This is how exertional angina—angina that arises from physical overactivity—comes on: fast, hard, very painful, and subsiding only when the exertion stops. Of course rushing from the bathroom into the living room would not normally constitute overactivity for most people, but for me, at that time, it was clearly overactivity enough, and the sudden agonizing manner in which my body told me about it was jarring in the extreme. In a sense, it was the first clearcut, indisputable warning that something in my body had indeed really and permanently changed.

The same kind of chest pain came on in the same way the next morning, when I took my first brief walk outside the apartment. That walk involved stepping down two steps from the porch, down another four steps to the sidewalk, and then very slow pacing about half a block up the street on a cold, raw morning. This time I knew the angina was coming on before it actually started because I was overexerting less abruptly and the pain appeared more slowly. As I walked down the steps, I could feel a sort of gathering heaviness in my chest, a feeling that I couldn't completely fill my lungs with air, not really a pain but a sense of disquiet, a sort of pressure. And then as I continued to walk, the pressure evolved into a deep-seated, angry, dull pain with the radiation to the shoulder and the left arm that I had noticed before. When I stopped walking, the developing pain subsided into the dull sense of pressure again, and then that, too, faded away. As I turned to walk back, more slowly than before, the pressure recurred, and the pain was just beginning as I got up onto the porch, walked into the apartment and sat down.

That night for the first time I experienced a different kind of angina—different because of the way it felt, and different because of the circumstances under which it developed. We had had a modest dinner that night—I wasn't very hungry and wasn't eating very well—and had watched a movie on TV before retiring at about nine o'clock. I was having no trouble whatever sleeping in those days— it was as if I was always exhausted—but that night at about 11:30 I woke up because something was wrong. I had been sleeping on my back and now realized I had a pain in my chest that had been there at least for a while before I woke. It was a deep, pressing pain, not terribly severe, but very real, very present, and it seemed to grow very slowly in depth and intensity as I became aware of it. I felt it only in my chest, not in the shoulder or the arm, and the pain was different in quality from the pain I had had on exertion before. It wasn't as severe but it was more of a nagging, persisting discomfort deep inside my chest. What was disturbing was that it obviously wasn't related to exertion in any way, since I'd been fast asleep when it developed and had not, that I could recall, been having bad dreams or anything of that sort.

I sat up on the side of the bed. The pain seemed to subside a little, but it didn't go away. I walked into the bathroom and took one of the nitroglycerin tablets that Fred had sent home with me. Nothing very much seemed to happen. Finally, more angry and disgusted at the disturbance than suffering from the pain, I turned on the living room lights and moved around the living room, back and forth for five or ten minutes. After a while the discomfort slowly subsided and disappeared. When I went back to bed and to sleep, the pain did not recur again that night. This was my first acquaintance with what I came to think of as "the other angina," an angina that occurred at rest and that didn't respond very well to ordinary doses of nitroglycerin.

This sudden introduction to two different forms of angina or "heart pain" came as a completely new experience to me. I could not remember ever having encountered either one of them before. Later, in retrospect, I realized that I probably had actually had one or two episodes of exertional angina in the years immediately before my MI and had either failed to recognize them as angina at all or else had recognized them on some level but had blocked or denied the recognition, so that no action was taken. There had been a time, two or three years before in North Bend, when I decided to walk the quarter-mile out to the rural route mailbox rather than driving, as I habitually did. On one or two occasions I had encountered some chest pain on those walks, but if I recognized them as angina, I had discounted them because they didn't appear with any regularity. I also now remember one episode a year or so before the MI, over at Thorp, when Becky and some of her girlfriends from college had found a dead cedar waxwing along the edge of the county road. I had hustled out to the road, to see the bird and confirm its identity, then hustled back to the house, and had severe chest pain by the time I got back to the porch. But it had been a single incident, nonrecurring, and again I had failed (or refused) to recognize it as possible angina. An investigation of those episodes of chest pain when they occurred, perhaps including a treadmill test, might have made a major difference in the course of later events, but it was never done.

Since these new episodes of chest pain were clearly angina, and nothing else, I called Fred Cleveland about them, as instructed. He doubled the dose of Inderal I was taking and ordered a new medicine: a relatively long acting nitroglycerin-type compound, *isosorbide dinitrite* (trade name Isordil), to be taken four times a day. (We'll discuss the usefulness and action of these and other drugs in combating angina in more detail a little later.)

Why all the emphasis here on angina pectoris? The reason is simple and basic: Angina is part and parcel of emerging coronary artery disease in the vast majority of cases. Angina is not a disease in itself; it is merely a symptom of a more basic, underlying disease process. But when it occurs, it is a flagrant and compelling symptom. What's more, unlike many vague, generalized symptoms of illness, such as fever, muscle aching, or coughing, angina is very *specific*. It is a signal of one thing and one thing only—coronary artery disease; and it tells both the patient and the doctor some very specific things about the nature and extent of the disease that causes it. In many cases it is nothing less than a ringing alarm bell, a recurring and persistent early warning of absolutely certain trouble ahead. In other cases, it is a continuing reminder of heart damage already done and impairment already accomplished.

Perhaps most important of all, it is a symptom that can exercise a staggering influence on the life of the person who has it. The extent of a person's angina and the degree to which it can be controlled can be a major determinant of precisely what a person with coronary artery disease can and cannot do with the rest of his or her life.

The What and Why of Angina

In order to see how a symptom can be so important and exercise so much influence, we need to understand something about a process known as *ischemia* and the role it plays in the body.

Ischemia is a fancy medical term, derived from Greek, meaning, "to suppress blood." It refers to the diminution of blood flow to any part of the body as a result of some obstruction of the blood vessels supplying the area. We've seen that all the cells, tissues, and organs of the body require a constant flow of fresh oxygen-carrying blood. The blood picks up oxygen in its passage through the lungs, then unloads it in cells and tissues far and wide. Anyplace where the steady supply of oxygenated blood is somehow obstructed, the cells very quickly become starved for oxygen—that is, they become *is-chemic*. And if they are deprived of oxygen for any length of time—even a matter of minutes, in some cases—the biochemical reactions in those cells that require oxygen come to a halt and the cells begin to die.

Obviously ischemia is a dangerous business anyplace it turns up—so dangerous, in fact, that the body has evolved a delicate, sensitive alarm system to call immediate attention to it. Any part of the body equipped with pain-sensitive nerve endings begins to carry pain messages to the brain whenever ischemia is prolonged in any area for more than a few moments. In short, any part of the body that becomes ischemic begins to hurt almost immediately.

You can observe ischemia, and the pain signals that result from it, by means of a simple experiment. Wrap a small rubber band around the tip of your ring finger—not too tightly, just enough so that you can feel the constricting pressure. The tip of the ring finger is normally a delicate pink color due to the bright red, oxygen-rich blood flowing through the capillaries in the fingertip. But within moments after you block that blood flow with the rubber band, you will see the color fade from a healthy pink to a dark dusky bluish purple color—the color of venous blood from which all the oxygen has been exhausted. At the same time, you will notice that that fingertip has become distinctly cooler than the other fingertips; not only is it no longer receiving fresh, warm, body-temperature blood in a steady flow, but the cells' capacity to conduct heat-producing biochemical reactions is already being impaired. Then, within a few seconds an even more striking change will occur: The obstructed fingertip will begin to feel uncomfortable, then actually painful, and the pain will get progressively worse as long as the rubber band remains around the finger.

Don't worry that you might forget and leave the rubber band in place—the pain in the fingertip won't allow you to do that for very long. It will quickly become excruciating unless you take the rubber band off (which, of course, you should do immediately). The very nature of the pain itself is significant. This is not the sharp stabbing pain you get from cutting your finger with a knife, or being stuck by a pin, or even like the throbbing pain of a headache. This pain is a sort of crushing, continuous, intolerable aching, a visceral or "deep inside" type of pain that grows progressively worse the longer the ischemic obstruction continues.

The moment you remove the rubber band, things change back with almost unbelievable speed. Within seconds the blue color changes back to a healthy pink. Almost at once the fingertip feels warmer again, and within a few more seconds the pain vanishes as if it had never been there.

All this is extremely characteristic of pain due to ischemia. The pain gets worse and worse as long as the ischemia continues, and then quickly fades as soon as blood flow is restored.

Unfortunately, ischemia does more than just cause pain in the obstructed area. *It interferes with the way the machine works.* If you had put the obstructing rubber band down at the base of the finger, for instance, you would have found that the finger refused to function normally while the ischemia was present—it would become more and more difficult to move it. In addition, the sense of touch and the sensitivity of the finger tip to heat would both have been impaired. This loss of function would very quickly be reversed as soon as the obstruction was relieved, so it might appear that no harm was done. But this would not be quite true. On a microscopic level, as soon as ischemia begins, a certain number of cells in the ischemic area are injured and begin to die. And once they die, those cells are *dead*. They never recover. They may be replaced by healthy cells around them, but they themselves will never recover.

Of course in the simple, brief fingertip experiment I just mentioned, not enough cells would be destroyed to make any significant difference or to be noticeable later. But if the obstruction were allowed to continue, for hours or days, for example, irreparable damage could occur, with obvious loss of tissue—loss of skin, peeling of the nail, and so forth. When extreme or prolonged ischemia arises in a foot, for example, as a result of frostbite or prolonged immersion, whole toes may become gangrenous and peel off after circulation is restored. As the great physician Sir William Osler once put it, "Ischemia not only interferes with the function of the machine, it wrecks the machinery as well." And the more severe and prolonged the ischemia, the greater the wreckage.

Obviously the pain associated with ischemia is not a disease itself: It is merely a symptom of an underlying disorder—obstruction of blood flow to part of the body. As soon as the obstruction is relieved, the pain goes away. While the obstruction is present, however, a certain number of cells will die from lack of oxygen; the more prolonged the obstruction, the more cells will die, and if the obstruction is recurrent, a few more cells will die during each episode.

Considering this, it is easy to see what *myocardial ischemia*—ischemia of the heart muscle—can do to the heart and why angina pectoris, the characteristic pain that arises as a result of myocardial ischemia, is so very important. A slow, steady, day-by-day, month-by-month obstruction of a coronary artery branch supplying a portion of heart muscle will lead to greater and greater impairment of blood flow to the part of the heart muscle that particular vessel supplies. As long as the obstruction is not too severe, the heart muscle can limp along doing its regular job, contracting and relaxing, pumping blood. As long as enough oxygen reaches it in spite of the obstruction, no symptoms will appear.

But as the blood flow is gradually restricted, a point can be reached at which the heart muscle cells involved can really only manage to do their job under quiet, inactive circumstances. What happens then when exertion of some kind places a sudden, unusual work load on that heart muscle, requiring the heart suddenly to pump faster (increased heart rate) and more effectively (with more forceful contractions than normal)? Clearly such a sudden, excessive work load can require the heart muscle to use oxygen faster, temporarily, than the partially obstructed vessel can supply it. In such a case the heart muscle that was barely limping along during quiet, inactive conditions becomes suddenly ischemic whenever exertion begins. This suddenly occurring ischemia in turn triggers a pain alarm that, in the case of myocardial ischemia, is the agonizing pain of angina pectoris.*

Characteristically and typically, angina sweeps in when exertion demands extra work from a heart whose blood supply is impaired, and then subsides when the exertion is terminated. A man who rarely walks any further than from his car to his office elevator in the course of a day may never have any angina, and, thus, may never know that his heart's blood supply is impaired in any way. But when that same man finds the elevator out of order and walks up four flights of stairs to his office, he may get halfway up and suffer an attack of angina. Another man may stroll along the sidewalk or road on the level and do just fine, but when he comes to a hill and has to exert himself a little, he may find chest pain occurring suddenly. Physical exertion is the typical trigger, and the appearance of episodes of angina during physical exertion is the most common early warning that something is seriously wrong with blood flow to the heart.

This is not the only situation in which angina can occur, however. Other things besides exertion can trigger it. In fact, *anything* that places an extra demand upon the impaired heart can trigger angina, whether it involves exertion or not. A man might return from a restful vacation, plunge abruptly into a high-tension business situation at work, and begin having spells of angina even though he doesn't walk, run, or exert himself at all. A woman may become angry over some acute injustice and be seized with chest pains in the middle of her anger. Sir John Hunter, a famous British physician and surgeon of the 1780s, was one of the first to realize that angina pectoris was related to coronary artery blood flow. He suffered severely from angina himself and clearly recognized that the surge of adrenaline occurring during a fit of anger could place just as much excess strain on the heart as running up three flights of stairs. As he once so eloquently expressed it, "My life is in the hands of any

---

* It's important to mention here that this is true in most cases, but not necessarily always. There are people, for example, who develop myocardial ischemia during the extreme exertion of a treadmill test but feel no anginal pain whatever. We know the heart muscle is ischemic from changes that appear on the EKG (about which more later), but no pain is triggered. Nobody knows exactly why this happens; perhaps it's just a matter of individual differences. But myocardial ischemia *does* trigger angina so very commonly in such a large proportion of cases that these few "aberrant cases" have to be considered unusual.

rascal who chooses to annoy and tease me." He was right on target, too: At the age of sixty-five, during a board meeting at St. George's Hospital during which he became angry, he incurred an attack of angina and died within a few minutes.

Still another person may walk to work each morning quite comfortably during warm, seasonable weather, yet begin to suffer chest pain while walking on icy cold mornings. Dampness and cold require increased metabolism and increased cardiac blood flow; in many instances cold weather can trigger episodes of angina when nothing else seems to. And sometimes the exertion of sexual intercourse can bring on an angina attack, especially under tension. (It has been documented that adulterous men with mistresses have a high rate of angina pectoris and myocardial infarctions.) Even a rich, heavy meal can precipitate angina by drawing so much of the body's blood supply to the gastrointestinal tract that the already impaired supply to the heart drops to the ischemic level.

Patterns of Exertional Angina

Whatever it is that triggers an episode of exertional angina, the attack itself is very often self-limiting because it literally forces the person to stop doing whatever he or she is doing to cause the angina. A person will not ordinarily keep on exercising when angina strikes, because the pain simply becomes worse and worse until the person is forced to stop. If angina comes on every time someone engages in a certain exertional activity, that person very soon learns to avoid that activity because he knows he is not going to like the consequences. The individual who suffers fifteen minutes of angina after a heavy evening meal is not likely to endure this experience very often before he consciously begins to temper the quantity and quality of what he eats for dinner. The person who develops angina while walking briskly on a cold morning will very soon get the message that he'd better not walk briskly on cold mornings or he's going to wish he hadn't. Indeed, recurring exertional angina can very quickly and sharply limit exactly what the victim finds he or she can or cannot do. Angina can become a real tyrant: It can *make* you do things—or avoid doing things—whether you want to or not.

I found this out very early in my experience walking on the street outside the Busbys' apartment. I very soon realized that my angina attacks were dictating just how far and how fast I could walk. If I walked too fast or too far, or both, I would first develop the heavy "intimation of approaching angina" feeling in my chest, and then the angina proper would come, and I would stop walking. At first it seemed to be very much as though there were a brick wall that I came to that I couldn't go beyond. *Whatever I was doing,* whether walking on the level, going up stairs or whatnot, when the angina came on, I stopped doing it.

This was not a matter of choice, or courage, or determination, or anything else; I simply could not press on with the exertion because the anginal pain would become worse and worse to the point of being intolerable if I tried to continue. At one point during that time I recorded in my journal that it seemed that this "brick wall" perimeter lay at a distance of about two blocks of moderate-speed walking on the level—that is, I couldn't walk farther than two blocks at moderate speed without running into the wall—into the angina. If I wanted to go any farther than that, I had to stop and wait for the angina to pass before going on. Later, as the oxygenation of my heart muscle improved, due to the medicines I was taking, and, perhaps, the slow development of new arterial blood vessels, called *collateral arteries,* in my heart, that "brick wall" perimeter was pushed back to perhaps three and a half blocks of moderate-speed walking on the level. It seemed at the time that this change was at least a rough measure of the help I was getting from the medication or of improvement in my heart's exercise tolerance, or of healing of injured myocardium, or whatever.

Later, as I became more intimately acquainted with this symptom, it seemed to me that the angina was not so much a matter of running into a rigid brick wall that was absolutely there or absolutely not as a matter of pushing a heavy ball up a geometric curve, with the curve starting out quite flat, then gradually, geometrically increasing, steeper and steeper. At some point along the flat part of that "curve of exercise," I knew that the angina was soon about to start. If I persisted in the exercise, pushing the ball farther up the curve that became steeper and steeper, the angina itself would begin, and the higher I pushed the ball up the curve, the more severe the angina. Thus, an arithmetic increment of moving the ball forward would cause a geometric increase in the angina, perhaps even an exponential increase in the angina, to the point that no further activity was tolerable. Up to a point, I could continue to push the exercise in the face of the angina, but very small increases in activity would bring greater and greater progressions of the angina.

Two other things typically mark the pattern of angina: the nature or quality of the pain, and its distribution—where it's *felt.* The pain of angina is very similar to the pain in the obstructed fingertip: a deep-seated, aching, continuous pain-pressure; a spreading, ugly sort of pain so very characteristic that once one feels it and identifies it as as angina, it can never be mistaken for anything else. In most cases it begins down in the chest under the breastbone or just to the left of it, first as a feeling of pressure or discomfort, then escalating into an aching, crushing pain. People often say it seems to take their breath away, and certainly it is often associated with a sense of shortness of breath or inability to fill the lungs completely. Part of the nature of this pain is its characteristic tendency, upon subsiding, to vanish completely, no matter how severe it had become at its peak, with no residual discomfort or aching. It subsides so completely that a person may well scratch his head and wonder, Did I really feel that? What happened to it? Where did it go?

As for the distribution of anginal pain—where it is felt—this is perhaps the oddest thing of all. Usually felt in the chest at first, it often spreads quickly to quite distant areas. Typically this so-called *referred pain* spreads up into the left shoulder or around under the left shoulder blade. Often it will spread into the left side of the neck and jaw. Equally often, it may spread on to the left elbow or wrist, perhaps into the left thumb or forefinger. But different people may feel the pain in other odd places. About 25 percent of victims feel the pain referred to the *right* side. A given person may feel angina only in the right shoulder, for example, or as a crushing ache in the small of the back, or as a terrible stiff neck. Another individual might have a very quirky angina felt solely and exclusively in one thumb, or just in the angle of the jaw on one side or the other.

Of course, there are reasons myocardial ischemia can cause pain felt in such a variety of locations. The referred pain is felt in the same general pain-distribution area served by the deep visceral pain nerve fibers that also serve the heart. And it may be that the specific nature and distribution of a person's angina may be related to the exact part of the heart muscle that is ischemic. But the nature and distribution of a person's angina do *not* necessarily say anything about the severity of the underlying coronary artery disease. One person, with a relatively minor blockage of a small coronary artery branch, may develop very severe angina, while another, with 90 percent obstruction of one of the main coronary arteries, may have only brief episodes of angina on extreme exertion, or maybe none at all, as we have noted.

The angina on exertion that we have been discussing is by far the most common and most easily identifiable form of angina there is. An astute physician may be able to make an almost certain diagnosis of severe coronary artery disease—or, at least, suspect such a di-agnosis—just from a patient's history of recurring chest pain. We now know that exertional angina is usually related to some fixed obstruction somewhere in the coronary artery system—at least one of the arterial branches is rigidly pinched by physical obstruction caused by atherosclerotic plaques, so that blood flow is diminished.

In addition, the affected artery has lost its normal elastic capacity to expand and allow more blood to flow through in times of exercise and demand.

In recent years, however, physicians have come to recognize a different sort of angina that can arise in a slightly different way. In 1959, a prominent cardiologist named M. Prinzmetal described an oddly different kind of anginal pain suffered by a number of patients he had seen. These patients reported episodes of angina appearing at times when they least expected them, for example, when they were completely at rest, even asleep, with no exertion, stress, or adrenaline stimulation involved.

These people might be awakened from a sound sleep by the sudden onset of this anginal pain or find it coming on while relaxing in the evening reading a book. Dr. Prinzmetal observed that people afflicted with this odd kind of "variant angina," "atypical angina," or "angina-at-rest," were often people who had very severe degrees of coronary artery disease, and this variant kind of angina (now sometimes called Prinzmetal's angina) came to be regarded as a bad prognostic sign. These were people, it was felt, who were much more likely to drop dead without warning than were people with ordinary exertional angina.

We know today that this is not necessarily true. Over the years a great deal has been learned about variant angina, and one of the things it has taught us is that coronary artery disease is often a much more dynamic, actively progressive disease than it was once thought to be. It has long been known that muscle tissue tends to contract or go into spasm when it is irritated in some way. When atherosclerosis begins to manifest itself in the coronary arteries, the fatty deposits and associated inflammation can be highly irritating to the muscle in the artery walls, causing that muscle to go into spasm. And in some cases practically all the blood flow through the vessel can be temporarily cut off just by the spasm alone.

Cardiologists today still aren't certain that this is exactly what happens to bring on an attack of variant angina. Some people have coronary spasm to the point of obstruction in apparently perfectly normal coronary arteries; others, with variant angina, are found to have moderate to severe atherosclerotic plaques in their coronary arteries, and the spasm does seem to occur in the areas where the arteries are diseased. But the ischemia that results from such coronary spasm is just as real as if the heart were working hard under stress and couldn't get enough blood for the extra work, and the ischemic pain reaction—the angina—is also just as real.

Obviously this kind of angina cannot be relieved by discontinuing exertion, since exertion isn't involved. It only goes away when the artery spasm gradually relaxes and allows blood to flow freely again, or when some medication causes the irritated artery to relax.

Back in the days of Sir John Hunter, angina pectoris must have seemed a very mysterious and ominous symptom, since physicians of those days really had no very clear idea of what exactly was causing it. All they knew was that angina meant that something was wrong with the heart and that people with angina were increasingly vulnerable not only to severe episodes of chest pain but to heart attacks and sudden death as well. What's more, in those days there was very little that could be done to control the angina except to stop whatever activity seemed to be triggering it. At that time the onset of severe angina must have seemed very much a pronouncement of doom for the patient. Many patients became virtual cripples, unable to do anything at all without the dreadful punishment of angina following immediately. A person was chained to his angina like Prometheus to the rock, with the crows pecking away at his liver.

Today we understand the nature of angina far more clearly and can see it more precisely for what it really is—a delicate, dynamic measure of myocardial ischemia. It has also become possible to deal with it far more effectively, at least to some degree, to control it when it occurs, and in some cases, even to turn it to the patient's advantage. Today when a patient comes to a doctor with a history of the onset of angina, one of the first things the doctor will do is to order an *electrocardiogram*—another important part of the coronary artery disease story.

The Remarkable EKG

In the very early years of this century, a Dutch physiologist named Willem Einthoven invented a device that must have seemed very much of a magical machine to physicians of his day.

Einthoven was trained as a doctor, but he was fascinated by the phenomenon of electricity. In 1903, he invented a simple instrument known as a string galvanometer. This was little more than a length of conducting wire, essentially, with a delicately balanced indicator needle attached to the middle of it. When the wire was connected to an electrical circuit, and a switch thrown, allowing electricity to flow through the wire, the needle would jump when the current began flowing and would jump again when the current was switched off. This device was simply a meter to indicate when a galvanic current started or stopped flowing through the wire, hence the name *galvanometer*. As Einthoven refined this device to make it more sensitive, it was able to detect the movement of extremely tiny electric currents—currents so weak that their presence could not have been detected any other way. Of course the galvanometer did not *create* an electric current, it had no generating power source. All it could do was measure with a flick of a needle when an electric current from some other source passed through the wire.

Between 1903 and 1907, Einthoven began using his device to study the tiny electrical currents generated by the human heart. His technique was crude by today's standards: He connected a galvanometer to wires attached to the patient's arms and feet; then he stuck the patient's arms and feet into buckets of saltwater and measured the electrical currents passing between them. When this was done, a remarkable thing happened: The galvanometer needle began twitching in perfect timing with the patient's heartbeat. Each time the heart contracted, a tiny electrical current passed through the galvanometer. At first this seemed impossible—where was the electric current coming from? Since there was no other possible source for the current, it obviously had to be generated by the heart itself, and the galvanometer measurement of that current came to be known as an *electrocardiogram*. (Electro Kardio Gram or EKG in German—and now universal—usage.)

Today, we know that the beating of the heart is quite literally triggered by electricity. In the normal, healthy heart there is a small patch of highly specialized heart muscle tissue located in the wall of the right atrium—the upper chamber of the right side of the heart. This lump of tissue is known as the *sino-atrial (S-A) node*, sometimes just called the *sinus node*. Special chemical reactions occurring in the cells of that node generate an electrical impulse. This impulse—a tiny current of electricity—is then conducted through other special nerve and muscle channels to other parts of the heart.

First the impulse spreads through the walls of the left and right atria, triggering a muscle contraction in that area of the heart muscle. At the same time, the impulse is conducted by special fibers composed of both nerve and muscle tissue down into the septum between the two ventricles. From there, the impulse spreads to the ventricles, stimulating them to contract. All this happens very quickly—within a fraction of a second. Once the stimulating electrical current has passed through the heart, and the atria and ventricles have contracted in turn, the heart muscle relaxes in a brief *refractory period* or resting period as the heart fills once more with blood. Then the whole cycle begins again. Some three-quarters of a second after the last electrical impulse was triggered, another one is triggered and the heart contracts again.

In a healthy heart this whole cycle of electrical triggering, heart muscle contraction and relaxation occurs regularly and repeatedly at an average rate of around 70 times a minute, creating what is called the *normal sinus rhythm* of the heartbeat. The rate varies, however, as the body's demand for blood and oxygen increases or decreases. During exercise, for example, the electrical stimuli in the sinus node speed up, leading to a heart rate as high as 120 beats per minute or more; during sleep, when the body's demand for blood is at its lowest, the normal sinus rate and heartbeat may slow to as few as 55 or 60 beats per minute.

The tiny electrical current that stimulates each heartbeat does not just vanish after it passes through the heart. It travels on out through the other tissues of the body, gradually dissipating but still strong enough to be picked up by electrocardiograph leads on the wrists, ankles, or chest wall. The current moves in a consistent manner from the top of the heart down, with the electrocardiograph needle deflecting at each step of the way. When the current causes the atria to contract, the needle makes a blip; as it passes down to make the ventricles contract, the needle makes a more complex series of blips. By recording these blips as up or down markings on a moving strip of specially treated paper, a permanent record or "tracing" of the heart's electrical activity is obtained—a record we call an electrocardiogram or EKG. A typical tracing of any normal, healthy heart will look very much like this:

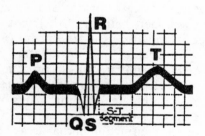

Traditionally each blip or "wave" on an EKG tracing is given a special letter name and represents a specific event in the course of a heartbeat cycle. The first little blip, called the P wave, represents the beginning of the contraction of the upper chambers of the heart or the atria. The small flat segment following the P wave represents the time necessary for the current to move down to the ventricles. As the current spreads through the ventricles and causes them to contract, there is first a weak downward deflection (called the Q wave), then a strong upward deflection (the R wave), and another downward deflection (S wave). As the current then begins to dissipate, there is another flat segment of the tracing and then a final upward blip (the T wave), which occurs as the ventricles relax. In most EKG tracings, the P wave and the T wave usually appear quite distinct and separate, but the ventricular contraction waves all run together in a sort of jiggle, sometimes called the QRS complex.

Actually, this EKG tracing is nothing more than a stretched-out picture of the movement of an electric current across an imaginary line drawn from a contact placed on one side of the heart to a contact placed on the other side. Early investigators found that by varying the position of the contacts, or "leads," they could obtain varying wave patterns as the electrical current crossed imaginary lines placed in different positions. In a sense, it was as though one were looking at slices of the heart made at different angles and showing different aspects of the same thing—much as one might take simultaneous pictures of racehorses crossing the finish line with cameras placed at different angles, so that each view of the same incident taken at the same split second would reveal different pictures or impressions of what was happening.

When a modern electrocardiogram is taken, leads are placed on both arms and legs, and at several positions across the left chest and under the left arm. By throwing switches so that the galvanometer measures the electrical "picture" between a succession of different leads, the cardiologist obtains "pictures" or tracings of the electrical waves in a total of twelve different "exposures," or "exposure angles," across the heart. In a normal, healthy heart, each of these exposures or tracing segments will have a characteristic normal shape or pattern. But if something alters the flow of electricity through the heart—an area of damaged heart muscle, for example, that doesn't conduct the electricity properly—the normal EKG pattern may change in one exposure or another to show a "current of injury."

At first the electrocardiogram was used primarily to diagnose abnormal heart rhythms. But very soon it was found that other changes in heart function could cause revealing changes in the EKG pattern. During a heart attack, for example, the EKG will often show an elevation of the normally level line between the end of the S wave and the beginning of the T wave. This "S-T segment elevation" practically never appears in an EKG of a healthy, normal heart, but often shows up almost immediately at the beginning of a heart attack, indicating some kind of sudden, acute injury to a portion of heart muscle. Somewhat later, under the same circumstances, the normal upward blip of the T wave may become reversed on the EKG tracing and appear as a downward blip—a so-called inverted T wave. These things don't *always* happen during a heart attack, but they happen so commonly under those circumstances that their very appearance on the EKG is a strong diagnostic indicator that a heart attack is probably in progress right then. This is the reason a doctor will order an immediate EKG anytime he or she even suspects a heart attack may be going on.

Doctors soon came to realize, however, that these typical changes in the S-T segment or the T wave on an EKG did not always necessarily indicate the total destruction of heart muscle. They could appear even when a portion of heart muscle was merely injured but not yet destroyed. The "injury," of course, was due to ischemia in a portion of heart muscle—the same ischemia that was causing the pain of the heart attack. When these currents of injury reverted back toward the normal pattern later, the change suggested that actual death, or necrosis, of the heart muscle cells had not occurred, and that the heart muscle was recovering from the injury.

Somewhat later, another discovery was made: when an EKG was done in the midst of an angina attack, S-T segment elevation or depression, or just T wave changes, would often appear temporarily, then revert to normal when the angina attack subsided. What was happening here? The EKG changes were similar to those of an acute coronary, but these people were not having heart attacks. They were merely having angina due to temporary ischemia of a portion of their heart muscle. Clearly, these EKG changes could sometimes occur from temporary ischemia alone and did not necessarily reflect any permanent, measurable damage to the heart muscle. The changes might appear briefly during angina, even though the electrocardiograph tracing might appear perfectly normal at any other time.

It was not long before the question arose, could such EKG changes be helpful in identifying individuals who already had very early stages of coronary artery disease but had not yet suffered the catastrophe of an outright heart attack? The answer was, yes, maybe, in certain cases—and a whole new approach to diagnosing early coronary artery disease was devised.

The Terrible Treadmill

As we saw earlier, atherosclerosis in the coronary arteries does not lead to a myocardial infarction overnight. It is a slow, progressive disease process that develops over the years. (Early, active medical treatment may slow, even stop the progress of atherosclerosis, at least temporarily, but thus far there is no solid evidence to suggest that the process can be reversed.) Once a heart attack occurs, however, the horse has been stolen in a very real sense. There is then no turning back the clock, no going back and fixing things up; one lives with whatever is left, if one lives at all. But if there were some way to discover this disease process early—some way to diagnose it before it reaches the point of imminent catastrophe—then at least there might be a chance to change *something* in a patient's way of life that would slow or stop the disease in midstream, avert later catastrophe and, conceivably, protect him or her from an untimely death.

Suppose, for example, that Ted Johnson, at the age of forty, already has atherosclerotic changes in his coronary arteries, getting inexorably worse all the time, and doesn't even know it. He feels fine, is apparently healthy and hearty, a man in the very prime of life. Maybe his coronary atherosclerosis is already severe enough that he is an absolute sitting duck for a future myocardial infarction and it just hasn't happened yet because the artery damage hasn't gone quite far enough. He is simply a walking disaster just waiting for the right time to happen.

Typically, Ted Johnson doesn't have a clue that this situation exists within his body, and neither does his doctor. What his doctor *does* know is that Ted is a heavy cigarette smoker; eats lots of marbled beef, butter, eggs, bacon; has elevated blood cholesterol and triglyceride levels; doesn't get much daily exercise; and that his father, grandfather, and an uncle all died of heart attacks.

So far, Ted has had no sign of angina, even when running for a bus, skiing in frigid weather, or hiking with a backpack. He experiences no shortness of breath, and both the baseline electrocardiogram his doctor took five years ago and the new one taken today are perfectly normal, with no sign of any trouble. But Ted's doctor knows that these "good signs" unfortunately do not necessarily mean anything. On the contrary, he feels quite certain that Ted probably has a moderate to severe degree of coronary atherosclerosis already in progress—he simply has no way to demonstrate it, or prove it. After giving Ted a careful and complete physical examination, all he can really say is that everything looks all right.

All the same, Ted's doctor considers what *may* be going on inside. He knows that Ted has a whole squadron of positive risk factors for coronary artery disease; there's a high probability that he's already in trouble and doesn't know it. If the doctor could actually look, he might find that one of Ted's main coronary arteries is obstructed some 40 to 50 percent by atherosclerosis. Farther down that coronary artery, a major branch might be obstructed 25 percent, another branch obstructed 50 percent, yet another 75 percent.

Now, what about that 75 percent–obstructed branch artery? It supplies blood to a moderately large segment of heart muscle. Under ordinary resting conditions, it is letting enough blood get through, so that segment of myocardium isn't terribly starved for oxygen. But when Ted is exerting himself, the blood flow through that branch artery just isn't enough to really do the job, so that segment of heart muscle is already having occasional brief intervals of ischemia impairing its function, and slowly whittling away at some of the muscle cells as well. Perhaps the ischemia isn't enough to bring on angina, but it's there, from time to time, all the same.

Suppose the doctor's guess is right on target. What can he do? As a physician, he has two choices: He can wring his hands and wait for a catastrophe that he is pretty sure is on its way, or he can use some diagnostic craftiness to try to trap that episodic ischemia into revealing itself. This doctor doesn't like the idea of waiting for the catastrophe, so he chooses the other course and recommends a treadmill test for Ted.

Essentially, a treadmill test is nothing more than a simple "human experiment" to try to detect by external measurements just what is really going on with a patient's myocardium. First, the patient is hooked up to an electrocardiograph machine with wires that are long enough so that he can move around more or less freely while the machine records a continuous EKG tracing of his heartbeat. In addition, a cuff is placed on his arm for continuous monitoring of his blood pressure. The EKG tracing, of course, records changes in his pulse rate as well as any changes in the electrical conduction through his heart. With all these recording devices in place, a "baseline," or resting measurement, is taken of pulse, blood pressure, and EKG pattern.

Then the patient is taken through a carefully graduated program of steadily increasing exertion. In the early days, this involved a modern-day torture known as the Harvard Step Test: A two-step wooden stile was placed on the floor, and the patient was instructed to step up the two steps to the top of the stile, then down the steps to the other side, turn around, and step back up the two steps to the top, then down to the bottom again. He would then gradually increase his speed going up and down the steps. The longer he continued going up and down, the faster he was urged to go, the more he exerted, and the more exhausted he became. Experiments had indicated that a healthy person with a normal heart could carry this on for a certain number of minutes on the average before he collapsed panting on the floor, with an ongoing EKG tracing recorded throughout the whole time.

It's easy to figure out how a normal, healthy person would respond to this test. With increasing exertion, the whole body would require more and more oxygenated blood. The respirations would increase sharply to bring in more oxygen to the lungs. At the same time, the heart rate would increase sharply as the heart pumped blood faster and faster. In addition, the blood pressure would rise as the heart's output of blood increased to deliver more oxygenated blood to the muscles. Then, when maximum exercise had been achieved, the patient would rest and the recording devices would show how fast his body recovered from all this overexertion.

It was soon discovered, however, that some apparently healthy people with apparently healthy hearts didn't do so well with the Harvard Step Test. In some people the EKG tracing began to change with increasing exercise, with the same kind of S-T segment and T wave changes that might appear with angina pectoris.

Sometimes these changes would appear on increasing exertion, but without any sign of angina at all; in other cases the patient might begin complaining of anginal pain just as the S-T segment began to sag on the EKG tracing, and the angina and EKG changes would continue until the exercise was stopped.

Clearly, some of these people who *appeared* perfectly healthy did not have such normal, healthy hearts after all. In fact, they already had some degree of unsuspected atherosclerotic obstruction in their coronary arteries or the coronary artery major branches.

Unfortunately, this early Harvard Step Test presented some practical difficulties and dangers. There was no good way to measure or control the exact amount of exertion any given patient was subjected to. A lazy patient might not exert enough, while another might exert himself more vigorously than was either necessary or wise. The test required a doctor in attendance, as well as some very tricky medical judgment to determine when to stop. Worst of all, a certain small number of patients, on reaching a maximum exertion level, would proceed to have a real heart attack in the middle of the test—and, now and then, one would drop dead on the floor.

The treadmill test was developed in hopes of overcoming these problems. The treadmill was simply a machine with a moving platform on rollers that could be speeded or slowed down at will, with handrails on either side for the patient to hold on to. The treadmill surface could also be raised from a perfectly flat position to any degree of upward tilt desired. With the treadmill flat and the roller moving slowly, a person on the treadmill could walk in place at a leisurely rate while baseline respiration rate, pulse rate, EKG, and blood pressure were recorded, After a minute or two at the baseline, the treadmill then could be tilted slightly upward and speeded up so that the person was walking more briskly in place on a slight incline, with continuous EKG and blood pressure monitoring. After a given amount of time, the incline would be increased steeper still, and the treadmill rate increased still further. Any time that S-T segment changes appear on the EKG tracing, or the patient notices angina, or blood pressure begins to fail, the test can be discontinued immediately.

This arrangement provides a far more sensitive measurement of the patient's response to increasing exertion than the older step test. Since the exercise level increases very gradually, with continuous monitoring of the patient's heart's response there is relatively little risk of untoward events occurring.

One of the more refined calculations made possible from the data gathered in such a treadmill test is a measurement of a person's *functional aerobic capacity*, or FAC—essentially an estimate of how well the person performs compared to normals for his or her age and sex. Normal people will reach a functional aerobic capacity of 85 to 100 percent of normal—their hearts' ability to deliver oxygenated blood is essentially unimpaired. Individuals with an FAC of 50 to 75 percent *are* impaired and will be capable of only sedentary activity, while those with an FAC of less than 50 percent will be severely impaired. In the absence of some severe lung disease, the main thing that determines a person's functional aerobic capacity is how efficiently the heart is pumping out blood, commonly spoken of as the *cardiac output*. Thus, in a sense, this calculation of FAC is a gauge of "cardiac horsepower."

With this kind of refined treadmill testing available, it became possible in many cases to identify the presence of coronary artery disease well in advance of the time that symptoms begin to occur. But what could be done with this information? Unfortunately, fifteen or twenty years ago the answer was, precious little. Because of this, and because the testing itself still carried a small risk of actually precipitating a myocardial infarction, treadmill testing was not at that time used widely for examining and managing patients. For a long time it was regarded as an interesting but fairly useless laboratory curiosity. It was not until medical and surgical advances began to offer some real hope of somehow *intervening* to alter the course of developing coronary artery disease—that is, in the last fifteen years or so—that treadmill testing began to prove its real usefulness.

What is that usefulness today? If treadmill testing can indeed pick up evidence of coronary artery disease before symptoms begin to occur, why not use a treadmill as a broad screening test on practically everybody at regular intervals? Unfortunately, the treadmill test is not a good screening test for the general population because it produces a high rate of false positive results—it often indicates trouble when there isn't any—in people who don't have coronary artery disease at all (which, after all, is the majority of the population). False positive results occur especially frequently in two large groups of people—in women, and in men with normal hearts. Thus, the treadmill test is mainly useful today with patients who already have other markers for coronary artery disease: those who have angina, for instance, or those who have had a previous myocardial infarction in the past, or people like our friend Ted who had many positive risk factors. For the most part, the treadmill is used today to confirm a tentative diagnosis, to demonstrate myocardial ischemia and roughly measure how much is present, and to determine a baseline measurement of an individual's functional aerobic capacity, for later comparison after treatment.

Meanwhile, there remained the real problem of what one could do to control the angina when it appeared. Just recognizing it as a symptom of advancing coronary artery disease wasn't enough. The ischemia that brought it on caused the machinery of the heart to function badly and began wrecking the machine—the heart muscle itself—as well. What was more, the angina could very sharply circumscribe how a patient might live, severely limiting his activity, forcing him to endure recurrent episodes of agonizing pain, and, in many cases, reducing him to an inert cardiac cripple if it could not be controlled.

Thus, even though angina was only a symptom, doctors came to recognize that everything about it was bad. It was not a symptom to be tolerated or put up with if anything at all could be done to relieve it, because while it was occurring, continuing damage to the heart was being done. *Any* method of controlling or preventing angina was clearly better than none at all.

Controlling Angina: Nitrates and Beta-Blockers

Fortunately, we have a number of medicines today that are extremely useful in controlling or relieving angina. Knowing what we know about this symptom, it is not hard to imagine two major drug actions that might help relieve angina anytime it occurred:

1. Any drug that might suddenly reduce the amount of blood returning to the heart, and, at the same time, relax or dilate the arteries receiving the blood the heart is pumping, should sharply reduce the amount of work the heart has to do, at least temporarily. This should help relieve myocardial ischemia and, thus, relieve the angina. Ideally, such a drug should act very quickly, so it could be used either in the midst of an angina attack, to bring swift relief, or be taken *before* exertion, to prevent the angina attack from occurring in the first place.

2. Any drug that might act on the heart itself to slow its activity and reduce the work it must do, without sacrificing its pumping ability, should help relieve myocardial ischemia and thereby reduce

the frequency or severity of the angina. Similarly, any medicine that might reduce the amount of oxygen required by the heart muscle cells to do their work should also help prevent ischemia and reduce the chances of angina.

Of these possible drug effects, the first was achieved many years ago with the use of various compounds known as nitrates. One of the oldest and most familiar of these drugs, used since the 1860s and still widely used today to combat acute angina attacks, is *nitroglycerin*.* A small amount of nitroglycerin introduced into the body has a remarkable effect: It causes the walls of veins, arteries, and arterioles all over the body to relax and dilate. This brings about two immediate results: first, blood tends to pool in dilated veins all over the body so that less blood is returning to the heart; second, blood flows out of the heart into the arteries faster and at lower pressure. The result is that the heart, suddenly and temporarily, has less work to do, which means that the myocardium needs less oxygen. This immediately decreases the myocardial ischemia and helps to speedily (if only temporarily) relieve the angina.

In its most familiar form, a tiny dose of nitroglycerin (1/150 of a grain, or approximately 0.4 milligrams) is packed into a small, easy-dissolving white pill. When the pill is placed under the tongue, the nitroglycerin is absorbed directly into the bloodstream within about ninety seconds, and the drug takes effect immediately. This speed of action is highly desirable, because a person in the middle of a severe angina attack wants something to happen *fast*. The effect also wears off rapidly—in a half an hour or less—but if exertion is terminated at the same time the nitroglycerin is taken, the angina may be quieted for quite some time. And if the pill is taken *before* exertion, prophylactically, it may prevent the angina attack altogether.

Why not just swallow the nitroglycerin? For one thing, the drug action would be much slower; for another, part of the drug absorbed in the stomach would first be routed to the liver and destroyed, so the action would be much weaker. Placing the drug under the tongue for immediate absorption avoids this so-called first pass through the liver, and it provides the advantage of very swift action (highly desirable), but at the cost of very short term action (not so desirable). This can be a problem for a person with severe angina that recurs with any small degree of exertion: He or she may have to take the medicine very frequently—as often as every fifteen or twenty min-

---

* Yes, this is the same nitroglycerin that is used to make dynamite, dispensed in tiny nonexplosive doses that are placed under the tongue for fast absorption. Some oldtimers still refer to them as "dynamite pills."

utes, for a total dosage of perhaps twenty or thirty pills a day in order to control the chest pain. Unfortunately, nitroglycerin's effect of dilating arteries in the brain also can lead to severe pounding headaches in some people, so frequent high dosage is not always a good answer.

This problem can be solved, at least in part, by using other nitrate or nitrite compounds with similar action but with more staying power. One such medicine is isosorbide dinitrite (trade name Isordil, and others), a first cousin to nitroglycerin, with a slower onset of action but a much more prolonged period of antianginal activity once the dose is taken. Also used as an under-the-tongue tablet, this substance begins to take effect in about five minutes, but then remains effective for some sixty to ninety minutes. This means that it isn't as well suited to swift emergency control of angina as plain nitroglycerin, but it is useful in helping to prevent angina attacks on a longer-term basis. An individual might take one of these tablets every three or four hours, for example, and have some measure of protection against angina all day long, except in the event of sudden extreme exertion.

Larger doses of Isordil are sometimes swallowed; they take even longer to take effect (perhaps thirty minutes), but they have a similar sixty- to ninety-minute range of action. Still other nitrate preparations, sold under such trade names as Nitrospan and Peritrate, are designed to be taken orally. They have even slower onset and an even more protracted range of effectiveness, so that for some people, two or three doses a day provide reasonably good control.

As an alternative, nitroglycerin can be taken another way, based on the fact that it can be absorbed directly through the skin into the bloodstream. Nitroglycerin mixed in a lanolin paste and dispensed from a tube like toothpaste can be smeared on an area of the chest and covered with a piece of parchment paper. This can provide a rapid blood level of nitroglycerin in a few minutes, with additional nitroglycerin soaking through the skin over a period of several hours, so it may be effective for up to five or six hours per application. This "nitroglycerin paste," unfortunately, is both extremely messy and somewhat unpredictable. One person may receive far more benefit than another. Part of the problem of messiness has been solved in recent years by the development of so-called transdermal nitroglycerin patches—small adhesive patches, containing nitroglycerin enclosed in a semi-permeable sack, for absorption into the body transdermally; that is, "across the skin." These patches don't smear clothing and bedclothes. Enthusiastic manufacturers proclaim that they can produce a smooth dosage over a period of anywhere from twelve to twenty-four hours, but clinical tests indicate that very few people have any such lengthy response. And, as opposed to plain nitroglycerin tablets, which are very cheap, the transdermal patches are extremely expensive.

For people with only occasional mild angina, different nitroglycerin or nitrate compounds can provide a good answer for relief. But for people with more severe, frequent angina, the control achievable with the nitrates is incomplete at best. A new medical weapon against angina for such individuals appeared in the late 1960s: the so-called beta-adrenergic blocking agents. As most people know, adrenaline (more properly known as epinephrine) is a hormone produced in the adrenal gland in response to such stimuli as danger, fear, tension, anxiety, stress, and so forth. Its first cousin, norepinephrine, is produced in cells of the nervous system under the same stimuli. These "adrenergic hormones" have a widespread body effect. The molecules of the hormones attach to special receptors on the cells in heart muscle and blood vessel walls, and, thus, gain entry into those cells to stimulate the heart rate, speeding it up, and to cause the muscular walls of the arteries to contract and the blood pressure to rise. These hormonal effects prepare the body to react more quickly to threats and are accompanied by other adrenergic effects, including increased respiration rate, greater keenness of vision, and a tendency to perspire. Sometimes these effects are called the fight-flight reaction since they seem to prepare the human animal either to fight for survival or to turn and run from danger.

Unfortunately, the adrenergic effects of epinephrine and norepinephrine are bad news for the person who has an impaired or damaged myocardium. They are just exactly the kind of physiological effects likely to precipitate myocardial ischemia and angina attacks— one of the main reasons that angina is triggered so often by anger or fear as well as by physical exertion. In the 1960s, a group of drugs was discovered that had the effect of blocking the special adrenergic receptors in heart muscle that respond to the adrenergic hormones and allow them to affect the heart. They were called beta-adrenergic receptors, to distinguish them from "alpha-adrenergic receptors" in such areas as the brain, the intestine, and other parts of the body. By knocking out these beta-receptors, the new drugs (now called beta-adrenergic blocking agents or just beta-blockers) help protect the ischemic heart from adrenergic effects.* They slow down the heart rate, for example, thus reducing the amount of oxygen that the myocardial muscle cells require in order to continue functioning. In persons with moderately severe coronary artery disease, the beta-

---

* They also help lower the blood pressure so effectively that they are widely used today for treatment of hypertension.

blockers could be used side by side with nitroglycerin or nitrates to provide much more effective, predictable, round-the-clock control of angina than was ever possible with nitrates alone.

The first beta-blocker approved for use in the United States was called *propranolol*, sold under the trade name of Inderal since the mid-1960s. Subsequently, a large number of similar compounds with essentially the same effects have been added to the list. These drugs are by no means perfect or free of side effects. They can cause gastrointestinal reactions in some people, extreme exhaustion or physical inertia in others, and reduced sexual potency in still others. But their great effectiveness in controlling angina has led to widespread use today. Many people using these drugs have been able to increase their physical activity quite markedly without having the limiting wall of angina constantly blocking them. What's more, later studies have revealed other important beneficial effects. For example, it was found that people using beta-blockers after suffering heart attacks were significantly less likely to have recurrent heart attacks or sudden death due to cardiac arrythmias. The beta-blockers seem to have a distinct protective effect in such people.

Finally, in the 1980s still another family of drugs appeared in the armamentarium against angina—the *calcium slow-channel blockers,* or simply "calcium blockers." It had long been known that calcium ions in the smooth muscle cells in the arteries have a great deal to do with the spasm and relaxation of those arteries; natural mechanisms pumping calcium ions through the cell walls into or out of the cells can influence whether the artery wall contracts or not. The kind of irritable muscle spasm we spoke of earlier that can lead to angina at rest, or "variant angina," was believed to be a function of this calcium ion control.

The calcium-blocking drugs have the effect of slowing or limiting the flow of calcium ions into or out of the smooth muscle of the coronary arteries, so that the arteries are less likely to go into spasm and cause angina when injured. They dilate or relax these arteries. One of these drugs, *nifedipine* (trade name Procardia), was first approved by the Food and Drug Administration (FDA) for use in the United States in 1982. It was followed by verapamil (trade names Calan or Isoptin) and diltiazem (Cardizem). These drugs can be used safely in combination with both nitroglycerin and beta-blockers to provide still another avenue of control over the root causes of myocardial ischemia and angina. They are widely used today for this purpose, although their effects can be less predictable and far more tricky than either of the other medicines, as we shall see.

One other medical weapon against angina should be mentioned for the sake of completeness: the use of inhalation oxygen. Since the whole name of the game in angina is not enough oxygen getting to the heart muscle, it makes sense that increasing the amount of oxygen available from the air that is breathed and thereby increasing the oxygen concentration in the blood should reduce the likelihood of angina—and so it does. In fact, during such emergencies as acute heart attacks or episodes of acute heart failure, inhalation oxygen therapy is a very important part of treatment. Indeed, there are people who keep an oxygen mask and tank around the house for use when angina won't quiet down any other way. The problems are obvious, however. Oxygen constitutes a real fire hazard; even a small 10-liter oxygen tank is clumsy and awkward to handle; treatment ties a person down to the tank and mask so that, for any prolonged use, it is both extremely limiting and extremely expensive. In addition, people can become so emotionally dependent upon the oxygen tank that they may soon feel they can't do without it. For these reasons oxygen therapy is generally confined to hospital use, usually not considered practical as an outpatient or in-home method for dealing with angina.

Angina pectoris is an extremely commonplace symptom in progressive coronary artery disease. Most patients have it to some degree or another, at one time or another. For some it is a "first symptom" that appears before any such catastrophic incident as a heart attack has occurred. For others it appears after a heart attack, due to the obstruction of circulation and damage to heart muscle that accompanies a myocardial infarction. Whenever it occurs, however, angina is no delight to live with. Angina means *pain*, and the person with severe angina is living with constantly recurring pain unless he finds some effective way to control it.

For this reason treatment of angina pectoris becomes an urgent matter whenever it appears, and dealing with my own angina became extremely important to me during those first few days I was out of the hospital and staying in the Busbys' apartment. What's more, it soon became clear that this was not some temporary condition that was going to correct itself and presently go away. According to Dr. Cleveland, chances were excellent that having appeared, it was there to stay and might well be expected to get worse rather than better.

Consequently, as soon as the angina first appeared, he prescribed medicine for me to take on a regular basis to control and prevent it: 40 milligrams of the beta-blocker propranolol (Inderal) four times a day, at mealtimes and bedtime, and four doses of isosorbide dinitrite (Isordil) daily under the tongue, with an effort to use it particularly at times before exercise in order to prevent anginal attacks if possible. I also had a supply of regular nitroglycerin tablets, to use as needed.

Fortunately, I never had any headaches or other side effects from nitroglycerin, but I found the regular tablets extremely frustrating to use: one of them at a time only did about half the job, so I had to use two at a time, and even then the effect wore off in a matter of a few minutes. With the Isordil and the Inderal, in addition to the nitroglycerin, I was able to establish reasonably good control over the angina most of the time, but I soon learned that hardly a day would go by that I did not have at least one severe angina attack that would come on unexpectedly and get its hooks in before I could slap it down.

Further, I found that the angina that occasionally awakened me from sleep at night just didn't respond very well to the nitrates or nitroglycerin, tending to hang on for an hour or more before finally subsiding. For this reason Dr. Cleveland prescribed the tube of nitro paste for me to use when I was bothered by such nighttime attacks. This did seem to help quiet things down after a half-hour or so and let me get back to sleep without being bothered by recurrences.

All in all, this program of medication controlled the angina well enough that I was able to get on with the process of recovery, gradually increasing my in-house activities, gradually decreasing the amount of time I had to rest in bed each day, and gradually beginning to develop a tolerable outdoor exercise walking program. But the control was anything but perfect, and there were bad days. A cold, windy or rainy day, for example, would often be a bad day. A day with more tension than usual, or more frustration, or more anger at some stupidity that I encountered in my work or in relationships with other people, would mean a bad day. An overindulgent evening meal could mean a bad night. Even on the days when I didn't actually encounter the brick wall of sudden angina in my daily activities, I would have near-brushes with it. There would be times when I could feel the premonitory fullness in the chest and slight shortness of breath that I came to recognize as absolutely certain indicators that an angina attack was about to begin if I didn't stop whatever I was doing and take some medicine *right then* to prevent it.

Throughout the rest of that stay in the Seattle apartment, it seemed to me that just getting hold of the angina monster and subduing it enough that I could get on with some sort of normal daily living was goal enough for the moment. The day that Fred would release me from the apartment and allow me to go home to Thorp began looming in my mind as a sort of end point to my illness—a closing of a door upon a dreadful, jarring, catastrophic accident that had struck my life. At the same time I became fundamentally aware of a terrible truth about angina: that however successfully one might treat it with medicines, subdue it, control it, even prevent it from occurring, for the most part all that treatment was doing absolutely nothing to change or improve the underlying heart disease. The damage that was done was *done*; the underlying disease was still there, just as bad as it ever was, no matter how symptom-free I might remain. In fact, that underlying disease process might well still be slowly progressing even as I breathed, no matter how I readjusted my life. The threatened imminence of another close encounter with death, perhaps an unrecoverable one, was still there.

But I was also aware of something else. Twenty years before this would have been all that could have been said: One would go home to a comparatively vegetative existence, and one would treat the angina in order to remain as comfortable as possible, and then wait for the next blow to strike. At that time the bald survival statistics for a person who had suffered a severe myocardial infarction were clear and unyielding. Fifteen percent—fifteen out of every hundred of those people—would no longer be alive one year after the first catastrophe. Another 5 percent would die during the second year, and 5 percent more during the third year, and so on down the line. One out of three would be dead within five years. Only about 35 percent would survive for ten years. And as for twenty years— forget it. If you think such statistics would seem appalling to a man at the age of fifty-two years, well, you're right.

Fortunately, however, some very startling things had been happening in the treatment and management of coronary artery disease during the twenty years between 1960 and 1980. New medicines were being developed that could profoundly alter those grim statistics. New ways of life, real changes in life-style, were beginning to hold out some hope of improving those statistics even more. And new, aggressive ways of treating the diseased heart itself were appearing—techniques that would have seemed utterly reckless and hopeless just a few years before. I clearly remembered attending a medical conference at Virginia Mason Hospital in the late 1960s at which the Mason Clinic's chief of cardiovascular surgery showed absolutely fantastic X-ray pictures taken of a patient's coronary artery system, identifying atherosclerotic lesions that were virtually certain to kill that patient very soon if left untreated, and then blandly described surgical techniques being developed at that very time to correct or by-pass those lesions. I was aware of what had been happening ever since on that pioneering surgical front and had heard of still other, newer techniques being explored even more recently.

Indeed, it seemed to me that if one had to have a heart attack, perhaps 1980 was a good time to have it. I knew that ever since the late 1960s we had been at the cutting edge of an incredible new technology that promised ultimately to give new and very real hope to hundreds of thousands of people suffering from this devastating killer disease. During those years, naturally, I had not expected to be one of those hundreds of thousands, but I knew that by the early 1980s that incredible technology was already paying handsome dividends, and I was there then, perhaps one of those who might really benefit.

As the end of the prescribed two-week posthospital stay in the apartment approached, Ann and I decided to call Fred Cleveland on his promise to let me go home to Thorp again. I had already seen him twice during that two-week interval, but very little had been said about any aspect of the future. Fred had seemed quite satisfied just to find me warm and pink on those occasions. Understand that my own feeling of closing a door on a dreadfully unpleasant episode in my life was very strong, and that I was not feeling like urging any very radical course of action with any degree of vigor at all. I, too, was satisfied just to remain warm and pink. But on the day before we were appointed to go home, Ann and I went in together to see Fred for a "last" formal clinic visit, and I knew that some questions had to be asked. In fact, I had written them on a piece of paper so I wouldn't forget them, and I brandished it at him when he came into the examining room, looking wide-eyed and owlish. "I need some answers to some things," I told him, "before we wrap this up and you sneak back into the woodwork again."

I meant wrapping up that particular office visit, of course, but he thought I was speaking of wrapping up the care of the illness. For a moment he looked startled, then he came forth with a sardonic laugh. "My boy, we are not anywhere near wrapping up the care of this illness," he said, "so don't get impatient. We are going to have many, many more visits together, and you're going to have many more opportunities to ask questions, and there are going to be many interesting things that have to be done before the care of this illness is anywhere near wrapped up."

It was not that I hadn't already asked Fred questions. But Fred had not yet provided any very specific answers about the illness and my future prospects. I had known him for many years and had always regarded him as an exceptionally sharp and canny physician, especially in the field of cardiology. During my hospitalization I also had come to recognize that Fred Cleveland made some of my craftiest and most evasive friends look like rank amateurs when it came to the game of artful dodging and responding with the ambiguous answer; his skill at never quite answering a question had absolutely amazed me on half a dozen occasions. That afternoon, however, when explicit answers were definitely called for, I found that Fred was good at that, too. After carefully examining me, and checking on my day-to-day progress since I had last seen him, Fred got down to specifics.

First he reviewed for me in very simple terms just what we actually *knew* about what had happened to me at the time of the heart attack and in the days that followed. It turned out that what we actually knew was extremely limited. We knew that just before midnight of Friday, October 24, after a long hard day of elk hunting, I had suffered a severe acute myocardial infarction that involved at least one major branch of one of the two main coronary arteries—probably a branch of the right coronary, which supplies the posterior and inferior portions of the heart, knocking out some portion of the wall of the right ventricle. This had not been just a transient episode. An artery had plugged up and stayed plugged up. Heart muscle was destroyed, and the destruction, to whatever degree it occurred, went through and through the heart muscle. All this could be determined, Fred pointed out, just from the electrocardiograms taken during and after the attack.

A heart attack involving that part of the heart muscle was not the kind most likely to cause instant fatality, but it could trigger cardiac arrhythmias—irregularities of heartbeat—or even cardiac arrest during the first few hours or days after the attack. This was consistent with what both Dr. Coppock in Ellensburg and Dr. Cleveland at Virginia Mason had observed during the first few days I was in the hospital: I did indeed have runs of arrhythmias as well as evidence of severe heart muscle damage and destruction. "You may well have Ann to thank for knowing what to do, staying cool and not delaying for more than a couple of phone calls before getting you to the emergency room to account for the fact that you are still among the quick," Fred said. "God knows those first days were confusing enough as it was."

This accounted for Fred's very cautious approach to treating me when I reached Virginia Mason, and for his determination to keep me close at hand in Seattle for two weeks after I left the hospital, until, in his judgment, I wouldn't be likely to have to be rushed back immediately.

We also knew that my hospital recovery had been complicated by two completely extraneous problems: First, I had a whopping attack of gout in both ankles; second, I apparently developed an acute toxic psychosis in response to one or another of the medicines I had been using before the coronary attack. For about a week, when I was awake at all, I was way out in Neverland somewhere, telling the doctors and Ann and everybody else all sorts of bizarre things. As for my own intense perception of a close encounter with death during that period, Fred had had no inkling about that, because I had never mentioned it to him. At that time I was not ready to talk about the experience, or even think about it very much.

In spite of these problems—really rather minor annoyances, as far as Fred was concerned—my recovery in the hospital at Virginia Mason had gone along without any major complications. The main problem that bothered Fred was the angina that developed later. I had no memory of having any serious angina in the hospital (although my hospital records certainly indicated that I had plenty of chest pain), but as soon as I got on my feet and moving around a bit, I developed a lot of angina on very little physical exertion and also had spells at night when at rest. "Of course, I expected that to happen," Fred said. "I would have been incredulously delighted if it hadn't, but it did. So now we must keep dealing with that so you *can* move around, so you *can* begin getting some daily exercise and rebuild your cardiac circulation to whatever extent is possible."

The problem we faced now, Fred pointed out, was what we didn't know about what was going on with my heart. We didn't know, for example, whether the whole right coronary artery was blocked, or only a major branch of it. We didn't know exactly how much heart muscle was infarcted, or exactly where. Above all, we didn't know just how extensive my coronary artery disease might really be. The fact that one coronary artery branch was "involved," as Fred so nicely put it, didn't necessarily mean that others were, too, but we had no way to know. "Which means," Fred said, "that you could well have another heart attack and infarction any old time. What we can do right now—use medication to control your angina, cut down on your dietary salt, keep your alcohol intake very moderate, watch your blood pressure like a hawk, get you to lose weight, gradually increase your exercise, and keep you off your cigarettes—will all help decrease some risk factors by some indefinable amount. But all that may not be good enough. Sooner or later we need to *know* what your coronary arteries are doing, instead of just sitting around waiting for the next disaster to happen. And that means we're going to have to go looking for trouble."

"You mean like doing a treadmill test?" I asked.

He looked pained. "What would that tell us that we don't already know? Right now that would just be an unnecessary risk. Treadmill tests are useful for people who have not yet demonstrated the presence of their coronary artery disease quite as spectacularly as you have. No, we already have the broad framework of your diagnosis. What we really need are specific details—a road map of your coronary arteries—and that means a cardiac catheterization and coronary artery angiograms—detailed X rays—of what is going on. There are also some other tricky studies that will tell us quite specifically how much of your heart you actually have left and what it's capable of doing."

"And you want to do this right now?"

"Not unless something forces my hand, I don't." Fred looked at me over his glasses. "I'd like to have you a little further down the road from this acute event before I allow someone to put a catheter in your ventricle. Maybe three or four months down the road—unless something happens that absolutely forces me to move faster."

That was certainly explicit enough. I had been quite certain that a cardiac catheterization was going to be in the cards sooner or later; I just hadn't known when. That procedure would permit coronary angiograms to be taken—clear, sharp, definitive X-ray pictures of the coronary arteries to show which ones were involved and how badly. Fred would not be pinned down precisely to the timing, or about what he thought those studies might lead to. He wanted to wait another three months or so before having them done at all, and then wanted to take his own stately sweet time considering those X rays and other studies with expert consultation before even thinking about consigning me to the surgeons. I seemed to remember that as long as I had known him, Fred had never been terribly enthusiastic about surgeons.

Meanwhile, he made it clear that there were specific things that I could do and other things that I couldn't, once I arrived home. I could not fly anywhere, for the time being. I could be driven places, but I could not drive the car myself, for the time being. In fact, I was not to travel any great distance at all by *any* mode of conveyance, for the time being. I could be up and around, reading, typing, dictating, doing office work, plotting novels, drafting books—no problem. "Writing? Sure, why not? Write anything you want to," Fred said. "Just don't do any hard work." I might even go duck hunting in the local area, he said: a. if it was a warm dry day, b. if I were carried to the blind, like the King of Siam, and c. if I refrained from leaping into the water after the ducks.

When a few other questions had been answered and Ann and I were rising to leave, Fred fired his parting shot. "You know," he said, "what might be the best thing of all for you for the next few months would be for you to try to stop being a doctor and just settle for being a patient. What do you think of that?"

I smiled at this innocent jest.

II

INVESTIGATIONS

— 7 —

The elk hunt for that year was already over and done with two days before we finally rolled into the place at Thorp late in the afternoon of Tuesday, November 18, 1980, and I remember wondering vaguely if the infinitely clever and prescient Dr. Cleveland had not deliberately planned it that way. Bob and Wilma Dlouhy, our neighbors up the creek, had both gotten skunked, which was not unusual. They had hunted most of the season in knee-deep snow way up on the Yahne Plateau, and had thoroughly exhausted themselves without so much as a single good sighting to show for it. Cow elk all over the place, but no bulls to be seen. Merle Gordon had also gotten skunked, which *was* unusual, since he almost always gets an elk. He had hunted with his cronies out of their camp up in the North Fork Taneum Creek drainage; two of the others had gotten bulls but not Merle, much to his obvious chagrin. They had hunted in snow, too, and now there was lots of snow in the hills, deep snow higher up, but no snow yet down in the Taneum canyon.

After our long interview with Fred Cleveland that morning, and upon receiving permission to go home, I had settled down for a two-hour wait to see Ken Wilskie about my ankles before we could leave. Ann had gone back to throw our bags in the car, close up the apartment, and return the rental TV. Neither of us wanted to hang around that place another night. Much to my disgust, I had a severe angina attack just sitting in the car as we drove east from Seattle across the Lake Washington bridge and Mercer Island and up through Eastgate toward the Cascades; probably a matter of predictable excitement, but I remember thinking, Christ, you don't suppose we're going to have to turn right around and go back again? We stopped for a late lunch, and the angina finally quieted down. We left the rain and drizzle behind us in Snoqualmie Pass and came down into Cle Elum to a bright, sunny late afternoon of clear, crisp, east-of-the-mountains autumn weather. It got down to twenty-four degrees that night. I was infinitely pleased to get back to my own warm bed again just twenty-five days after the night of my heart attack. Gypsy, our spaniel, snored all night from her place on the floor on Ann's side of the bed. She, too, was happy to be home.

Those first few days back at Thorp were a revelation, returning as we were to a place and a life-style that would never again be the same. The two weeks at the apartment in Seattle had been a sort of a holding pattern for me, largely confined to a tiny living room and a tiny bedroom, an absolutely torpid existence involving such exhilarations as watching "Good Morning, America" for an hour and a half every morning on TV, reading a little, napping morning and afternoon as well as sleeping all night, writing an occasional letter, drafting a few (very few) pages of manuscript on the typewriter, and, for the high points of the day, two sedate fifteen-minute walks of four or five city blocks each, on the level. During those days, I hadn't been able to stir up sufficient interest or attention even to read a good murder mystery; the only book I actually *read* during those weeks in Seattle was Craig Claiborne's new low-salt recipe book.

Now, back at Thorp, things were different. There was no more "Good Morning, America"—we had no TV capability there at all—and suddenly I found myself faced with all the piled-up labors-in-waiting of the old life. There was the demanding imperative of an unfinished first draft of a novel (*The Fourth Horseman*) on my desk, and me without a glimmer in the world of where to go with it next. There was a month's worth of mail piled on the kitchen table, waiting to be sorted and responded to. There was a new *Good Housekeeping* column deadline looming within a few days, and, above all, the need for a lengthy and long-overdue report to my agent, Carl Brandt, about what had happened, where things had been and where things were going, in order that the two of us together could begin to make some sort of business sense out of what was going to happen next. And then there was a program of physical exercise and rehabilitation that was going to take a ninety-minute bite out of every day that I had never in my life yielded up to exercise before.

At least half of my mind recognized all these things as imperatives, but the other half balked. That half said, "Forget it, Alan. What gets done gets done and what doesn't, doesn't, and don't worry about it." Actually I had a very clear idea of the *real* imperatives that were facing me: resuming a style of life and a level of work that I could actually live with through a long recovery period; moving slowly and resting a lot; somehow learning how to ignore pressures and tensions; and working to rebuild the capacity of a damaged cardio-vascular system, to help my heart build new arterial blood vessels, to provide better circulation to the part of my heart that was still undamaged, to the greatest extent possible, by the time, somewhere down the road, that detailed diagnostic investigations and prognos-tications were to be made. It simply didn't make sense to slide instantly back into the same pressure tank of self-imposed worries and goals, intemperate eating, heavy smoking, and militant lack of exercise that had paved the way for this mess in the first place. Clearly, decisions had to be made to change things.

Certain things made those decisions much easier than I expected them to be. In those first weeks back at Thorp, my body's energy was the great leveler. I simply did not have even one-quarter of the energy to devote to daily activities that I had had before the heart attack. In the first week or two, I seemed limited to accomplishing just two beautiful things a day—and that was all. I could read and respond to two letters, or write two pages of manuscript, or write the checks to pay two bills, or read two pages of a book, and that was it for the day. I had a good hour or two each morning after breakfast, and then I was bushed and had to rest. A two-hour nap after lunch restored energy for another hour or so in the afternoon, and then again I was bushed. It did no good whatever to try to push things beyond this level, because nothing happened: The energy was not there. All that trying to push things did was make me worry and fret, which depleted my energy level all the more and accom-plished nothing, so I simply refused to worry and fret. After a lifetime of intensely obsessive-compulsive behavior, a typical type-A-personality life-style, that change took quite some doing, a total reversal of attitude. Instead of stewing away fruitlessly over all the things that weren't getting done, I learned to force myself to be grateful for the two beautiful things that *were* done each day. At times it seemed like climbing painfully up out of an enormous pit—but at least I was climbing, however slowly.

One thing that helped was to force myself to set priorities re-garding the work that I thought had to be done, to do what I could off the top of the pile each day, and then just not worry when I reached the day's limit. It was amazing how many things really didn't have to be done today, and even more amazing how many things didn't really have to be done at all. But by spreading the work out over a full two weeks and ignoring virtually everything else, I managed to come up with a respectable column for the upcoming March issue of *Good Housekeeping*, only a few days beyond dead-line. It wasn't a particularly distinguished column, but it wasn't a bad one, either, and my editor, Bob Liles, called on the telephone when he received it, obviously delighted. I suppose he had anticipated a terrible bummer and was just as relieved as I was to see something plausible turn up on his desk. The novel in progress could—and did—wait; likewise, correspondence: I began using the telephone more, writing letters less.

Through all this I was fully aware how fortunate it was that I was a free-lance writer working at home with no time clock to punch, no rigid office hours to meet, no fixed daily volume of work that absolutely had to be turned out in order to keep my job. If I had been engaged in such work, I think I probably couldn't have done it; my return to a formal employed work pattern would surely have had to be delayed for two, four, maybe six months, and I began to understand how it could be that so many postcoronary patients never did get back into regular employment again, even when their physical recovery had progressed enough to make it possible. Once out of the habit of regimented work, it could easily become virtually impossible for such people to get back into it again, especially if everybody around them, including their doctors, urged them not to. And meanwhile, what could they do for money? In this respect I was very, very lucky. Lots of people aren't.

Diet control didn't require any great energy, but it did require some changes and some compromises. At that time (1980) Fred Cleveland was not terribly sanguine about the value of abrupt dietary changes in terms of recovering from an MI or preventing further progress of coronary artery disease. The whole matter of how fast or how inevitably coronary atherosclerosis would progress, once it was well started, or whether the process could be stopped by any measures whatever, or whether it could ever be reversed or not, simply wasn't clearly understood at that time (and still isn't today, I might add). But it seemed to him, Fred said, that all the studies he had seen on dietary risk factors, and especially cholesterol level as a risk factor, among people with already established coronary atherosclerosis, were as full of holes as a Swiss cheese and didn't support making extreme demands on a patient. "Do what you can comfortably do," he had told us, "but don't do anything that's going to make you absolutely miserable. And above all, for God's sake, don't worry about it a whole lot."*

One of the main dietary changes that we found we could comfortably make involved altering the kinds of food we ate and the

---

* As we will see later, attitudes have now changed to the point of quite a good deal of concern over cholesterol, but that was what my cardiologist believed at that time, and that was what guided us.

ways we prepared it. I had always been a red meat–potatoes–gravy person, without much enthusiasm for vegetables or salad; fish or seafood turned up on our menu as rarely as once a month. Now we set up a regular four-day rotation system: red meat one day, chicken or poultry the next, fish or seafood the third day, and some kind of pasta main dish the fourth. We tried this, and it worked splendidly. Suddenly, we found ourselves eating fish twice a week, chicken twice a week, red meat only once a week, as opposed to four or five times a week, before. We saw the effect of this program demonstrated during the winter by the fact that we had two whole freezers full of beef, lamb, pork, venison, and veal that just sat there, while we seemed to be constantly shopping for fresh fish and looking for special prices on those nasty little Arkansas rubber chickens. In addition, we made a conscious effort to back off from deep-frying or sautéing our food and began leaning more heavily on steaming, poaching, braising or roasting for food preparation.

Eggs, cheese, and breakfast meats, especially bacon and sausage, were something else altogether. These were foods I prized above almost anything else, and I could not (or thought I could not) give them up. I had always eaten a very hearty breakfast to get through a long morning's labors, the part of the day in which I had always done my best, most concentrated work. If I didn't have a hearty breakfast, I would find myself going around at 10:30 in the morning looking for food. Now a bowl of shredded wheat and a glass of orange juice just didn't hack it. Consequently, we did not abandon my usual eggs-sausage-and-toast breakfast completely, but we managed to whittle it down a little: one breakfast egg instead of two, using egg substitutes instead of real eggs one or two mornings a week, two slices of bacon instead of four, half an English muffin instead of a whole one, and so forth. I even resolved to suffer through a cereal-and-toast breakfast twice weekly, and stuck by this for at least two or three weeks before it went by the board.

Finally, we cut back on the frequency of heavy cheese meals and worked at limiting such things as cheese-and-cracker hors d'oeuvres to a couple of nights a week instead of all seven. I was permitted my customary drink or two at cocktail hour and a glass of wine with dinner—"but perhaps not eight or ten double martinis a day," Fred had told me sourly. We also experimented with salt substitutes at the table and in cooking for a while, but found the results pretty undistinguished, so finally that largely went by the board, too.

I wasn't really satisfied with this sort of dietary control, at least not at first. I suspected it was more a matter of spitting into the wind than any really effective preventive effort, but at least I conceded it was a move in the right direction. The smoking was a far tougher problem. As a lifelong, two-packs-a-day cigarette smoker since about age thirteen, I had stopped smoking two or three times in my life, a couple of months at a time, but had always fallen back into the trap. Now, on getting out of the hospital and getting back home, I found that the period of abstinence in the hospital hadn't helped much, and, presently, I was smoking cigarettes again—not many, maybe two or three a day, at first, and never escalating beyond seven or eight, but this was obviously not "stopping smoking." Fred was clearly disgusted with me about this, and so was I, but this is an account of how it actually was, not how it ought to have been. Just as my dietary control program fell short of the ideal, so did my control of smoking. It was not until the summer of 1982 that I finally made another determined attempt to discontinue smoking completely, and ultimately succeeded.

The exercise program demanded more attention than anything else and was by far the most successful of my "lifetime reforms." Some of it was easy. Since our house is located on the banks of a creek an eighth of a mile in from a county road, there was a daily, quarter-mile walk out and back to the mailbox for the outgoing mail every morning, and another round trip to collect the mail in the early afternoon. A writer never knows when there may be a thousand-dollar check in the mail. The first few days, these short walks just about exhausted me, especially when I had a heavy load of mail to carry back, but this gradually improved. In addition, each morning I also made the rounds of the place, checking the creek, watching the ice forming as the nights got colder and colder, watching for deer on the hillside beyond, and so forth.

All this was enough exercise for the first few days, but as medication brought my angina under better control, I started organizing short daily walks, sometimes twice a day, gradually escalating to longer walks once a day in the afternoon. By using the car and checking the odometer, we were able to mark the county road from our door in quarter-mile segments with little purple plastic ties as markers. Going up the canyon, we found that Mrs. Lankin's road was almost exactly half a mile, Gene Brain's farm was a full mile, Josh's camp up the canyon was 1.6 miles, while the Yahne meadow was just over 2 miles from our back door. Going down the canyon toward the interstate highway between Loel Knudson's lower pasture and Loel's bare hills, it was just exactly a mile to the irrigation ditch, and a mile and a half to the highway overpass. With these measurements taken, I set daily walking times and began taking daily walks.

I should make it entirely clear that I was anything but enthusiastic about this totally unwelcome addition to my daily activities. All my life I had loathed physical exercise, especially the whole idea of make-work exercise—exercise taken just for the sake of the exercise. During deer- or elk-hunting season, I would cheerfully walk ten or twelve miles a day, up and down steep brushy mountainsides, and enjoy it, because I enjoyed the hunting. In the summer I would carry a forty-pound backpack seven or eight miles up a mountain creek trail to get to a good fishing spot. This kind of "motivated" exercise was fine, except that it was totally irregular and intermittent.

Now, it seemed to me, I was faced with regular daily increments of the most boring exercise in the world—walking along a fairly level road—on a "do it or else" basis under doctor's orders with no reward in sight other than the rather vague promise of some possible long-term benefit to my cardiovascular system. All the same, I initiated the program and followed it doggedly day after day. The first few days, I made two half-mile round trips a day, then two daily three-quarter-mile round trips. I soon discovered that this program, although physically tolerable (I could do it without very much angina), was devouring my most productive working hours in both the morning and the afternoon. Since I didn't think that I would really continue that for very long, I began doing my walking all at one time, in the late afternoon, and set up a two-mile round-trip course. Then, rather than extending the distance as a means of increasing my cardiovascular conditioning, I worked to step up the briskness of the walking.

One of the two courses that I set up took me up the county road a mile to Gene Brain's ranch gate and back again. The other took me down the canyon, on the county road past Loel Knudson's ranch, to the irrigation ditch and back. During the first two weeks or so, these walks seemed to be absolute crashing bores. Then something very odd began to happen. For one thing, I began to relax and quit fighting the exercise as exercise. Simultaneously, for perhaps the first time in my life, I began noticing things that I had never seen before because I had never moved slowly enough to see them.

One of the first things I noticed was a fascinating variety of microclimates that I encountered on these walks of mine. Our house sat in a small flat clearing along Taneum Creek, with the mountain foothills rising sharply across the creek to the south. The place was surrounded by tall cottonwoods and ponderosa pines on all sides; it was very much protected. Although we had some wind from time to time, it was only intermittent, and much of the time during fall and winter the air was very still. Out on the county road, however, just an eighth of a mile from the house and situated in an open sweep down the canyon, there was almost always a wind—not just a breath of air, but anything from a husky breeze to a stiff enough wind that you had to lean into it to walk. Whichever way I walked, up-canyon toward the Brains' or down-canyon toward the irrigation ditch, I had that wind with me one way, against me the other way.

I found it much easier to manage my walk, going quite slowly, if I walked into the wind on the first half, then had the wind at my back to carry me home. I got trapped a couple of times. Once or twice, early on, I walked up to the Brains' very briskly, feeling that things were going just fine, and burning all my energy walking as fast as I comfortably could, only to discover that I was walking briskly because I had an unnoticed breeze to my back, and then had to face into it all the way home. This did not work so well. Therefore, I took to picking the route up-canyon or down according to which way the wind was blowing that day. Later I discovered that even the wind quality was different on the two routes. Walking toward the Brains' was walking up the canyon into the mountains; whatever breeze was present on a given day was quite steady and even for the entire distance. Walking down the canyon past Knudson's ranch, however, the road took a turn around the knob of a hill where the floor of the canyon was quite narrow (an area I came to think of as Knudson's Pass), then opened out to bare prairie hills to the north. A terrific blast of wind invariably came down off the prairie at just that point, and it was almost always down-canyon. That route, I found, almost always carried me with a very brisk wind to my back as I walked down to the irrigation ditch, and then faced me with an equally stiff headwind on the way home until I reached Knudson's Pass. Not infrequently that particular route would bring on an angina attack, so I would have to slow my pace, or take nitroglycerin, or pause to rest several times along the way, in order to get home again. These considerations took on more and more significance as the winter got deeper and more bitter.

Another development that took me quite by surprise—and still amazes me—was how rapidly I developed my powers of microobservation, the ability to see minor and fascinating details in the most mundane, everyday surroundings. In retrospect, I think that many people spend most of their lives ignoring, or just not seeing, practically everything that goes on in the world around them. They are going to this place, doing that thing, thinking about something else, and they just plain *don't look*. As my walking program developed, I was forced to devote time to it—up to an hour and a half a day—and there was nothing much to do during that time, and I often didn't have much to think about, or didn't particularly feel like thinking seriously, so I fell into the practice of looking around me as I walked. And the things I saw with this kind of close, repeated observation, proved perfectly fascinating.*

I suppose I shouldn't have been so surprised at this, because Ann and I had both remarked on the power of microobservation many times during the long days we spent each year in the woods and ridges around us while we were deer or elk hunting. Naturally, during those times we were primarily looking for deer or elk, usually walking very slowly, stopping and looking, walking a little farther, stopping and looking some more, sitting down on a stump quietly for a while, then going on just as quietly as we could—a perfectly ordinary still-hunting technique. On many of those days we would never actually see a deer or an elk all day even when we hunted from dawn until dark. But we never once went out on such a day without seeing or hearing *something* we would never have seen or heard if we had not been out there doing what we were doing. Some of the things we saw or heard were simply interesting; some, puzzling; still others, downright funny—but always they taught us something new about the natural life in that country. It was one of the fascinations of hunting.

Take an example or two. One autumn, Ann and our oldest son, Ben, were hunting together on a wooded ridge on a bright, cold, sunny day in early November. They had followed a game trail through the woods to the edge of a small grassy clearing. An old windfall log lay out in the middle of that clearing, and on it was an enormous snowshoe rabbit busy sunning himself and sleeping. He had turned completely white for the winter, except for his legs and his ear tips, which were black. Both Ann and Ben expected the rabbit to bolt as soon as they stepped out into the clearing, but as they approached, the rabbit just lay there on the log, obviously sleeping. How close could they get without disturbing him? They spent five minutes tiptoeing up to this enormous bunny until Ben was almost close enough to reach out and touch him, and the rabbit snoozed on. Then Ben said, "Boo!" in a very loud voice. That rabbit leaped three feet straight up in the air, landed on the ground on all fours, and was out of that clearing and into the woods with three enormous bounds. He probably went right on into the next county and never knew what startled him.

On another occasion, Ann and I were hunting together up above Josh's camp, working our way through a wooded area toward the Lost Forest, before the loggers had chopped all the trees down: a

---

* Maybe this capacity for microobservation is just another of the polarities in humankind. I have had friends tell me that they have been microobservers all their lives. Maybe so, but it was a whole new experience for me.

rolling area of small hills and ravines leading to a vast somber stand of huge, flooded-out aspen trees at the foot of a great scree slope. We were going along together very quietly up one shoulder of a ravine when, suddenly, we thought we heard someone laughing and talking quite loudly some distance up the ravine. We stopped and listened, but the sound was not clear enough for us to be sure whether it was human, so we worked slowly up the ravine's shoulder in the direction of the sound.

As we got closer, we realized that these were not human sounds. We were hearing *coyotes*: yipping, barking, chattering sounds interspersed with little yelps, occasional croons, and numerous friendly growls. As we listened, it became obvious that the sounds were coming from more than one coyote; two or three were talking simultaneously, making different kinds of noises, and we could actually identify five or six individual voices. Neither was there any kind of fighting going on—they were simply having a coyote convention in that ravine, electing officers and amending by-laws, or whatever coyotes do at coyote conventions.

We wanted desperately to actually see them, so we moved very slowly and quietly toward the sounds. Then, abruptly, as though somebody had thrown a switch, all the sounds came to an end. We froze and waited. Perhaps three minutes later, as we stood there, we saw a very large, very furry gray coyote come loping down the bottom of the ravine, his huge bushy tail waving behind him, all gray except for black markings around the eyes and some black on his tail. He was in no hurry, just trotting down the ravine, such a very large animal that we would have sworn he was a timber wolf had we not been earnestly advised by various members of the Game Department over the years that we had no timber wolves anywhere in Washington State. At one point we must have moved, because the coyote stopped, looked directly at us, drew his head back, then turned and loped away into the thickest brush there was at hand.

We worked our way on up the ravine, hoping to find some evidence of where the convention had been, but search as we would, we couldn't find a single sign to indicate a recent large congregation of coyotes. Not one sign. Since that day we have seen many coyotes in the woods and prairies around our place, and have heard numerous coyote conventions and songfests over the years, but never since have we seen any coyote as large, gray, and handsome as that princely creature we saw loping down the ravine that day. We still wonder if we had not actually sighted one of the last remaining timber wolves in Kittitas County, Washington.

Still another time, Ann had a fascinating encounter with an owl. It was during elk season, and she was hunting alone, following a major game trail through the woods, going slowly, quietly, as we usually did. Presently, she sat down on a stump to watch and wait for a while. She had only been sitting there a moment when a small twig fell and hit her on the head. She looked up and was startled to see a great horned owl sitting on a branch high up directly over her head, staring down at her. She was fascinated because she had never seen a horned owl that close, but her attention was really on the woods and the game trail, so she continued sitting on the stump, assuming that the owl had just inadvertently knocked off a twig or a piece of bark. A few seconds later, however, another twig fell and hit her on the head.

Ann decided to take the hint; clearly that owl did not *like* her sitting under his tree. She stood, shouldered her rifle, walked on up the game trail about fifty yards, and found a windfall to sit on, again turning her attention to the woods and the trail. She was undisturbed for no longer than two minutes; then she saw the owl lift its wings and glide silently through the air to perch on a branch of the tree directly over where she was now sitting. After a moment or two, another twig fell, hitting her on the head. She sighed, got to her feet, and went on up the game trail. She had simply misunderstood the first time: That owl not only didn't like her sitting under his tree; he didn't want her anywhere in the neighborhood!

We had learned that these kinds of observations and encounters were commonplace during our hunting forays. Those woods and hills were teeming with life, going its own way, doing its own thing. All you had to do to bear witness was be there, and move slowly and quietly, and observe. As my walking program began to develop, I found that exactly the same thing applied to the county road I walked on, to the ditches on either side, to the rocky bare hills rising up to the north of the road, and to the meadows and woodlands to the south. My eyes were really opened on the third or fourth day that I walked up toward Brain's ranch, at that time just a few days after the elk hunting season had closed. At one point, on the right of the road, the bare hills rose up to a high rocky promontory, and as I approached along the road, something on the skyline caught my eye. A huge bull elk walked out onto that high rock and stared down at me, fully outlined against the sky, a great five-point rack of antlers rising above his shoulders into the sky. It was a typical, classical bull elk profile: the large blocky body, the powerful shoulders, the neck, head, and antlers curving out and up in front. I stood still and watched, and he watched me back, totally unconcerned. He knew perfectly well that elk season was over. He leaned his head down to take a mouthful of dinner, then raised it up again and looked at me some more. Then, without the slightest sign of haste or alarm, he turned and walked back up over the ridge, showing me his white rump as he went, and disappearing from the skyline. I felt a chill go down my back as he walked away so nonchalantly. I felt that I'd seen that elk before very recently, and that his appearance there that day was somehow prophetic.

Most days my sightings were not that spectacular. Frequently on my walks I would see deer, now that the season was over, appearing on the high meadows to graze, and, then, when the weather got colder, down in the lower meadows along the creek. Many things seemed minor or would have been missed altogether: a flock of half a dozen lovely pink-and-gray pine grosbeaks pecking away at last year's seeds in a field at the edge of some snow; three large orange-yellow amanita mushrooms with their oatmeal-sprinkled tops appearing suddenly alongside the road, unseasonably late, enlarging each day until they were spread out like dinner plates; a skunk that made a den in the rocks near the road and made frequent promenades along one of the Brains' fences from time to time. Every day I would make some different microobservation. I never knew what I would see from one day to the next, but I came to know that every day I would see something I had never seen before.

I dwell on this matter at such length simply because I began to realize that the success of this exercise conditioning program, extended a little bit further each day, was very deeply influenced—and, perhaps, even made successful—by such a simple thing as anticipation of these microobservations. For me a daily exercise program was a truly radical change in life-style, a change that could have great bearing on how I was going to fare in the future. But I do not believe that most people can make such changes in life-style simply by forcing themselves to do something they hate every minute, kicking and screaming all the way. I think that one must search out something new, something unexpected or unsuspected, something surprisingly rewarding in itself, in order to make the change truly viable and sustained. I think many people attempt life-style changes "for their own good"—diet controls, exercise programs, giving up smoking, reducing alcohol intake—in terms of the negative, as a sort of martyrdom, giving up old comfortable pleasures and habit patterns they really don't want to give up at all. Too often these changes soon fail. I'm convinced that such changes can have a far better chance of being sustained if, instead of hating them, one can seek out some new richnesses, satisfactions, or rewards that are inherent in the changes. Life-style changes have to be enriching, not impoverishing, if they are to have any chance of enduring. The enrichment of microobservation made the difference for me; it could work as well for anyone else faced with the problem.

Of course, as time went on, I found other rewards also. Gradually my energy level began to creep back, not immediately to normal, but increasingly better than the absolute rock-bottom level I felt when we first returned to Thorp. The shortness of breath that I had experienced at first grew less and less, and the angina, although it was still present, appeared less frequently and was less bothersome—perhaps, I hoped, because the undamaged part of my heart was recovering from the shock of the illness. I found, to my delight, that I did not instantly gain back the fifteen pounds I had lost in the hospital during the acute illness. And, as a bonus, an element of gloominess, of dwelling on the idea of perhaps dropping dead any minute, began to fade away, and I began to think in terms of possibly living for two or three months longer. And, in fact, the more distance I put between myself and that close encounter with death, the more I felt the distance widening between crippling illness and real recovery.

There were other adjustments that had to be made during those early days back at Thorp, some fairly minor, but some very major. During this time Ann and I both had the very major problem of feeling our way into some sort of living relationship other than that of a half-dead, debilitated husband and an ever-apprehensive wife. So far in this account Ann may seem to have come across as a sort of stalwart, ever-faithful, cardboard cutout of a Good Soldier Sam, but that wasn't quite the way it was. During the critical period, Ann had done largely what she had to do; she was stuck, without much choice. Surely she must have resented that sometimes, but she couldn't allow herself to resent it, and she couldn't be free of the fearful awareness that her husband of twenty-eight years might just suddenly drop dead at any moment. The nurses at the hospital complained that she "hovered" too much—and hover she did, during the critical days. But back home at Thorp, with a long pull ahead, something better than hovering had to be made to work. She knew that, and so did I.

Unfortunately there were some realities that had to be faced and dealt with. In those early days there were a multitude of things that I simply could not do, and I hated it. I hated being unable to do them, and I hated having to have Ann do them for me. I couldn't carry a bag of groceries in from the car. I couldn't split kindling for the evening's fire. I couldn't walk upstairs to the bedroom and back down again more than a couple of times a day—it brought on shortness of breath and angina. I couldn't drive the car to speak of; the doctor had said, "Let Ann do the driving." When the heavy snow started, it was Ann who had to get up in the dark at 5:30 in the morning and plow out to the county road with the little tractor and blade—I couldn't take the cold, and I couldn't handle the machine. I hated all this, and, perversely, resented having to watch Ann do it all. Ann hated it, too, and resented the fact that I couldn't do it, but there she was, doing it just the same.

The problem reached into far more subtle areas as well, and placed even greater physical and emotional burdens on Ann. With me running out of energy an hour after arising in the morning, somebody had to take over a dominant role in running the whole household operation. When things were left up to me, they just didn't get done, so it was Ann again who got stuck. If the porch got shoveled, it was Ann who shoveled it. When the car wouldn't start, she had to take care of it, get it in to the garage, pick it up, plan her time around it. She took over the financial responsibilities—paying the bills, keeping the accounts, balancing the bank statements— because it took me all day to write three checks. If we wanted to go somewhere for a weekend, she did the planning and preparation, because if the planning and preparation were up to me, we wouldn't go. More and more she got into the habit of taking over such things— she had to—and to me it seemed more and more belittling to have to let her. There were abraded feelings, sharp words, tense feelings, long silences. She was stubborn, sometimes abrasive. So was I. We both planted our heels in the ground, and it sometimes took days to quiet things down after a confrontation.

To make things worse, Ann had to work out her role while being constantly hemmed in by a bunch of medical "mustn't do's." For example, Fred had vigorously enjoined us to avoid stress at almost any cost. I made a fairly straightforward (and successful) effort to reduce stress in my approach to my work, and that was fine, but for Ann it wasn't that simple. She felt she had to tiptoe around, trying to avoid anything controversial. Sometimes that meant avoiding discussion of "heavy" items, which, therefore, just remained hanging. Sometimes it meant grabbing the bull by the horns and just arbitrarily making disagreeable decisions—disagreeable to me or disagreeable to her—because they had to be made, only to have me get angry at being preempted.

Obviously these were no-win situations, far more emotional than rational. As a single example of the distress that they caused, there was the matter of my angina. The angina was painful and debilitating and frightening and infuriating to *me* when it came on, especially the attacks that came on at night and didn't want to subside, but I soon found—irrational or not—that I just couldn't bear having Ann worrying about them when they came on. I tried, therefore, to hide them when they occurred. I wouldn't tell Ann about them, which naturally made her worry about them all the more. Unfortunately, the nighttime attacks were hard to disguise, but they just got worse if she got stirred up as well as me. Ultimately, her role at such times became defined as turning over in bed, saying nothing, and pretending nothing was happening.

As time passed, this business of sitting back and saying nothing extended to other things. I felt, sort of fatalistically, that I had to go my own way as recovery progressed. I would walk, but after the first week or so I wanted to walk by myself. Much later I wanted to do things that I "shouldn't do" while she was away; during later hunting seasons I wanted to hunt alone. This was irrational, of course, and worried her; we both knew that in the event of real trouble, CPR might be the only thing that would save me, and what if no one was there? Presently I learned to put my intimations of imminent mortality aside. I *had* to; you can't sit around and brood about this sort of thing indefinitely. But Ann couldn't set her fears aside. There was always the possibility that an attack of angina might not go away. There was always the possibility of waking up one morning, any morning, and finding the other one simply *departed*, and all the important things never communicated.

Ultimately, of course, it was a battle between emotion and reason. Fortunately, time works on the side of reason, and as it happened, we did have time. I cannot tell you precisely how we worked these problems out, and I don't think Ann can either, but with time, and jousting, and accommodating, and plain doggedly blundering through, we gradually reached new footings and made things go, maybe not ideally, but at least reasonably well. Love and caring had a lot to do with it; you just can't beat them.

Throughout all this, of course, I was constantly thinking about the upcoming, in-depth diagnostic investigations that Fred Cleveland had in mind for me when I was "a little further down the road" into recovery. I was all in favor of those investigations, and I wanted to be in as good physical condition as possible by the time they were undertaken. I wasn't concerned that the results of those studies would necessarily lead to any other treatment program than the one I was already on. Fred had made it clear that he didn't regard them as a mere *pro forma* prelude to some different kind of treatment, such as by-pass surgery, but simply as a necessary means to find out what options might exist. Instead of flying along blind, we would then proceed with our eyes open, with all the solid knowledge and information that might then be available.

On the other hand, I was perfectly aware that the investigations might well reveal that we had options or choices—maybe even imperatives—that we simply couldn't assess or consider without looking. I knew quite well that coronary artery by-pass graft surgery had been performed since the early 1960s and had been applied widely to many patients with coronary artery disease. Now, in 1980, that kind of surgery was in the process of high technical refinement in the operating room and careful statistical reassessment in the great clinical medical centers. There were many doctors, including myself and possibly Fred as well, who had felt that this surgery had in the past been used far too widely and aggressively on far too many patients without any real proof that it actually achieved anything. Many of these patients, I suspected, had been subjected to the very significant risk of the surgery without any clearcut potential benefit being demonstrated. But then I also suspected that for certain selected patients such surgery might be definitely beneficial, at least helping to make their lives more livable and, perhaps in some cases, increasing their longevity as well. I didn't think that I regarded the prospect of such surgery with any great enthusiasm for myself, but if I turned out to be one of the patients who might really benefit from it greatly, I at least wanted to know it. My attitude was really very simple: Let's proceed with the investigations when the time comes and see what they turn up. Then at least I could make a rational decision of whether to have the surgery or not.

For these reasons it seemed very important to me to get in shape for the investigations, and I was cheered by what I sensed as a steady process of recovery going on. I was not so cheered, however, at one complicating factor that appeared along the way. On Thanksgiving weekend we had family festivities at Thorp. My brother, Bill, came over from Spokane on Wednesday evening to join us (his wife, Mo, had gone out to spend Thanksgiving with a sister in Minot who was having some kind of problem), and my daughter, Becky, came in from Walla Walla with a Japanese girl from Hawaii as her weekend guest. Thanksgiving afternoon we had fancy hors d'oeuvres and cocktails, then our traditional Thanksgiving dinner, so I overindulged to a certain degree, although I wouldn't say that I abandoned all efforts at keeping myself pure. After we retired for the night I slept just fine, but woke up about five in the morning with an awareness that my heart seemed to be hopping all over the place. There wasn't any sign of angina, just a gross arrhythmia.

At first I thought I had just developed a hell of a bradycardia (slow heartbeat), since my pulse rate seemed to be down to about thirty, and I immediately assumed that the four-times-a-day dose of Inderal that Fred had me taking was playing hob with my heart rate. When I got up and walked around a bit, the arrhythmia seemed to stop, but then it recurred periodically again and again throughout the rest of the day. Nitroglycerin didn't seem to affect it in any way. In fact, the only thing that seemed to make it stop jumping around for a while was to get up and move around. When I went out to walk, the arrhythmia shifted back to a perfectly normal sinus rhythm of about 80 beats per minute, as long as I was walking, but then it would start jumping around again when I got home and sat down to rest. I had no idea why it was behaving like this.

I didn't know quite what to do about it, or whether I needed to do anything at all. There seemed to be no tiredness, shortness of breath, or chest pain associated with the arrhythmia—it was just annoyingly *there* much of the time. I didn't mention it to Ann; there didn't seem to be any point. I hated to bother Fred Cleveland at home over the Thanksgiving weekend; I wasn't even sure there was anything to bother him *about*. But the arrhythmia continued on and off for the next couple of days, and it was extremely irritating when it occurred, since I was very much aware of it: thump, thump— thump, thump—thump—thump, thump, thump—thump—thump, thump, thump. It felt as if my heart were jumping around in my chest. On Sunday evening I got the bright idea of listening to my heart with my stethoscope, while checking my pulse at the same time, and I found that I didn't really have a bradycardia at all. I would have one good strong pulse beat, followed by two or three funny, shallow-sounding heartbeats that I couldn't feel at the wrist at all.

Monday morning I called Fred at the Mason Clinic and told him what was going on. He immediately wanted to know if I was fibrillating; that is, was I experiencing an extremely rapid heartbeat so that the pulse just wasn't coming through part of the time. I said I didn't think I was fibrillating exactly, just having a whole bunch of premature or ectopic heartbeats strung in between a few normal pulses. "All right," Fred said, "have Ann take you in to Ellensburg to a clinic or emergency room or someplace and have somebody run a rhythm strip on the EKG. Then ask them to look at it and call me immediately to tell me whether this thing is atrial or ventricular in origin." What he wanted to know, of course, was whether the irregular beat was originating in the atria (which would mean that it was probably pretty benign) or in the ventricles (which might be a serious threat).

Ann drove me into the Valley Clinic in Ellensburg, and there we encountered young Dr. Horsley. He thought it was probably just an atrial arrhythmia, after listening a moment, but he had a nurse run a rhythm strip—a simple, one-lead EKG intended to show P waves, QRS complexes, and T waves, in order to determine just where in the heart the arrhythmia was originating. After glancing at the strip, he looked a little less self-assured and had the nurse run a full twelve-lead EKG, while he stood watching the tape as it came out of the machine, saying that it was the strangest rhythm he'd ever seen on a tracing. I seemed to be having about one normal, effective heartbeat out of every three or four; all the others were ectopic (triggered from the wrong place or abnormal in EKG pattern) and appeared to be ventricular in origin.

Horsley called Fred and described his findings while I sat there in his office. Fred asked him to prescribe some Norpace, one of the powerful antiarrhythmic drugs that work somewhat like quinidine, in 100-milligram capsules for me to take four times a day, starting as quickly as we could get them at the drugstore. He also asked Horsley to mail him the rhythm strip and the full EKG as well, or copies, and to ask me to call Fred first thing in the morning to report in.

Ann and I got home with the medicine about five o'clock and I took one of the Norpace right away. We had a small drink and thought pure thoughts about dinner, and then the arrhythmia suddenly converted to a normal sinus rhythm within an hour after I'd taken the first dose. I took another dose at bedtime, with my pulse still running a nice orderly eighty beats per minute. Next morning it began flip-flopping again for a while but stopped an hour or so after medication, and after two or three days' dosage even these brief runs of arrhythmia stopped completely.

Later on I began to wonder if maybe something odd hadn't been going on with my heart rhythm for several days before I even noticed it, since within three or four days of starting the Norpace I found myself to be feeling generally better than I had at any point since I got home from the hospital. I seemed to have noticeably more energy, less tendency to tire quickly, better exercise tolerance when walking, and less angina. Certainly I was relieved that my ventricle had stopped twitching around in this fashion, but it was clear from Fred's attitude that he did not consider this late appearance of an arrhythmia suddenly turning up, weeks after the heart attack, to be particularly good news.

One other development during this time caused just enough irritation that it kept calling itself to my attention: the matter of the angina while I was at rest. When I had first started the regular Inderal and Isordil antiangina medication, the nighttime angina at rest had subsided completely for a week or two. Then it began to reappear one or two nights a week, not as severe as it was originally, but enough to wake me up at one or two in the morning with a dull, aching pain in my chest. This did not seem to be related to anything I ate for dinner, or having too much to drink, or extra exertion during the day, or anything else. It just seemed to appear when it felt like it and didn't when it didn't. But unlike the angina that appeared during exertion, this nocturnal angina didn't quiet down readily with medicine. A regular nitroglycerin tablet would make it feel a little better for ten or fifteen minutes but not go away completely, and then it would get worse again. The Isordil didn't seem to affect it at all for fifteen minutes or so, and then would only quiet it down about 75 percent for half an hour before it would resume. The pain itself wasn't terribly distressing, it simply meant that I seemed to be doomed to a couple of hours of sleepless discomfort in the middle of the night when it occurred.

Finally, I found that placing a gob of the nitro paste on my chest at the same time that I took the Isordil under the tongue was the best answer. The angina would gradually subside completely over the next half-hour and then wouldn't recur, so that I could get back to sleep. I discovered this purely by trial and error. All in all, this nocturnal angina was more worrisome than painful, but it led me to what I considered a rather startling insight: that whatever was going on with my heart, whatever degree of healing of past injury was taking place, whatever recovery and rebuilding was taking place, there was still an extremely changing, dynamic process going on.

Of course, I knew that the part of the heart muscle that was destroyed would never recover or rebuild. That area would simply become a tough, fibrous scar over the weeks and months. But the parts of the heart surrounding that scar—heart muscle that was injured and ischemic but still alive—*could* recover and rebuild. That heart muscle, for example, could become progressively stronger and better conditioned; and meanwhile, new collateral blood vessels could grow and develop in that area, providing better oxygenation and reducing the ischemia. But I had originally assumed that once the injury had occurred, the process of healing and recovery would all be upward, a slow, inch-by-inch progressive process, perceptible, perhaps, only after weeks or months, but steadily getting better and better.

Now I wasn't so sure of that. Things seemed to be changing in a dynamic, up-and-down fashion, day by day, and whatever it was that was changing was causing fluctuating symptoms or sensations of which I was very viscerally aware—as, for example, the coming and going of the arrhythmia, or the coming and going of the resting angina. I was quite certain, for example, that the arrhythmia had nothing whatever to do with having two cocktails and a big Thanksgiving dinner. Why would it go on for days and days if that were the case? The arrhythmia was caused by some physical change in the electrical conducting system of part of the heart muscle, either the part that was scarring or the part that was healing, and it was a threat because it might evolve into a life-threatening ventricular fibrillation without warning at any time.

I couldn't identify any particular outside influences that might be triggering those changes, but I did begin to realize, perhaps for the first time, that a terribly dynamic process was at work that might well be influenced by any one of a whole squadron of factors—day-by-day diet, day-by-day exercise, constantly fluctuating hormonal influences, constantly fluctuating emotional influences, maybe even the varying diurnal blood levels of the medicines I was taking. Any one or all of these factors could be exercising a dynamic influence upon exactly what was happening to my heart at any given moment. Any one individual influence might be too subtle to sort out, but what I perceived happening in terms of visceral sensations or symptoms was the aggregate of all these influences.

This idea was not particularly comforting. Certainly it didn't seem that the dynamics of the thing were necessarily all in the direction of healing and recovery. It seemed that I was constantly in the process of climbing up a hill three steps and sliding back two, maybe sliding back all three on some days, maybe even sliding back four, sometimes, depending upon precisely what was happening at a given time. I would really much rather have felt that it was all smooth and steady, either staying the same or moving slightly upward toward healing and recovery all the time, but it seemed more and more apparent to me that this was not the way it was working.

I didn't call Fred Cleveland to communicate any of this. He would simply have sighed and told me to quit trying to second-guess my doctor. But I had an appointment to see him at the Mason Clinic on Monday, December 10, forty-seven days after my heart attack, so I made a note of this as one of the things to call to his attention. Meanwhile, Ann and I decided to make the trip to Seattle our first Grand Adventure since returning home. We would go over to the city on Thursday evening, stay at a downtown hotel, and enjoy our annual Christmas shopping weekend and pre-Christmas pig-out. For some years we had been taking such a holiday weekend in Seattle early in December to wrap up our Christmas shopping, let the kids see Santa Claus, and sample some of the newer restaurants that we seldom got an opportunity to try. This, however, was the first year that we would have such a weekend all to ourselves, with no children along, since they were now all scattered. We started anticipating the trip as another small step toward normalcy, a pleasant change of pace after almost a month of rather bland, uninteresting routine at Thorp, a fun outing, just like old times.

As it turned out, it wasn't such a bright idea. It wasn't all that much fun, and it brought us both sharply to the reality that ''getting back to normalcy" and the recreations of old times were not precisely in the cards. The time back at Thorp had been bland, dull, and unstressful, all right, and that was probably just as well. The shopping weekend was too much of a shift, too much too soon. The hundred-mile drive to Seattle was uneasy in itself, with rain and snow through Snoqualmie Pass. The Seattle weather was cold, wet, windy, typical of the damp, raw Decembers so common there. The hotel was highly convenient to all the stores, but the excitement of the trip was a sharp change and there was not much time for resting.

Friday morning we went our separate ways for shopping. I had heard of the fine Christmas atmosphere at the just-opened, three-level shopping mall in the new Rainier Bank Building, and headed up there in mid-morning after paying courtesy calls on all the downtown book departments and loading up a shopping bag with twenty-five pounds worth of books. It was uphill into the wind and rain all the way, and halfway there I had the worst exertional angina attack that I'd had since the first day out of the hospital. It wasn't the continuing pain of another heart attack; it quieted down completely with nitroglycerin, but then recurred and recurred again; once I achieved the Rainier mall, I had to find a bench and rest for three-quarters of an hour, listening to the Christmas music in the grand lobby, before I could even poke around the stores.

After meeting Ann for lunch, I had more angina on the way back to the hotel for a two-hour nap. Out again later into the wind and rain, I had still more trouble with angina and shortness of breath. This seemed to set the pattern for the whole weekend: As long as I didn't go anywhere or do anything, everything was fine, but the moment I ventured outside into the weather or into a crowded store or anyplace more than two or three blocks away, the angina was back and progress was slow. By Sunday I had thoroughly had it and spent the day in the hotel, loafing and watching television, wishing we could go back home then and there. I was not feeling at all chipper by the time my appointment with Fred Cleveland rolled around on Monday morning.

Fred had ordered a new EKG and chest X ray to be done before I saw him, and they were both on hand by the time of the appointment. He checked me over carefully, asked specific questions about the amounts and times of angina, about the arrhythmia, about the levels of activity I was able to achieve, and about how I felt things were going in general. He even listened to my theory of dynamic changes without any evidence of impatience, just shrugging and saying, "Well, of *course* it's a dynamic process. After all, it's living tissue trying to keep its head above water." He seemed particularly interested in how much shortness of breath I had, and he was interested in the problems I had been having on this first outing weekend. Then he patiently tackled my list of questions, foremost among them being whether the EKG showed any evidence of new infarctions or extensions of the old infarction.

"None whatever," he said. He hadn't expected any, and anyway, he said, that wasn't what was worrying him. "Of course the risk is always there, and we have to live with that, but that's not the problem that bothers me. What I don't like is all this angina. It's actively bad for you, and we must reduce it if we can. I'm going to have you double the amount of Inderal you're taking; that should help control the angina, and you seem to be tolerating the medicine pretty well. I also don't like the arrhythmia, it shouldn't *be* there at this point, and you must plan to stay on the Norpace to control that for at least three months. The arrhythmia may have resolved itself by then; if not, we'll keep you on the Norpace for at least a year or more. These things are annoyances and threats, maybe even ominous, but if you want to talk about your most immediate prime prognostic hazard, the real screaming danger that you face, it isn't those things, or another infarction either."

I was startled. "Then what is it?"

"Heart failure," Fred said. "Of course, another infarction would be a terrible blow, and we have to be concerned about the possibility, but at least you could survive another infarction. The Inderal itself may already be protecting you there, or maybe we'll be able to do something about it ahead of time to reduce the risk, or even right in the middle of it. You could survive another infarction—but you would not survive heart failure."

For a while Fred scribbled some notes on my chart, while Ann and I waited. At one point he picked up his phone, punched an extension, and carried on a brief, largely unintelligible conversation with someone. Finally, he put down his pen and turned to us both with an air of finality. "Last month I told you I wanted Alan further down the road, maybe into March or April, before we started our detailed investigations. Now I've changed my mind. I don't like some of the things that are going on; they're making me nervous. We've been flying blind so far, and I think it's time to stop that. I want you to go home now and increase the Inderal and have a *very quiet* Christmas. I want to see you here again on Monday, January 5th, and then I want you to come into the hospital the morning of Tuesday, January 6th, for heart catheterization and coronary artery angiograms, to be followed by some other studies a week later. Flying blind isn't good enough anymore. We need to have a road map."

— 8 —

One winter evening in Berlin, during the waning months of 1929 (just a year after I was born), a young German surgeon named Werner Forssmann conducted an experiment so totally remarkable and revolutionary that it was destined to go down as one of the great steps forward in medical history of the Twentieth Century. It was also an experiment so hair-raising that Forssmann's colleagues thought he was a lunatic: For the first time in history, he introduced a catheter into a living human heart—*his own* heart—and took a picture of it.

Of all the disorders known in those days, none seemed more tragic and frustrating than the congenital heart defects that appeared occasionally in newborn babies—abnormalities in the way the heart and great blood vessels developed during embryonic life. At that time there was no clear idea why such defects occurred. Often they resulted in the death of the baby within hours or days after birth; in other cases, a child might limp through half a dozen years as a terribly debilitated cardiac cripple before death finally came. There was nothing much that medical science could offer these unfortunate children other than to stave off heart failure for as long as possible with medications. Surgical correction of these defects seemed totally beyond reach. By doing autopsies on the bodies of such children, anatomists had identified a dozen or more different kinds of defects, ranging all the way from dextraposition of the heart (placement of the heart toward the right side of the chest, rather than the left) to all manner of structural defects and obstructions to the normal flow of blood through the heart, the great blood vessels, or the lungs. Some of those defects might conceivably have seemed repairable, except that in those days the heart was considered totally off limits to the surgeon. Although the refinements in surgery from the mid-1800s through the 1930s had made it possible to do surgical repairs and intervention on other parts of the body—the stomach, bowel, kidneys, or the bones, for example—the most eminent cardiologists were opposed to the very idea of surgical treatment of the heart. It was assumed by everyone that any approach to the heart with a scalpel would either induce massive, uncontrollable bleeding, or that it would simply cause the heart to stop beating altogether.

One problem was the matter of diagnosis. Cardiologists and surgeons had no reliable way of determining which of many different kinds of defects might be present in a congenital heart abnormality. X-ray examination helped elsewhere in the body; it could detect a fractured bone or a malformed joint, for example. By using contrast agents—radio-opaque materials introduced to outline the interior of various organs—many internal organs could be visualized. But none of these techniques helped in the least as far as the heart was concerned. A liquid iodine contrast agent might be injected into a vein, but by the time the substance reached the patient's heart it would be so diluted by the blood that no clear picture of the interior of the heart could be obtained. In order to obtain any such picture, it would be necessary, somehow, to introduce a contrast agent directly into the heart itself. But how could you do this without disturbing the function of the heart in the process?

Ideas had been proposed—some rather startling, even frightening. As early as 1844, the great French physiologist Claude Bernard had inserted a long, narrow rubber tube or *catheter* into the jugular vein of a horse, then threaded the tube down the superior vena cava into the horse's right auricle, then on through the tricuspid valve into the right ventricle. Similarly, he placed a catheter in a horse's carotid artery and then threaded it down against the flow of blood into the aorta and on into the left ventricle. By attaching pressure-measuring devices to the ends of the catheters, Bernard was able to measure blood pressures in the vena cava, the aorta, and both ventricles during both contraction and relaxation phases of the heart.

These experiments had provided a great deal of information about the amount of force the heart exerted when it contracted, and, indirectly, they offered a way to measure the *cardiac output* of the horse's heart—the actual quantity of blood pumped out of the ventricles with each heartbeat. The procedure, which Bernard spoke of as *cardiac catheterization*, didn't seem to cause the horse any great difficulty—but nobody was terribly enthusiastic about trying it out on a living human being.

Werner Forssmann walked in where angels feared to tread. Working with human cadavers in his anatomy laboratory, Forssmann had found that a long, narrow urinary catheter made of pliable rubber could be inserted in a vein in the cadaver's arm, then threaded up the vein into the superior vena cava, thence into the right atrium of the heart. Since the catheter he used was opaque to radiation, it showed up as a dark tube on X-ray film. He could follow the progress of the catheter up the vein and into the heart, either by taking intermittent X-ray pictures or by observing the procedure "live" under a fluoroscope. By twisting and turning the catheter from the one end, he found that he could maneuver it through the venous system until it reached the heart.

This was all very well with a cadaver, but there was no proper way Forssmann could risk such an experiment on a living patient. There was no reason, however, that he could not perform such an experiment on himself, if he chose to. In 1929, at the age of twenty-five, Forssmann decided to try to repeat his cadaver catheterization experiment on himself, with another doctor reluctantly assisting him.

On that first attempt the other doctor lost his nerve halfway through the procedure and pulled the catheter back out. Forssmann repeated the effort the following evening by himself, with only a nurse standing by to run and get help if something went wrong. Using a little local anesthetic, he opened his own arm vein and inserted the catheter, using a fluoroscope and a mirror to follow the catheter's progress up the arm into the shoulder region. When the tube had been inserted a total of about twenty inches, the tip of the catheter entered his own right atrium. Forssmann knew it was there because he could see it on the fluoroscope screen, but he realized that no one would ever believe him unless he could somehow produce absolutely unquestionable evidence. With the catheter still in place in his heart, Forssmann got up from the chair in his laboratory, walked down a long corridor and up two flights of stairs to the X-ray laboratory where he had permanent chest X rays taken in order to provide absolutely unassailable proof of what he had achieved.

Forssmann knew exactly what this self-experiment implied: If a catheter could be placed in the right atrium of a living human heart by passing it up through a vein, perhaps it could be passed on into the right ventricle of the heart as well. If this could be done safely, perhaps a catheter could also be introduced into an artery in the arm and threaded up to enter the ascending aorta and also down into the left ventricle. This would allow living measurements of blood pressure inside at least three chambers of the human heart. It would allow the measurement of cardiac output from each of the two ventricles. In theory, it would also allow radio-opaque iodine solutions to be introduced directly into the heart so that interior heart X-ray pictures could be taken. Last but not least, it would make it possible to introduce medications directly inside the heart chambers.

Forssmann wrote up an account of his experiment, which he repeated on himself at least six times to verify that his first success was not a fluke. His paper was published in an obscure German medical journal, going unheeded for a dozen years, during which time Forssmann became a surgeon in the German army with the outbreak of World War II. Toward the end of the war, he was captured by American forces and spent some time in a prison camp. Meanwhile, it was not until 1941 that two doctors in America, André Counand and Dickenson Woodruff Richards, recognized that Forssmann's catheterization of a living human heart was the absolutely essential diagnostic technique that was needed if surgical correction of congenital heart diseases was ever to be possible.

These two men, following up on Forssmann's pioneering experiment, applied the technique of cardiac catheterization first on laboratory animals and then on living human patients. They improved on the technique and vastly expanded its power to actually diagnose a wide variety of congenital heart diseases. For the first time, it began to appear that surgery involving the living human heart might actually become a practicality. And, in 1956, Forssmann, Counand, and Richards all shared the 1956 Nobel Prize for physiology and medicine for their pioneering work in developing cardiac catheterization.

Even by the late 1940s this diagnostic technique had been refined into a commonplace procedure for patients with congenital heart disease. With the subsequent invention and engineering perfection of the heart-lung bypass machine in the 1950s, one of the surgeon's greatest dreads—uncontrollable hemorrhage during heart surgery—was laid to rest. This machine made it possible literally to disconnect the heart and lungs from the rest of the circulatory system for brief periods of time, using the machine to aerate incoming venous blood and pump out the aerated blood into the great arteries.

With the use of this machine, the actual practice of heart surgery began to blossom. For the first time, patients suffering from many formerly hopeless congenital heart lesions* were enabled to lead normal lives through open-heart surgery. Openings between the right and left ventricles, for example, could be closed. Stuck heart valves could be restored to function and later even replaced with artificial valves. Displaced great blood vessels could be returned to their proper anatomical position and their proper physiological function. These operations were by no means universally successful: Many early procedures carried extremely high mortality rates and could only be justified if there was virtually no hope for survival without the operation. Even the technique of cardiac catheterization itself carried certain significant risks. There was the risk, for example, of bleeding from the incision where the catheter was introduced into the vascular system, the risk of triggering dangerous or fatal arrhythmias, the risk of perforating the heart or the blood vessels with

---

* A "lesion" is simply a defect or abnormality of some kind somewhere in the body.

the catheter, and so forth. These procedures were considered very high-stakes surgery. Even after months of planning and medical management to prepare a patient for the operation, with every effort made to select only those patients with the greatest chances of benefitting, and after hours of meticulously delicate surgical work in the operating room, many patients were still lost.

It was for this reason that an odd tradition arose in medical and surgical circles in dealing with these patients, who were at that time usually small children. No pediatric cardiologist wanted to be accused of recklessly referring a desperately ill infant to the surgeon unless everybody concerned would agree that the surgery offered the baby its only hope—or, at the very least, had more to offer than doing no surgery at all. As a result, in the great medical centers where these children were treated—places such as the Johns Hopkins Hospital in Baltimore or Boston Children's Hospital—it became traditional that no one doctor or surgeon should be entrusted with the decision of performing surgery on a given patient. Rather, everyone at the institution who had any expertise whatsoever in children's congenital heart problems, be they medical doctors or surgeons, would gather in a "clinic" or "cardiac conference" to review every patient's case, together with all the diagnostic studies that had been proposed or accomplished, to determine, as a group, what they all concurred would be the best approach to treatment for each patient.

Of course, this might seem to be an eminently sensible procedure, but it led to an odd phenomenon. Whatever decision was reached was not necessarily a "democratic" decision, because in coming to a decision, a *minority*, or dissenting, opinion might often carry extraordinary weight. A group of fifteen cardiologists and surgeons might agree that a given child, whose case had been carefully studied, should have the benefit of corrective surgery. But if two or three physicians vigorously objected in a given case and could present good reasons for objecting, the conference would at least proceed very cautiously, and might, in fact, decide *not* to recommend the procedure.

The consensus opinion of such a doctors' conference was much more of a recommendation than an edict. The final decision *always* rested with the patient's personal physician or cardiologist. Such a "cardiac conference" or "clinic" approach to planning a patient's treatment was obviously extremely conservative, yet it had real advantages. Clearly it protected the patient from the ambitious or possibly reckless enthusiasm of the surgeon—or from the cardiologist who pushed for operations whose risks he might not fully understand. It guaranteed that surgery was done only when most of the best medical minds available agreed that it ought to be done,

including a number of physicians who were not involved economically in the case in any way. It protected the individual physician
from any appearance of personal aggrandizement as an underlying
motive for recommending surgery (or not recommending it), and,
above all, it relieved the physician from the sole burden of making
a terrible decision in a case in which no one could foresee the outcome
with absolute certainty.

Such cardiac conferences began to appear in the late 1950s and
early 1960s in major medical centers involved in the treatment of
congenital heart disease. But the establishment of such consensus
groups for dealing with one kind of heart problem led logically to
the establishment of similar conferences when other forms of cardiac
surgery began to be done, including coronary artery bypass grafting.
We will have more to say about such cardiac conferences later on.

During the 1950s, the technique of cardiac catheterization came
into its own as a lifesaving diagnostic procedure. Pressure gradients
in the interior of the heart could be measured; liquid contrast agents,
discharged through a catheter into the heart ventricle, could show
a clear picture of the ventricle's interior, and could demonstrate all
sorts of structural defects of the heart and the great blood vessels.
But there was one thing this technique could *not* do at that point:
It could not permit physicians actually to visualize the circulatory
pattern of the coronary arteries feeding the heart itself. Even if the
contrast agent was discharged when the tip of the catheter was just
outside the aortic valve, only about the first half-inch or so of each
coronary artery could be seen. And nobody dared approach a coronary artery itself with the tip of a catheter; it was firmly believed
that any manipulation of these vital arteries might immediately
precipitate a myocardial infarction and possibly kill the patient right
there in the Cath Lab.

This notion—that the coronary arteries could not be manipulated
in any way without risk of immediate death—persisted for fifteen
years. Then, in 1959, a fortuitous and almost unbelievable laboratory
accident demonstrated that it wasn't true at all.

The accident occurred at the hands of Dr. F. Mason Sones, Jr.,
an American cardiologist working at the Cleveland Clinic. Dr. Sones
was doing a procedure that, by 1958, had become almost routine in
the investigation of certain kinds of congenital lesions. The patient
was a seventeen-year-old boy who was thought to have a small defect
or hole in the muscular wall of the septum separating his right and
left ventricles. Such a septal defect could allow oxygen-poor venous
blood from the right ventricle to pass through to the left ventricle
and mix with oxygenated blood there—not enough to cause classic
"blue baby" signs and symptoms, but enough to put a continuing

strain on the heart so that the patient was edging into heart failure.

This was the kind of defect that might be correctable by open-heart surgery if the diagnosis could be confirmed by cardiac catheterization and X ray. Dr. Sones was doing the cardiac catheterization in order to obtain a *left ventriculogram*—an X ray, using a liquid contrast agent, that would show blood leaking directly from one ventricle to the other through a septal defect. The catheter was to be inserted in an artery in the patient's arm, threaded "upstream" through the artery into the aorta, then through the aortic valve into the left ventricle. There, a quantity of an iodine-containing solution would be squirted through the catheter and an X-ray picture taken.

The X-ray equipment required for this kind of exam in those days was ponderously large, installed underneath the operating table where the patient lay. The operator had to step down from floor level into a recessed cubbyhole in the floor in order to fire the X-ray camera at precisely the right moment to "freeze" the contrast agent in the ventricle before it dissipated into general circulation. Dr. Sones had carried the catheterization to the critical point. He could see on the fluoroscope screen that the tip of the catheter had reached the bulb of the aorta just where it rises from the heart, just above the aortic valve—the portion of the aorta from which the coronary arteries arose. Climbing down to monitor the X-ray machine, Sones instructed his assistant to advance the catheter tip through the aortic valve into the ventricle (a distance of about ½ inch) and then squirt in the contrast agent while Sones took the X-ray picture.

The film that was taken was developed immediately while the catheterized patient rested quietly on the table. But when Sones looked at the developed X ray, he could hardly believe his eyes: It was totally unlike any other ever taken before of a living human being. Instead of showing an outline of the interior of the patient's left ventricle, as expected, the film revealed a clear picture of the patient's left coronary artery and all of its branches down to the point where the smallest arterioles disappeared into the heart muscle—and nothing else.

An ordinary investigator might have dismissed this finding as unexplainable, and gone back to manipulating the catheter tip a bit and trying again. But Mason Sones was not an ordinary investigator; he instantly realized that the unthinkable had happened. Somehow the tip of the catheter, instead of passing through the valve into the ventricle, had lodged in the orifice of the left coronary artery instead. Then the entire dose of contrast agent had been ejected straight into that artery. It was Mason Sones's genius that he understood at once the significance of this bizarre accident. The catheter had inadvertently been placed in the patient's left coronary artery and produced a wonderfully clear *left coronary arteriogram*. But inserting the catheter there had not fatally blocked the patient's coronary artery, as everyone had assumed it would—blood continued to flow around it—nor had the contrast agent surging through that artery triggered a ventricular fibrillation, as many had predicted. The patient, in fact, had suffered no trouble whatsoever; he was pink, warm, snoozing quietly on the operating table, his heart still beating in a perfectly normal sinus rhythm.

Sones immediately realized that all the dire predictions of the terrible effects of coronary artery catheterization might be nonsense; he had *seen* that it could be done safely. With his next patient for cardiac catheterization, Sones deliberately manipulated the tip of the catheter first into the left coronary artery, then into the patient's right coronary artery, and obtained startlingly clear "road maps" of each of those arteries using only one-tenth the normal amount of contrast agent. Thus, Mason Sones proved that coronary angiograms could safely be taken—and that meant that individual, specific atherosclerotic lesions and obstructions of the coronary arteries and their branches could be visualized, identified, located, and measured.

Sones subsequently improved and refined his coronary artery catheterization technique. He developed a special catheter with a slight curve at the tip, so that it would virtually seek out the coronary arteries once the catheter tip reached the aortic bulb. He developed great skill in timing, taking and interpreting coronary angiograms. Perhaps most important of all, he recognized that this incredibly valuable diagnostic technique did not require some kind of virtuoso, one-of-a-kind cardiologist to perform it. Virtually any competent cardiologist could do the procedure, and Sones himself devoted years to personally teaching hundreds of cardiologists how it could be done.

There *were* occasional complications, of course. Once in a while, a patient would have bleeding at the site in the arm or leg artery where the catheter was inserted. Some patients suffered attacks of angina at the moment that the contrast agent surged through the coronary artery system, since the contrast agent itself carried no oxygen at all. On very rare occasions—perhaps one case in a hundred— a patient might indeed suffer a coronary thrombosis or stroke following the procedure, or a dangerous arrhythmia might be triggered. And in possibly one case out of a thousand, one or another of these complications proved fatal. It was clearly not a procedure to be undertaken lightly or frivolously, but as doctors became more experienced doing it, the risk of complications became smaller and smaller, the potential benefit of the information gathered greater and greater. Skill, experience and timing became highly important.

Early catheterizations and coronary angiograms required as much as an hour and a half of invasive manipulations with the catheter; today, in experienced hands, a catheterization and angiogram can be finished within ten or fifteen minutes from the time the catheter is inserted until it is removed.

There obviously wouldn't be much point in performing this kind of examination unless the information obtained could actually be put to use for the patient's benefit. The man who has severe angina pectoris already knows he has a potentially fatal problem with coronary artery disease—or, at least, his doctor does. He doesn't need coronary angiograms to tell him that, unless those angiograms might also point the way to more beneficial treatment than was possible without them. If nothing useful could be done anyway, why take the risk just to obtain a more elegant and detailed diagnosis?

As Fred Cleveland had pointed out, I had already demonstrated my coronary artery disease quite spectacularly enough when I suffered my heart attack. I didn't need a treadmill test, or angiograms either, to tell me that those arteries were in bad shape. More detailed, possibly dangerous investigations wouldn't make sense unless they might actually be useful in improving treatment or thwarting the inexorable progress of the disease. But today, the truly overriding importance of cardiac catheterization, coronary angiograms, and other investigations lies in the simple fact that they can open the doors to totally new horizons of treatment never before possible without them—treatment that might improve life quality, reduce the crippling effects of the disease, and offer real hope of increasing longevity.

Mason Sones's introduction of cardiac catheterization came at just the right time. By the early 1960s surgeons had the means, with the heart-lung machine, to temporarily reroute the circulation and provide a "dry heart" empty of blood on which to operate. They also knew by then that it was possible to stop the heartbeat deliberately for a brief period of time, thus providing a quiet as well as a bloodless heart, and they had learned how to later restart the heartbeat, with almost complete reliability, by means of electric shock. Now, with cardiac catheterization and coronary angiography possible, surgeons had a way to obtain a literal road map of the entire coronary artery circulation in any given patient, showing where it was obstructed, where it was narrowed, where it was diseased. And with all this available, it suddenly became quite thinkable that a potentially fatal obstruction of those arteries might conceivably be *bypassed* so that the heart could be provided with a fresh, reliable supply of blood *in spite* of the presence of diseased, scarred, or obstructed coronary arteries. For the first time, it became imaginable that *something might actually be done*—some active steps taken—to intervene in the progress of this terrible disease.

Within a very few years such intervention became not only imaginable but achievable. Revolutionary procedures were attempted—and succeeded. And, in a single decade, the whole approach to treatment of coronary artery disease emerged into a new era.

At two in the afternoon, on January 5, I appeared in Fred Cleveland's office for a checkover, prior to the scheduled cardiac catheterization and coronary angiogram that were to be done the following morning. Fred examined me and listened to my complaints, then spent a few minutes in a more or less perfunctory explanation of the procedure I was about to undergo. He said that one of the younger cardiologists on the Mason Clinic staff, Dr. Robin Johnston, would do the cardiac cath and coronary angiograms. He told me that Dr. Johnston had done approximately two thousand such examinations to date, and that, so far, he had had only about 0.15 percent major complications—such things as new myocardial infarctions triggered by the manipulation of the catheters, strokes following the completion of this invasive procedure, and so forth. The mortality rate for these complications—that is, the percentage of patients who actually died as a result of the procedure—was much lower, about one-twentieth of one percent. In short, Fred seemed eager for me to realize that the risk was very small, but there still was a very real risk involved.

That was fine, as far as I was concerned, considering that I had been living for the last three months with the perfectly clear recognition that I might drop dead at any moment from a recurrent myocardial infarction, cardiac arrest, or some other disaster. But Fred's description of what exactly was to be done, and how, was much more sketchy. He may have assumed that I, being a doctor, knew all there was to know about cardiac catheterizations. The truth was that, at that time, I knew very little indeed about the procedure and that I was going ahead with it largely because Fred rather urgently thought that I ought to.

Now, in retrospect, I suspect this is the case with the vast majority of patients facing cardiac catheterization and coronary angiograms: Despite their doctors' attempts at preparation, they really *don't* understand much about the procedure beforehand. And this is unfortunate, because I can think of no other diagnostic procedure in which it is more important that the patient understand exactly what is going on, and exactly how and why the procedure can open the door to a lifetime of effective treatment.

Everybody by now has heard or read about two or three vessel disease or double, triple, or quadruple bypasses. Superficially, these terms seem to be very significant; yet the fact is that none of them means anything at all unless one understands *specifically* what they mean. And for this understanding, you need to know a few brief basic facts about the anatomy of the human heart and the coronary arteries.

Many people don't really understand how the heart works—even what size it is or what the coronary arteries are. We know that the heart lies in the chest, thumping away day and night, but that's not enough. We can learn a great deal about the nature of the heart by means of a very simple illustrative experiment.

Take a medium-size Turkish or terry cloth hand towel and soak it in a basin of water. While it is still in the water, fold it in half once, top to bottom, then again. Next, roll it up from one side to the other and wring it out thoroughly. You will now have a twisted lump of wet Turkish towel more or less the size and shape of your fist.

Now place this lump of wet towel on your chest, with the upper end about midway up your breastbone in the middle and the other end canted slightly downward to the left. You will now have a plausible though inaccurate anatomical model of a normal human heart. It isn't nearly as large as most people imagine. The muscular fibers of this muscular organ are twisted, much the same as the wrung-out towel is twisted, around a central axis that extends from your right shoulder down through the middle of your breastbone and on down through your lower ribs on the left.

The heart muscle tissue that makes up the right ventricle lies twisted around this skewed central axis toward the back of the chest, twisting down against the diaphragm toward the tip of the heart. The part that makes up the left ventricle lies in the front of the chest, twisting down and around to the left side and under. We can see this demonstrated diagramatically in Figure 5 (page 128). What we do not see, of course, is a thick muscular wall inside, separating the right and the left ventricles, twisting up through the middle of the heart—the *interventricular septum.*

The job of the left ventricle is to receive freshly oxygenated blood from the lungs, and to push that blood out with each contraction of the heart into the aorta, thence on to all parts of the body in the arterial flow. To prevent backflow of the blood during relaxation of the heart, the aortic valve lies between the top of the left ventricle and the first part of the aorta. This first part of the aorta just above the aortic valve forms a sort of expanded bulb, an enlarged area known as the *sinus of Valsalva.* Above this bulb the aorta rises up

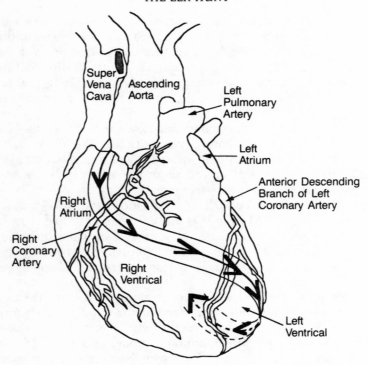

Figure 5   The front surface of the heart, showing how the organ is twisted around a central axis.

and back from the heart in a great arch, giving off arteries to the arms (the subclavian arteries) and to the head and brain (the carotid arteries) before arching back against the backbone and descending into the abdomen. Obviously these arteries to the upper extremities and the brain get an early chance at the highly oxygenated blood the left ventricle is pumping out, but they do not get first grab. First grab of this highly oxygenated blood goes to two arteries that branch directly from the aortic bulb itself, just above the aortic valve: the *right main coronary artery* and the *left main coronary artery*.

At their exit from the bulb of the aorta, each of these arteries is perhaps one-quarter to three-eighths of an inch in diameter, with the left usually slightly larger than the right. Interestingly enough, these arteries and their main branches lie largely on the outer surface of the heart, with smaller branches digging down to feed the heart muscle itself. The right coronary artery goes along the posterior or back-side surface of the heart, feeding branches into the right ventricle. It extends down from the upper right back-side surface to the lower left back-side surface, sending some branches up into the

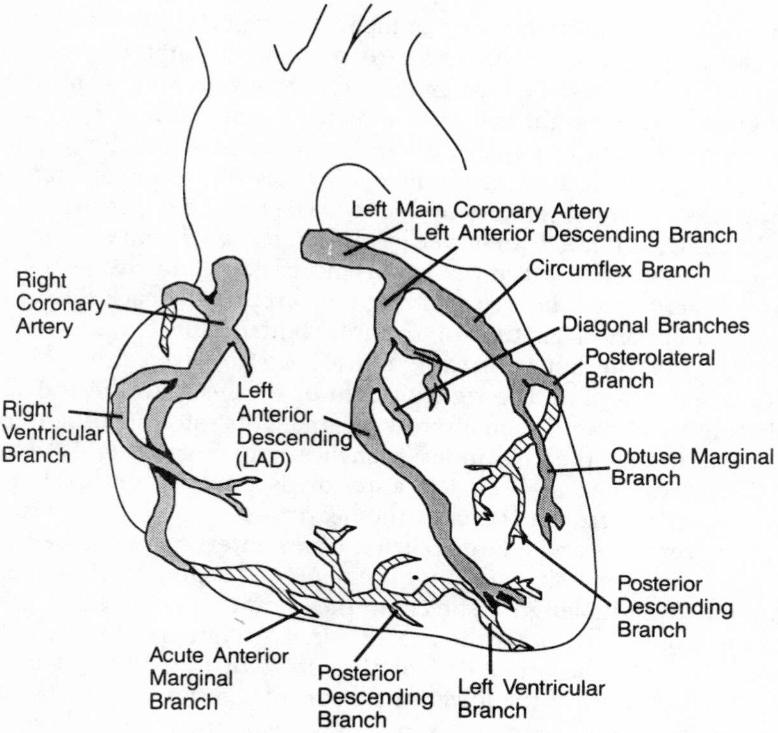

Figure 6 The four major coronary vessels—right coronary, left main coronary, circumflex, and left anterior decending (LAD)—and some of their main branches.

muscular septum between the ventricles and some other small branches around the tip of the heart. (See Figure 6.)

The left main coronary artery remains a major artery only for about an inch or two after taking off from the aortic bulb before it branches into two approximately equal-size main branches: the *left anterior descending artery* and the *circumflex artery.* The left anterior descending artery, or LAD, throwing off branches as it goes, moves down the anterior or front portion of the heart to feed a portion of the left ventricle and send branches down into the septum; the circumflex artery moves around to the left side of the heart in front, feeding the rest of the left ventricle and the upper part of the septum muscle between the two ventricular chambers, as Figure 6 shows.

The main branchings of these two major coronary arteries are simple, straightforward, and easy to understand. Although there is no point remembering every branch, it's important to be oriented to the major branches in order to understand later what bypass surgery is all about. The two main coronary arteries differ from each other in that the right coronary remains a major artery for several inches of its length, while the left does not. As the right coronary curves around the back of the heart, it gives rise to major branches known as the *right ventricular branch* (serving the upper part of the right ventricle), the *acute anterior marginal branch* (curving around under the heart to serve the lower and back side of the ventricle), the *left ventricular branch* (curving *way* around the back side of the heart to supply a portion of the interventricular septum and the lower tip of the left ventricle), and a *posterior descending branch* (going down around the right margin of the heart to the tip). The left coronary artery, soon after its origin, splits into the left anterior descending and the circumflex branches, which go roughly where their names suggest. The left anterior descending, or LAD, goes down over the front portion of the heart to serve one whole half of the left ventricle and a large portion of the interventricular septum, with several good-size *diagonal branches* and *septal branches* splitting off along its length. The circumflex branch, on the other hand, curves around the top of the heart toward the left and down the left side to supply the other half of the left ventricle, the rest of the septum and some of the lower or tip part of the right ventricle. One major branch of the circumflex branch is the *obtuse marginal branch*. Further around, the *posterior lateral branch* and the *posterior descending branch* fork off to disappear into the depths of the heart muscle. We can see these major branches of the two arteries pictured schematically and labeled in Figure 7. This diagram shows the *usual, average* configuration of the two coronary arteries and their major branches for the vast majority of human beings.

This should help clear up some of the terminology that you may have heard or read about. "Single-vessel disease," for example, simply means that there is atherosclerotic narrowing or partial obstruction in just one of the three most important arteries—the right main coronary, the left anterior descending or the circumflex—or one of the major branches of one of these arteries, but that the other major arteries or their branches are unaffected. Obviously, if that single vessel suddenly plugs up the resulting infarction will involve only the part of the heart supplied by the plugged-up artery or branch. "Two-vessel disease" usually means that two of the three most important arteries have obstructive disease in them—often a much more threatening situation to live with than single-vessel disease. "Triple-vessel disease" means that there are significant obstructions in all three of the most important arteries or their major branches.

From in Front and Above

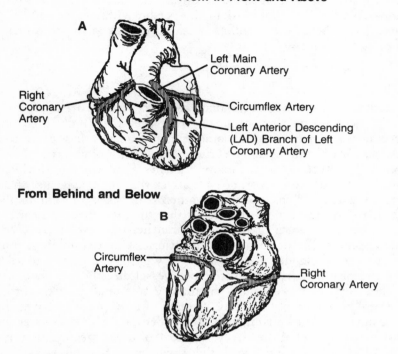

A

Left Main
Coronary Artery

Right
Coronary
Artery

Circumflex Artery

Left Anterior Descending
(LAD) Branch of Left
Coronary Artery

From Behind and Below

B

Circumflex
Artery

Right
Coronary Artery

Figure 7   The major coronary arteries.

With "quadruple-vessel disease," all three of the major vessels are involved as well as a major branch of one of those arteries.

What do these terms actually mean in terms of life and death? The fact that one person may have triple-vessel disease does not *necessarily* mean that he or she is going to suffer more disastrous trouble from a myocardial infarction than a person with single-vessel disease. The person with triple-vessel disease might go along for years without the catastrophe of a total obstruction in any one of those three vessels, while the person with single-vessel disease might have that one vessel obstruct completely tomorrow and drop dead. But doctors have learned that the number of vessels involved is, at least statistically, a determinant of mortality rate among these patients, ranging from 2 to 3 percent mortality per year for those with single-vessel disease, to 5 percent per year for patients with two-vessel disease, to 7 to 9 percent per year for those with triple-vessel disease. In addition, severe obstruction of the left main coronary artery alone carries an even higher mortality risk of about 12 percent yearly. And certainly the person with triple-vessel disease has a greater amount of total available cardiac circulation impaired—and vulnerable to catastrophe—than the person with single-vessel disease. To see what this signifies, we need to look at those coronary arteries in a bit more detail.

The Size and Shape of the Arteries

Although the right and left main coronary arteries are fairly good size vessels where they originate from the aortic bulb, each one becomes smaller in interior diameter as it branches, first down to a quarter inch interior diameter, then to an eighth of an inch, then a sixteenth, and so on, as the many branches disappear into the heart muscle. But atherosclerosis doesn't attack the whole length of these arteries evenly. Typically, when atherosclerosis is present in the coronary arteries, it tends to affect either the main arteries near the outlet from the aorta or the larger branches of these arteries; the smaller, more distant portions of the arteries tend to remain in good shape. The whole idea of coronary artery bypass surgery is to graft one end of a healthy substitute blood vessel directly into the aorta at the "top" of the coronary circulatory tree, and graft the other end into a smaller, still healthy segment of a coronary artery at the "bottom" end, thus forming a bridge or detour—a bypass—over the obstructed portion of the artery. The skill of the surgeons doing this kind of bypass grafting is such that they can graft the lower end of the bypass vessel into a coronary artery branch as small as one millimeter in inside diameter—a vessel slightly less than one-sixteenth inch in diameter.

Each major branch of each coronary artery supplies blood to a relatively small segment of the heart. It is that segment that suffers from blood hunger, ischemia, when the particular branch supplying it has become narrowed or partially obstructed by atherosclerosis. Of course, if the obstructive lesion involves either the right or left main coronary, then all the segments supplied by all the branches of the affected coronary artery will suffer impaired circulation, but atherosclerosis tends to be spotty rather than evenly distributed, blocking this branch artery here, that branch artery there. This means that one segment of heart muscle may have very poor circulation because of narrowing of its coronary artery branch, while the next segment may have perfectly fine circulation because there is no obstruction in the branch artery serving it. In short, there can be extreme individual variation in the degree and location of coronary artery disease from one person to the next, and some means is necessary to pinpoint *exactly* where each and every identifiable atherosclerotic constriction is located.

The Critical Collaterals

When we speak of a branch of one coronary artery supplying blood to one segment of the heart, and a branch of the other coronary supplying an adjacent segment of the heart, it sounds as if there were some kind of a stonewall barrier between the two—that what one coronary artery touches the other does not, and vice versa. If this were really entirely true, it would be bad news indeed for the person who suffers complete obstruction of a coronary artery branch, because it would mean permanent destruction, complete and total, of the segment of heart muscle that that branch supplied. Fortunately, nature in fact has been a little more generous than that in arranging the blood supply for such a vital organ as the human heart. There are actually many areas of the heart in which a segment of myocardium receives its blood flow from two different sources: the main supply coming from one coronary artery branch, but *some* portion coming either from another branch of the same coronary artery, or from a branch of the other coronary artery. Thus, even if a myocardial infarction cuts off the *main* blood supply to a large segment of heart, there may still be at least a trickle of blood still being supplied by another, unobstructed artery—and that trickle can mean the difference between life and death.

This kind of double blood supply to a vital area is known to doctors as *collateral* or "side by side" circulation. There is probably no place in the body where it can play a more important role in preserving life than in the case of the heart muscle. What's more, in a seemingly miraculous way, the sudden reduction of blood flow to an area from one source of blood, and the ischemia that results can actually stimulate growth and enlargement of small vessels from the other or collateral source. In practical terms, this means that if a victim of coronary artery disease can survive the catastrophic insult of an infarction, and if part of the heart muscle in the damaged area can manage to stay alive long enough, its blood supply may improve presently and the damaged area be strengthened with the passage of time. In the sketches in Figure 8 (page 134) we can see a schematic diagram of how two kinds of collateral circulation work—collateral circulation supplied by two branches of the same coronary artery to the same segment of muscle, and collateral circulation supplied by branches of two separate coronary arteries to the same segment of heart muscle.

Obviously, collateral circulation to the same area from two different arteries altogether is a better state of affairs than collateral supplied by two branches of the same artery, if the obstruction of the artery occurs above the point where the branches fork. It's this

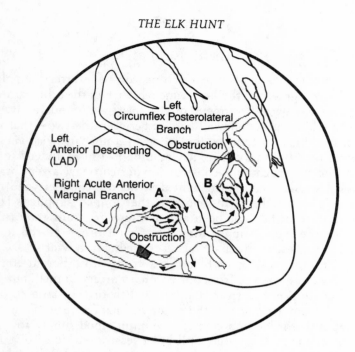

Figure 8 Collateral circulation (A) supplied by two branches of the same coronary artery to the same segment of muscle, and (B) supplied by two separate coronary arteries to the same segment of muscle.

arrangement of collateral circulation that helps explain how a person can suffer a severe myocardial infarction due to complete obstruction of a whole main coronary artery and still manage to stay alive through the crisis, with a heart still functioning well enough at least to maintain life. As we will see later, it is also extremely important when a surgeon is attempting to supply additional healthy blood flow to the injured area by means of a bypass graft.

The Artistry of Coronary Angiography

Of course, these details of the anatomy of the heart and the coronary arteries had been known to physicians for a long time. There simply hadn't been any practical use for this knowledge as the death rate from coronary artery disease continued expanding. It's easy to understand, therefore, why cardiologists were so excited when cardiac catheterization and coronary artery angiography proved to be possible. Here at last was a way to identify individual coronary artery lesions and pinpoint their exact location in individual living patients—a way, in fact, to produce specific, detailed maps of the disease with an almost unbelievable degree of accuracy and detail.

The ability to produce good, readable angiograms of the coronary arteries depended not only on skillful catheterization but also upon highly refined X-ray techniques. First, it was necessary to introduce a contrast agent into each main coronary artery by means of the cardiac catheter. An *ideal* contrast agent would be something like metallic lead, which is so extremely dense that X rays literally cannot penetrate it at all, but obviously molten lead would be tough on the coronary arteries. Today, there are a number of safe and effective liquid contrast agents suitable for injection into a patient's bloodstream—colorless liquids or syruplike agents that contain quantities of iodine, an element that has a high atomic number and a dense nucleus, and, therefore, when concentrated in an area, will stop X rays and show up on X-ray plates as a shadow of the inside of the blood vessel. The iodine atoms are bound to organic compounds and are simply carried along in the bloodstream and rapidly cleared out of the body through the kidneys into the urine without allowing the iodine to react with or damage any of the body's cells.

The technique of taking a coronary angiogram is simple and straightforward. The catheter is inserted either through an opening in an artery in the arm or the femoral artery in the groin and advanced against the arterial blood flow to the bulb of the aorta. The progress of the catheter is followed by direct visualization through an *X-ray image intensifier*. This is an electronic fluoroscope that produces an image three thousand times brighter than an ordinary X-ray fluoroscope, thus allowing safe, low levels of X ray to be used. Once the catheter reaches the aortic bulb, its tip is maneuvered into the opening of a coronary artery. Then a small amount—perhaps 6 or 7 ccs—of the contrast agent is injected through the catheter into the mouth of the artery and swept along with the blood flowing down the artery. Immediately, a cine–X-ray camera prefocused on the area is started. This is essentially a 35-mm movie camera that takes rapid-fire X-ray pictures through the image intensifier at a rate of about thirty exposures per second during the time that the contrast agent is coursing down the coronary artery, down all its branches, and eventually disappearing into the fine capillary bed that permeates the heart muscle.

Either the camera, the patient, or both may be tilted from one side to another so that repeat injections of the contrast agent can be cine–X-ray photographed from different angles. The cine–X rays that have been taken are then processed into a motion picture film, which can be projected onto a screen for study by the cardiologist— literally, movies that show the contrast agent concentrated in the coronary arteries and their branches. Particularly revealing single frames can be stopped during the course of projection for more detailed examination or reproduced as permanent X-ray plates.

These moving-picture X rays reveal to the cardiologist precisely where the coronary artery narrowing or obstruction is located—in which segments of which branches of which arteries. When the artery or branch of the artery is perfectly normal, without any atherosclerotic change, the flow of the contrast agent through the artery is seen as perfectly free, evidence of a smooth interior artery lining. Where early atherosclerotic changes are present, the angiogram of that artery area will show characteristic scalloping at the outer margins of the image of the vessel but no clear evidence of narrowing or obstruction yet. On the other hand, if a main coronary artery or one of its branches is completely obstructed by atherosclerosis, the shadow image of the contrast agent will simply stop at that point, showing no flow through the vessel at all. Between these extremes, progressive narrowing of a segment of artery due to atherosclerosis, wherever it may occur, will show a localized narrowing of the image of the flowing blood mixed with the contrast agent at that area.

By careful examination of these pictures, the cardiologist can make an accurate estimate of *what percentage of obstruction* or *what percentage of limitation of flow* is observed through what length of a segment of artery or branch.

In a way, coronary angiograms are simple to read. If a coronary artery has a gross obstruction in some area, any untrained layman can see it there on the X ray, once it is pointed out to him, and would agree that, yes, that little ribbon of shadow does indeed seem to be pinched down to a very narrow point at that one place. This, however, is not good enough for the cardiologist or the coronary bypass surgeon. A general impression won't do; rather, the angiogram requires an extremely careful, detailed, precise reading, and this is very difficult. It requires the skill acquired from reading thousands of such moving-picture X-ray tapes, and much experience, to interpret what appears on them. The cardiologist must be able to describe *exactly* what lesions exist, *exactly* where, in *exactly* what vessel or branch vessel. What is more, he must be able to describe the lesion that he sees in *precisely the same terms* that another cardiologist reading a similar angiogram would use to describe a similar lesion in another patient.

Location of the lesion and *degree of obstruction* of the vessel are the two critical sticking points. It wouldn't help much, for example, for one cardiologist to say, "Well, I think that lesion is reducing the flow by 30 percent in that vessel," and then have another doctor saying, "Oh, no, I think it's constricting the flow 60 percent." Who then would be right? What difference would it make?

These problems were resolved when cardiologists throughout the world generally agreed upon a series of conventions to guide them in interpreting and reporting findings on coronary angiograms. First, to indicate the location of lesions seen in coronary arteries on angiograms, the right coronary artery is divided into three segments— an upper segment, a middle segment, and a lower one, defined according to where major branches take off from the main artery. The left main coronary artery, which is usually very short, is regarded as a segment by itself. The left anterior descending branch of the left coronary artery and the circumflex branch of the left coronary are each divided into three segments—an upper, a middle, and a lower segment. Thus, by convention, a cardiologist can describe the location of a lesion in any of ten segments of the left and right coronary artery tree in the same terms that any other cardiologist would describe the same lesion, so that any cardiologist reading the report will understand precisely where in that coronary artery circulation the lesion is located.

The severity of the lesions is also recorded according to a convention. Cardiologists realized that it might not make much sense or difference whether an artery segment was blocked 30 percent or 35 percent. Measurements that fine might not be possible with any accuracy. But it was possible to recognize an area of an artery that was blocked 25 percent, or 50 percent, even 75 percent, simply by observing the amount of narrowing seen on the angiogram of a segment of artery. Similarly, it was possible to tell when an artery was 100 percent blocked, since no blood flowed through at all. Finally, between the 75 percent figure, where the opening through the artery is reduced to one-fourth of its former width, and the total 100 percent obstruction, either one of two purely arbitrary figures may apply. If the vessel appears more than 75 percent obstructed yet still allows some blood to flow through, that segment is reported as 90 percent blocked. In an extreme case, in which the vessel appears to be almost totally blocked and yet a tiny thread of contrast agent can be seen passing through to the other side, that vessel is said to be "99 percent blocked." The figure is in quotes simply because there is no practical way to tell whether it is 97 percent, 94 percent, or 98 percent blocked, so by convention 99 percent simply means almost completely closed but with a trickle of blood still going through.

Judging lesions according to such conventions has a very important practical purpose. If a segment of a coronary artery is only 25 percent obstructed, that observation tells the cardiologist that, unmistakably, the patient has coronary artery disease in that segment of the artery, but, in fact, such a small degree of obstruction doesn't make any difference *at the moment* to the function of that person's heart. The myocardium supplied by that slightly obstructed vessel is still getting enough blood and enough oxygen so that there is probably no ischemia, no damage to muscle cells, no angina involved. In fact, hemodynamic studies of the actual effect of restricted blood flow through the arteries have demonstrated that there is usually no serious functional effect on the health and activity of heart muscle until the segment of coronary artery supplying that muscle is observed to be obstructed by 70 percent or more.

In other words, if a patient has a less than 70 percent obstruction in the coronary artery, the artery is certainly diseased—a bad sign for long-term prognosis—but the patient is not likely to be suffering from any ill effects of the disease *right now*. It is only at the point of about 70 percent obstruction of a vessel, for example, that a patient might begin to suffer mild ischemia in the affected segment of the heart and possibly suffer mild angina on extreme exertion. Under normal nonexertional circumstances there probably wouldn't be any functional evidence of the disease at all. Another way to say this is that the person with up to 70 percent obstruction of a coronary artery appears to be in still reasonably good shape. It is just in the future that he or she is going to be running into trouble.

The difference between 70 and 75 percent obstruction of a coronary artery or branch, however, can be profound. With 75 percent, the myocardium supplied by that artery is in trouble. Perhaps under resting conditions it is getting enough blood supply and enough oxygen to limp along without impairment. But in the presence of physical exercise, tension, emotional stress, anger, or other conditions, the heart muscle becomes ischemic, and in the face of prolonged exercise that ischemia may well lead to the appearance of angina. A cardiologist would say that that segment of myocardium was *functionally impaired* part of the time. If the obstruction were as much as 90 percent, that functional impairment would be enormously magnified, and constant. Now, even mild degrees of exercise or the adrenergic effects of the emotions or tension would bring on severe angina. What's more, with 75 percent or more obstruction, the risk of a blood clot forming in the narrowed lumen of the artery, especially if the interior wall of that artery is roughened and ragged on account of the atherosclerosis, is greatly increased, so that the patient is far more vulnerable to a coronary occlusion and myocardial infarction, and with 90 percent obstruction the patient is literally a sitting duck for a catastrophic MI. Just a little bit of debris peeling off from an atherosclerotic plaque in the remaining 10 percent lumen, with a little bit of accompanying clotting, could block that artery completely.

We can see how these kinds of lesions can lead to exertional angina warnings of trouble. But we can also see how they can help to explain some of the vagaries of variant or resting angina as well. Remember that we are talking about living tissue in these damaged coronary arteries themselves, with a dynamic process going on and with constant efforts of the body to heal the damage at the same time that further damage is occurring. It is easy to see that such a diseased area of artery might be, in effect, "sore as a boil": If it carried any pain nerve endings and was constantly irritated, spasm of the muscular wall of healthier artery on either side of the irritation might well occur. We know now from angiographic movies that this kind of spasm can indeed cause almost complete obstruction of an otherwise apparently healthy artery for minutes, even hours at a time, until the spasm relaxes and allows blood to flow through again, and that this can occur without any exercise at all.

Reading and interpreting coronary angiograms with the use of the conventions we have described can provide a precise road map of the location and extent of coronary artery disease. This kind of diagnostic information can be invaluable in selecting the optimum form of treatment for any given patient. Twenty-five years ago, without the benefit of cardiac catheterization and coronary angiography, the cardiologist treating a patient with coronary artery disease was virtually flying blind. But today, such blind flying is not only unnecessary, it's downright reckless; now, if need be, a road map can be derived for each patient and a truly rational treatment plan becomes possible.

When I saw Fred Cleveland in his office that Monday afternoon, the day before my coronary angiograms were scheduled to be done, he did not take the time for the kind of anatomy lesson we have just outlined. It's my hope that this book will help fill in some of the holes.* Fred did briefly outline the risks of serious complications or mortality. In addition, he took time to make clear one very important point: that we were embarking on a diagnostic investigation

---

* In all fairness, it probably isn't reasonable to expect *any* doctor to prepare an individual patient for cardiac catheterization and coronary angiograms with this kind of anatomy lesson in the midst of a busy office schedule, particularly if the patient has no medical background. Yet I think this kind of information in some depth is vital to the patient for any real understanding of what is going on, especially the need and value of such diagnostic studies and their immense importance in future planning. If this information isn't available from the doctor on an individual-patient basis, it needs to be available in some form that is easily accessible and understandable to the patient—which, of course, is why I'm writing this book.

and nothing else. "This is just one of several diagnostic studies I want to do to help define where we stand with regard to your illness," he said. "And it's just that—a diagnostic study. It's not just some kind of formality we have to go through to set you up for a bypass operation, for example. Right now, nobody knows whether you are a candidate for a bypass operation or not, least of all me. We need to know what options we have for treating you in the future, so that we can then give you some kind of sane and reasonable advice as to which options we think you ought to choose. These angiograms will help us identify, locate and assess the severity of any obstructive atherosclerotic lesions present within the arteries of your heart. Other studies will help us assess how adequately your heart is functioning now, in light of the severe myocardial infarction you've already had. So maybe all this will tell us whether you're a candidate for bypass surgery or not, but that's not the purpose of tests. The purpose is to gain knowledge that will help manage this illness the best possible way for you, surgery or no surgery."

Before I left that afternoon, Fred took me down to introduce me to Robin Johnston, a short, bouncy man in his late forties with thinning brown hair and hornrim glasses. Dr. Johnston told me the plan of attack. I should continue the medicines I was taking on schedule, have a light dinner that evening, and take nothing by mouth, not even a morning cup of coffee, after midnight, except for a swallow of water to take my morning pills. I was to appear at the short-stay surgery department at Virginia Mason Hospital at seven o'clock in the morning, where I would be admitted and prepared, and the catheterization would be done some time between eight and nine. He would want me to remain in the hospital throughout the rest of that day and night, discharging me the following morning if everything was fine. He, too, read me the litany of possible complications, emphasizing that although they were uncommon, they did indeed sometimes happen, and that when they did it was generally an event that nobody could help. He also provided me with an informed-consent form for the procedure for me to sign. This form seemed to suggest that probably everybody had disastrous complications and that by signing it you were throwing yourself on the mercy of the gods with no recourse. Never mind that this didn't exactly jibe with what the doctor had actually told me; this is what informed-consent forms are for—to protect the doctor and hospital in case of any untoward happenstance—but I signed the form without a second thought. After all, I figured, if God had wanted me, he had missed a perfectly good opportunity to take me two months ago, and I was probably in as good hands with these doctors and this institution as I was ever going to be anywhere. At least there was not going to be any danger of complication from general anesthesia, I reflected, because, as I was somewhat startled to learn, no general anesthesia would be used. I would have some mild sedation upon admission to the hospital, and a local anesthetic would be used to place the catheter, but they wanted the patient to be wide awake, alert, and communicating with them during the course of the catheterization.

Ann and I went back to the Busbys' apartment that night, ate dinner in, and retired early. I didn't sleep particularly well, with some angina waking me up about two A.M. I remember wondering which branch of which artery was causing it—and then couldn't get back to sleep after it eased up. Of course I was nervous about the upcoming procedure—not nervous so much about the procedure itself as nervous about what the angiograms would reveal. It occurred to me that pinpoint diagnosis was all very well, but we might not be all that happy about what these studies might tell us. Except for the angina and the arrhythmia, and a few things like that, it seemed to me that I'd been doing reasonably well during the two months since the heart attack, just beginning to feel somewhat like my normal self again, and I was not particularly eager to find out that I wasn't doing as well as I thought. When ignorance is bliss, 'tis folly to be wise and all that.

We got up early, I ate my morning pills for breakfast and Ann whisked me over to Virginia Mason Hospital, arriving just before seven. It was a gray, windy, rainy morning—a good day, I thought, not to have to do anything vigorous. Ann stayed at the admitting desk of the short-stay surgery section to fill out the admitting information while I was trundled on a wheeled cart into a preparation room full of bright lights. The nurse brought me three little yellow Valium pills to take—mother's little helpers, she called them—and then started the inevitable IV going into my wrist. A young male orderly came by and shaved my groin on both the right and left sides, "so that they can have a choice of femoral artery in case one doesn't work as well as the other." I dozed off then for a while, until a couple of people in caps and masks were wheeling me into some other place and telling me to look alive, now.

My overall impression of the catheterization procedure and the angiograms was how absolutely simple the whole thing was—how swift and efficient, and how totally painless. Robin Johnston was in the cath room in surgical cap, mask, and gown, peering down at me from the overhead lights and sounding extremely cheerful. I was shifted over onto the table used for the cath and straps were placed over my shoulders, belly, and hips, "so you won't slide off when we tilt the table under you." Somebody poked for a minute at my right groin—"just a little Novocaine here now"—and there was a little pressure in that region, then, quite suddenly, Dr. Johnston told me everything was fine, the catheter was in my aorta. He told me I would feel a strange flushing feeling from the contrast agent when it was injected, and that I might feel a little angina at this time, too, since the contrast agent, unlike blood, didn't carry any oxygen with it as it passed through the myocardium. He also told me that if he were to instruct me to cough at any time, I should cough hard and immediately. I felt the flushing from the contrast agent three or four times, held my breath when they told me to, felt the table being tilted with me on it for different X-ray angles, and felt two or three brief twinges of angina, but I was never asked to cough.

Then, in what seemed an incredibly brief time, I was back on the wheeled cart again. Dr. Johnston confirmed that the catheter was already out and a nurse at the lower end of me was pressing on my groin for dear life, to prevent bleeding from the catheter insertion site, as she walked along beside the cart as it was wheeled into the recovery room. The whole procedure had taken about twenty-five minutes; it had seemed to me like about ten. The nurse kept hand pressure on the place in my groin where the catheter had gone in for twenty minutes by the clock and then put a pressure dressing on. I was instructed to stay flat on my back until the following morning so as not to stimulate any bleeding from the puncture wound in the artery. (This led to the only "complication" I suffered from the procedure, namely that I was too nervous and tense to relax my sphincter and empty my bladder. Considering that about a quart and a half of glucose water had been dumped into me by IV since I first turned up in the hospital, I was filling up fast. Ultimately, I had to be catheterized and relieved of 2200 ccs of urine, and later I talked the house staff into letting me stand at the side of the bed in order to urinate that evening.)

Dr. Johnston made perfunctory evening rounds—no, he didn't have the report on the angiograms yet, but Fred Cleveland would report in the morning. He mostly seemed concerned that I not do something to start bleeding from the catheter puncture site. Ann stayed around after supper to watch a TV show with me, then went back to the apartment, and I got a good night's sleep.

When Fred turned up next morning for rounds, he didn't seem to be in any hurry to report anything until I prodded him. "Well, the picture is not all good and it's not all bad," he said finally. "On a first look at the films, it appears clear that your right coronary artery is completely occluded—nothing is going through it at all—so that's why you don't have much right ventricle left, to speak of.

The left anterior descending artery is about 40 to 50 percent occluded, which isn't too bad. But your circumflex artery is 90 percent blocked off, and it happens to be an unusually small artery as well. All this helps explain why you're having angina—and why your left ventricle is not doing as good a job as we would like."

"That complete blockage of the right artery," I said, "is that something that could be bypassed?"

"Bypassed to what? It wouldn't do any good to perfuse blood into dead myocardium, or into scar tissue. But we're not ready to tackle the question of whether *anything* should be bypassed just yet. You have not only lost your right ventricle; there's evidence that your left ventricle is also impaired, and we need to find out how much. I'll want you back here at the clinic in a week to go through a very cautious treadmill test, together with some radioactive tracer studies of the heart that will give us a much clearer picture of what we can expect your left ventricle to do under the best of circumstances. Then, the whole picture goes to the cardiac conference for review— the angiograms, the treadmill test, the radionuclide studies, and all— and after that we will see what looks best for you for the long pull."

That still didn't explain to me how I could be doing as well as I seemed to be if most of my right ventricle was knocked out. Later, Robin Johnston put the picture in somewhat different words. "The right ventricle is badly damaged by the MI, but it's the left ventricle we're worried about. The right coronary artery supplies not only all of the right ventricle but a significant portion of the under surface and septum of the left ventricle as well. We know that the right ventricle only has to pump blood against fairly low pressure; it can take a tremendous amount of damage before pumping efficiency drops. The importance of a person's coronary artery disease is almost exclusively a matter of how much the *left* ventricle is impaired. The left ventricle has to pump blood against high pressure, and the loss of 40 percent of the left ventricle myocardium, whether all at once or a little at a time over a decade or more, will be fatal. Another way to put that is to say that you can't withdraw more than 40 percent from the left ventricular myocardial bank, because when you do, you've bought the farm."

More investigations, without any answers yet that I could see. The treadmill test, performed in the cardiology lab at the Mason Clinic one morning a week later, turned out to be more of a trial— and an eye-opener—than I had anticipated. Fred had decided against a treadmill test shortly after I got out of the hospital for very sensible reasons: We didn't need the test to diagnose that I had coronary artery disease, because I had already demonstrated that I did, to everyone's satisfaction. But now, two months and two weeks later, the test was necessary for different reasons. I had survived the catastrophe of a severe myocardial infarction that had caused permanent damage to a large section of my heart, particularly the right ventricle. Essentially, the left ventricle had been doing the right ventricle's work as well as its own since the time of the MI. I had undergone a two-and-a-half-month period of recovery and healing, and it was necessary now to know how effectively the left ventricle was performing its double work.

There were two good ways to pinpoint precisely how well that left ventricle was doing, and those two studies were done in combination: a treadmill test and a radioactive thalium uptake study. Both these studies had to do with the measurement of something known as the *left ventricular ejection fraction*, a term that had always puzzled me before but now began to take on some semblance of meaning. In essence, the concept was simple enough: In order to move oxygenated blood through the arteries of the body, the left ventricle has to contract and eject the blood into the aorta with sufficient enough force to keep it moving until the next contraction comes along. The left ventricular ejection fraction is a measurement of how well and efficiently the left ventricle is doing that job. It tells what percentage of blood in the ventricle is ejected with each heartbeat. A normal ejection fraction is 50 to 75 percent. An ejection fraction of 30 to 50 percent shows significant impairment of left ventricular function, and below 30 percent indicates very poor left ventricular function, with a poor prognosis for continued survival.

Thus, this figure is more than just an interesting number; it has real prognostic value, predicting at least roughly what a patient's heart is likely to be capable of doing—or not doing—in the future. A person recovering from a severe myocardial infarction with a measured ejection fraction of 60 percent, for example, would be far more likely to enjoy a long period of uncomplicated recovery than a person with a similar sort of injury who has an ejection fraction of just 35 percent. The ejection fraction is also extremely useful in studies of the effectiveness of new drugs or new procedures, because it enables the doctor to place similar patients in similar test groups, so that he can be reasonably sure that a given study is really comparing apples with apples, not apples with pumpkins. And, in particular, the ejection fraction is a helpful predictor of how well a given patient is likely to tolerate some extreme procedure such as coronary artery bypass surgery. A patient with a high ejection fraction, for instance, may be far more likely to tolerate such surgery well, with less risk of complications or death, than the person with a low ejection fraction. And this was where my treadmill testing and radionuclide uptake studies came in.

I was as "up" for these tests as I could be on the day I came in to have them run. I wanted to put on as good a showing as possible. For one thing, I hoped to learn how well I was really doing at that point. Would I run smack into the angina wall the minute I began a high-exertion test on the treadmill, in spite of all the medicine I was taking? Fred told me not to worry about this, just take all the medicine I had been taking on my usual schedule and come in for the test. He said he was not the slightest bit interested in putting me to Herculean labors and having me drop dead on the treadmill; he simply wanted to get my left ventricle working to the highest comfortable capacity it could, and then inject a radioactive tracer substance, some thalium 201, into my vein at the peak of performance. The thalium would then, in the first five minutes or so, be taken up to the fullest degree possible by the healthy heart muscle cells in my myocardium. I would next be laid out on a table in the Radiomedicine department at the Mason Clinic, and a gamma camera—a sort of high-tech Geiger counter—would pick up the radioactivity from those heart muscle cells and would create a computer image showing what parts of my myocardium had taken up the thalium (and were, therefore, presumably healthy) and what parts hadn't (and, therefore, presumably represented either ischemic or dead myocardium). In the course of this procedure, other computerized measurements would also be made to help determine what parts of my heart were working well and what parts were not.

Fred was not on hand in the cardiology lab when I arrived for the test, but another cardiologist was. A nurse and an EKG technician acquainted me with the treadmill machine and how it worked: a motorized strip of rubber-coated "moving sidewalk" with handrails on either side, with a variable speed switch, and a mechanism that could tilt it up from a flat position through various degrees of incline to a maximum of about 20 percent grade. After being hooked up to EKG leads and a blood pressure monitor, the patient starts walking on the level at moderate speed for a minute, then continues at a 10 percent grade and a slightly increased speed for three minutes, then a 12 percent grade and a still faster speed for another three minutes and so forth. The treadmill test is continued to the point of maximal performance or exhaustion, but the doctor may stop it earlier for dangerous arrhythmia or a falling blood pressure.

As I went on a brief test run to get the feel of the machine, a young doctor from the Radiomedicine Lab came in with a small syringe containing the radioactive thalium, all ready to go. This stuff has a very short half-life, something like seventy-two hours, and has to be manufactured and calibrated to order for each patient in some laboratory in Massachusetts and then flown to SeaTac Airport in Seattle and brought to the Mason Clinic by special courier the morning of the test—one of the reasons that this particular diagnostic study costs something like $450 to perform. Presently, then, with everybody assembled, they punched the time clock and started me walking on the treadmill.

I didn't do terribly well. There was no problem with angina, but I began to get short of breath on the first tilt during the second minute, and then even more short of breath on the second tilt during the third minute. It was much harder work keeping up with that treadmill walkway than I had imagined; my pulse rate was held down by the Inderal, but it did work its way up to 80 or 90 beats per minute. There seemed to be no particular ominous change on the electrocardiogram, but somewhere toward the end of the third minute, my blood pressure began to fall rather precipitously instead of continually rising (which is normal), and the supervising doctor said, "Okay, that's enough." The man from Radiomedicine injected the radioctive thalium, and they kept me walking for another thirty seconds. Then they disconnected the EKG and blood pressure monitors, planted me in a wheelchair and wheeled me out to an elevator they had been holding throughout the treadmill test, and whisked me one flight down to a table under the gamma camera.

I then spent what seemed like hours lying under this enormous toy and watching a video display tube as a succession of radioactive "pictures" were taken, run through the computer, and reflected as little pinpoints of light on the screen. Two or three radioactive doctors and technicians kept hustling in and out, muttering this and that, and since I didn't understand either what I saw on the screen or what they were saying, the whole thing was pretty much of a bore. Fred Cleveland stuck his head in the door at one point, and somebody asked him if he wanted them to do a cold-pressor test (in which a patient's whole forearm is dipped suddenly into ice water and kept there for five minutes, an extremely stressing situation) and Fred said, "No, not with his blood pressure acting like that, I don't. Let's just skip that," and wandered off.

Finally, somebody came in and said the test was over, and I could get dressed and go on home. I was to call Fred's office in the morning for further instructions. They didn't tell me if I was supposed to glow in the dark or not, but I made a mental note to check on that if I woke up during the night.

When I called Fred Tuesday morning he said that he thought they had all the information they needed. My case would be presented that morning to the cardiac conference, and, no, I wasn't invited. He wanted to see me in his office the following Monday afternoon for reports and planning, and, no, he didn't have any preview to offer me, so I was just going to have to mark time a little longer. I gathered that the cardiac conference met once a week and reviewed all the patients who had been "worked up" since the last meeting. The conference was composed of all the Mason Clinic cardiologists, other cardiologists who admitted patients to Virginia Mason Hospital, the cardiac surgeons associated with Virginia Mason, and any others who chose to come, as well as any other doctors in the city with special interest in cardiac problems. The idea was to gather a consensus about how each individual patient might best be treated, whether with bypass surgery, a purely medical regimen, or whatever else might be available. These meetings were also an educationally broadening experience for doctors caring for patients with coronary artery disease, since they had the opportunity to share opinions with other experts on a wide variety of cases, whether their own personal patients or somebody else's.

By the next Monday morning, when we drove over to Seattle again, I had had enough of waiting and delay. I was now more than ready for some kind of answers. I remarked to Ann that no one could claim that I was being rushed into any kind of precipitous decision, and that maybe it was just as well that I was not gasping my last breath.

Fred didn't examine me that day. He merely sat me down opposite his desk, with Ann sitting next to me, and leaned back in his chair to review where things stood. The angiograms had shown that the right main coronary artery was totally obliterated. That meant that most of the right ventricle was permanently gone. There was nothing to be done to correct that, Fred said, "unless, of course, that ventricle wall gets very weak and thin and begins to balloon out to form an aneurysm. We don't see any evidence of that happening at this point, but it's something that could happen, and if it does, the surgeons can go in and remove that wedge of weak scar so that it doesn't blow out on you. That's something you would just have to face when the time comes, if it ever comes."

As for the other arteries, the left anterior descending artery was about 50 percent occluded, and the circumflex artery 90 percent. In addition, it was a very small artery, so I was depending largely on the left anterior descending artery to supply the left ventricle and the interventricular septum, and the left ventricle was doing most of the work of the right ventricle as well.

As for my current left ventricular function, Fred sighed. "It isn't

147

as bad as I was afraid it might be, but it isn't nearly as good as I'd hoped. You have a left ventricular ejection fraction of around 46 percent. That may improve with time, as healing proceeds, but it may not improve all that much."

"So what does this all boil down to?"

He looked distressed. "It boils down to a group of facts we can't get around." he said unhappily. "You suffered a terrible injury, and nothing will ever reverse that. You've recovered nicely from the insult, but you haven't recovered as much as you may feel you have. In addition, the plain anatomy of your coronary arteries, or what's left of them, is not particularly promising, from a surgeon's point of view, especially considering that small circumflex artery. Any attempt to bypass your coronary lesions with grafts would be technically quite difficult for the surgeons. What's more, your left ventricle is impaired a lot more than the surgeons would like. You would be a high-risk patient for surgery. On the other hand, we know you're getting along reasonably well with medical treatment alone, doing a good job of healing whatever can be healed, maybe building some collaterals that could help later on. And your prospects with medical treatment aren't all that bad. These new Swedish studies that have just come in indicate that the beta-blockers you're currently taking do more than just control angina; they have a positive protective effect, actively reducing the likelihood of a recurrent myocardial infarction. And there are new drugs on the horizon—the calcium slow-channel blockers, for example, that the FDA may be approving in a year or two—"

"So come to the point," I said.

"The point is that the cardiac conference does not believe that you are a good candidate for bypass surgery," Fred said. I was startled at the anger and disappointment that I seemed to hear in his voice. "The consensus was that we should proceed with the medical treatment we've already started, and see what you can do to reduce the risk factors on a daily living basis. I don't entirely agree with that recommendation, but I think we have to be guided by it for now. Our surgeons think you would run far too high a surgical risk to justify the possible benefit from bypass surgery. I may not entirely agree with that, either, but I'm not going to try to cram you down their throats. Of course, there are other institutions in town, and other surgeons. I daresay that you could find some surgeon in this city to do a bypass on you without having to look too hard."

Yes, we all knew that there were surgeons around who would attempt a bypass operation on any man or woman who was still breathing and wanted one done. But I knew, and Fred knew, too, that I was not going to see one of those surgeons. I was going to do exactly what Fred recommended I do. Yet the fact that I wasn't even being offered a choice, that I simply was not considered a candidate for surgical treatment, came as far more of a blow to me than I ever would have imagined. It seemed to me that a whole area of option and decision making had suddenly vanished, that whereas before there had been some prospect that something active and corrective might be done, it now seemed we were going to be confined to the narrow limits of what we were already doing, imperfect as it obviously was. Without even realizing it, I had been hoping desperately that some real alternatives might exist to be weighed and then accepted or rejected. Now Fred was saying that there weren't any alternatives, and this, to my surprise, came as a severe and unexpected disappointment.

I must have said something to that effect to Fred as I rose to leave, although I don't remember exactly what I said. I couldn't have looked very happy, because I suddenly didn't feel very happy. Maybe what I said, or the way I said it, somehow suggested to Fred that I was disappointed in him as well, although nothing of the sort had crossed my mind. Maybe, in plain fact, Fred was just as disappointed as I was at the word he had to convey. Whatever the reason, for the first time Fred Cleveland's perfect control and aplomb seemed to crumble a little as I started out of his office, and he fairly shouted at me, his voice high-pitched and harsh: "I'm sorry that it ever happened, Al, but it *did*, and you've got to live with it. I can't help that. And I can't help the conference's recommendation, either. You're going to have to go home and live with that too."

Ann and I left the clinic then, in the gray and the rain. The investigations were over and the verdict was in. We retrieved our car from the parking lot and started home to Thorp, preparing ourselves to live with the decision.

III

BENCHMARKS

— 9 —

The late winter at Thorp that year of 1980 crossing into 1981 was long and cold, with extra snow piling down in February, but spring came early and fast. Instead of spending all of March and April, as usual, watching the snow melt from the yard—like watching grass grow, somebody once said, but not as dynamic—that year we saw warm, bright days in March and bare ground by early April, and found ourselves busy with things to do.

In late November of 1980, once I seemed reasonably stable a month after my heart attack, Ann had accepted a proposal from the Home Health Care unit of St. Elizabeth's Hospital in Yakima to serve as a sort of free-lance home health care physical therapist throughout Kittitas County—Ellensburg, Cle Elum, Easton, Roslyn, Ronald, and environs. In addition, she was spending two mornings per month in each of two nursing homes in the county as physical therapy supervisor, and was seeing physical therapy patients referred to her by a group of doctors in Cle Elum, right in their own clinic building.

This combination allowed her to establish a part-time, four-days-a-week physical therapy practice without having to set up and equip a formal office. She liked it especially well because the practice was heavily patient- and treatment-oriented, with very little administrative work to be done. She spent the spring and summer getting the guidelines established and getting started working again. Meanwhile, as I found myself able to cope with more than just the magazine column each month, I began to pick up the pieces of the *Horseman* novel and beat my way through to the end of a first draft by late summer.

During the rest of January, however, after the investigations were over, I spent my time trying to adjust to what the investigations

153

had revealed and trying to develop some directions and goals—benchmarks, you might say—by which I could judge the sort of nebulous things I thought of as "recovery." Before the investigations, I had simply gone along day by day, satisfied to get through a day satisfactorily, while looking forward to the alternatives that the investigations might reveal. That had been a sort of a holding period, a matter of just staying alive and gathering strength until the time came that we would know *what could be done.*

Now we *knew* what could be done, and it had turned out that what could be done was nothing very dramatically different from what I had already been doing, backed by a sinking awareness that that was all there was going to be. I was disappointed and depressed by this; I realized that I needed some kind of direction and goals, some place to be heading toward. Then, late in January, we did something that seemed to make sense to me other than just sitting around the house and taking my medicine, something that seemed to point out a clearcut goal for me to aim for.

It wasn't anything very dramatic: We simply took a day trip over to the Columbia Basin to go hunting. Not elk hunting—elk season was long since past—just duck hunting, since the duck season that year in eastern Washington did not close until the thirty-first of January.

I double-checked with Fred Cleveland first to be sure it would be all right, and he said, heavens, yes, go ahead and go duck hunting, just as long as I didn't do something stupid. It was very cold, with subzero weather at the time, and we suspected that the lakes might be frozen in the area we liked for duck hunting, but we bundled up for the Russian winter, Ann and I, and packed off in the Bronco long before dawn on a Friday morning for the fifty-mile drive east to the Columbia River and the desert lakes beyond.

Actually, we didn't hunt from a blind. We hunted, when we were duck hunting, on the largely barren Quincy Game Range with its rock-bound lakes and potholes. The hunting turned out to be terrible that day, with a leaden sky over the Columbia Basin and a chill wind, so we were cold and damp. Most of the waters were all frozen over and there weren't very many ducks still hanging around anyway. I think I got in four or five shots all day and didn't hit a thing. There were Canada geese in the air that day, however, moving south, and we saw one lovely V-shaped flight, about sixty of them, come across the barren hills toward us, honking away, so low as to be almost within range, flapping their great wings into the wind. For a while we thought they might come just close enough to try a shot, but they saw us and veered off to the north, out of range, so we watched those splendid birds go on past undisturbed, honking and gabbling as they went.

We headed back to the car just after noonday, thoroughly chilled, our bag empty, but I was exhilarated just the same. This was the first day since the day before my heart attack that I had really been out in the wilderness, sort of recreating old times again: the icebound lakes, the gray-brown open desert hills, and that bleak winter sky over there were all fantastically beautiful to see and to be out in. We got home by mid-afternoon, built up a huge fire in the fireplace, and had an early dinner.

I was tired from the outing, but I was pleased to see that nothing dreadful had happened. The nitroglycerin had successfully staved off the angina, the arrhythmia seemed under control, and all was right with the world. I knew then that I had at least one benchmark clearly in mind: the elk hunt that would be coming in the fall of the year. I had been cheated out of the elk season just past, but I was jolly well not going to be cheated out of the next one. I had nine good months to bring myself back by whatever means I could, in order to walk the woods and hills again in style by November.

During the spring I applied myself toward this benchmark, faithfully staying with a diet plan designed to reduce fat and cholesterol, increasing the length and vigor of my walks, whatever the weather might be, desperately holding my smoking in check (although I could not seem to shake it completely), doggedly pacing my writing work at exactly the level that felt comfortable, and refusing to worry about how slowly it progressed.

During those winter and spring months, I went over to see Fred once a month, and he fiddled with my medication. I asked him about going off the Norpace for the arrhythmia, since I didn't seem to have it anymore, but he said, no, not yet. I could try to discontinue it in another few months, but if the arrhythmia then recurred, I would have to stay on it for a full two years. He apparently knew what he was talking about; some time in mid-February, when I was over in Seattle doing some library work, it seemed to me that the arrhythmia was beginning to break through the Norpace dosage I was taking. I talked to Fred on the phone and he increased the dosage from 100 mg to 150 mg, four times a day, and the arrhythmia immediately quieted down again. Something dynamic was obviously still going on; something was still changing.

Fred also sought to achieve complete control of the angina by increasing the Inderal, while I, on my own, began using two of the Isordil tablets before exercise instead of one, since one did not seem to be holding so well. I didn't like the Inderal—it made me feel depleted and also seemed to have a definite negative effect on the libido, but when I complained of this to Fred and suggested that maybe we could lower the dose, he turned hands down. "I daresay it's not helping your sex life any," he said, "but controlling the angina is more important." What about trying different beta-blockers to find one with less deleterious effect? "Forget it," he said. "The Inderal covers the angina very well in your case, and you can live with the side effects. It's keeping things on an even keel; let's keep it that way."*

We didn't achieve perfect control of the angina; it kept turning up at odd and unexpected times. A simple stroll out to the mailbox to deposit the morning mail after breakfast would occasionally catch me with angina halfway back to the house, even though that same afternoon I might walk a brisk mile and a half on the highway without any trouble at all. It just wasn't predictable. Fortunately it wasn't terribly frequent either—I might have only one or two brief spells in the course of a day—but it was always there to remind me.

As for the resting angina at night, that was even less predictable. I would go for two or three weeks without a single sign of it, then have two nights in a row with lots of trouble. Something dynamic was still going on. Things were not stable, they were constantly changing. I was viscerally aware of this, and yet I could see how a physician following a patient along with occasional office examinations might see nothing but a stable pattern developing. Fred could look at my EKGs and listen to my heart and check my cardiac shadow on a chest X ray, and he could listen to what I told him, but he could not *feel* the visceral awareness that I had of day-to-day shifts and changes.

Some odd things came to my attention as time went on. During the depths of that cold winter I found that I was far more sensitive to temperature than ever before in my life. I had always been a "warm person"—an inside room temperature of 65 degrees was just fine for me, although it drove Ann crazy until it got up to 68 degrees. I could tolerate 68 degree but was too warm at 70 degrees, and when we went over to visit my brother in Spokane in a house that was kept at 75 degrees all the time, I'd always nearly baked and suffocated.

---

* It's pretty widely known by now that having a heart condition doesn't in itself necessarily interfere with sex, either with erection or orgasm. Sexual intercourse is usually permitted as soon after a heart attack or bypass operation as the patient feels recuperated enough to engage in it—assuming that the exertion in itself doesn't bring on angina. But some medicines heart patients must take for their heart conditions can indeed cause impotence—either lack of interest in sex, or loss of erection during intercourse or lack of erection at all—and this can be a real problem.

Now I found that even at 70 degrees inside I was always cold. The light weight wool trousers I had weren't warm enough, or the Orlon shirts that I had always worn before. I got a pair of Filson all-wool whipcord trousers, thick and heavy, and they were a little better, but not very comfortable for indoor use. Finally, I decided to quit fooling around: I found a pair of very dense, heavy, soft wool, "extreme-weather" trousers advertised in an L. L. Bean catalog, and I ordered a pair. They were absolutely perfect. They were *warm*—warm in the house, warm out walking on the road. They were heavy, had to be dry-cleaned, and they became lumpy and made me look like a logger, but they were *warm*. I followed this up by ordering some corduroy and heavy flannel shirts from Bean, and they were an improvement, but the upper half of me still got cold all the time. I finally added a wool sweater on top of the corduroy shirt and found that that, with a room temperature of 70 degrees, kept me warm. From then on I wore a shirt and sweater around the house from the first of October to the first of May every year, just to stay comfortable.

Also during this time I found it amazing how easy it was to slip into an unhurried, even downright leisurely, pattern of daily activity. Ever the worrywart before, I was long habituated to early rising, plunging into a long morning's work, since morning was by far my brightest working time, accepting a midday sag, and then turning out another good afternoon's work from two-thirty to five or six. I always had to be busy, and there was always a pile of things left undone for me to worry about; I would never actually find the top of my desk under all the rubble from one year to the next.

Now, all that changed. I found it easy to sleep in till seven-thirty or eight in the morning, especially if I had had a bad night with angina disturbing me for an hour or so at two in the morning. I became more and more resistant to being hurried in the morning. Ann's customary three-minute warning for breakfast, always before an acceptable goad to me to get my shirt on and get myself downstairs, now began to scrape a raw nerve. I didn't *want* to be rushed in the morning anymore. That seemed to be a time when an angina attack was easily provoked or when shortness of breath appeared for no particular reason.

To escape that three-minute warning (an irritation that Ann didn't seem to understand, or regarded as unreasonable), I started getting my own breakfast, especially on mornings when Ann had to be off by eight or eight-thirty to see patients. For me, if I didn't get to my desk until nine or nine-thirty, that was just fine. The mail would arrive between eleven-thirty and twelve, so this made a good excuse to break from whatever work I was doing. Reading the mail, eating lunch, and listening to the noonday news would take up an hour and a half, and this would be followed by an hour's nap, so that more and more I found myself doing only an hour or so of work in the afternoon after naptime before religiously taking off at four or four-thirty for an hour of walking. Back from my walk, Ann or I would get the fireplace going if it wasn't already, have a drink before dinner, catch up on the newspapers and the day's events, and then spend the evening mostly reading or listening to music, usually turning in by nine or nine-thirty in the evening.

The net result of all this, for me, was a much more leisurely work day, with considerably less work actually accomplished each day and a calculated sense of shiftlessness about almost everything. As a result, tensions were down, pressures off. I would never have believed that it could work, but to my amazement, it did. The column got written perfectly well every month, even though it took a larger bite of my working time each month, and since *Good Housekeeping* gave me a modest raise now and then, I could hardly complain about that. I also got book manuscripts worked up and finished. The first draft of *The Fourth Horseman* was wrapped up by the end of August. A small book on viruses for Franklin Watts's junior high school list was ultimately finished, followed by another small book on the immune system, also for Watts, then another book for junior high girls about menstruation, and so on. For all the new low-key approach to the work, the work did get done, and, most cheering of all to me, didn't seem to suffer any in quality. If you can't teach an old dog new tricks, I thought, perhaps you can't make him forget old tricks, either.

Sometime in this period I began to rearrange my thinking about the purposes and goals of my exercise program. Before I had considered it just a matter of getting out and moving around for an hour every day, doing penance for having been so stupid as to have a myocardial infarction in the first place, putting in a sedate mile or two of walking each day, largely because that was what the doctor had ordered. I now began to see daily exercise much more as a rehabilitation challenge, a program for real recuperation and rebuilding.

Instead of just walking quietly along on the level, I began increasing the length and vigor of my walks. I began taking a half-hour warm-up walk in the early morning as well as the regular hour of walking in the afternoon. Instead of knocking off after one mile when the weather was foul or the footing slippery, I made at least two miles every day. And instead of just strolling along, I took on far more brisk walking, pressing myself to the point of shortness of breath. I had the notion that the walking wasn't going to help me any unless it raised my pulse rate a significant amount for a significant period of time at a stretch.

Ordinarily, this might be true, but unfortunately I had the artificial pulse lowering effect of the Inderal beta-blocker to contend with, and found that if my resting pulse rate was about 60 per minute, I could walk myself to breathlessness and only get my pulse rate up to about 75. I pressed myself to breathlessness just the same, dreaming up all sorts of delightful fantasies about the dear little twigs of the collateral arteries extending and flourishing into the edges of compromised heart muscle like the roots of a tomato plant, visions of good myocardium growing stronger and more powerful, as I began pushing it on a regular daily basis.

To be sure, I was not, like Norman Cousins, gaily batting a tennis ball around the court every day, but I *was* by God moving the body up and down that highway at a fairly good clip, and it really irritated me when Ann wanted to accompany me on my walks, because she didn't want to hike along as fast as I did, and she soon gave that up.* Each day, reaching the county road, I would check the wind and try to plan my walk so I walked facing the wind on the way out, with the wind to my back on the return trip. When wind wasn't a factor, I would alternate direction, heading down the road through Knudson's Pass and the open fields to the irrigation ditch one day, up the canyon to the Brain's farm the next.

All this seemed to work reasonably well, since I took pains to take the Isordil under the tongue fifteen or twenty minutes before starting my walk. Presently, I began taking Gypsy, our elderly springer spaniel, along with me for company, and soon she became just as habituated to the daily walk as I was, maybe even more so. Whereas I walked largely because I felt I had to and thought it accomplished something, she really *liked* it and would start agitating to go walking along about two o'clock in the afternoon, planting herself outside my study door with her head between her paws and her tail wagging furiously. Then, when I finally, *finally* got ready to go, she would do joyful pirouettes in front of the door while I got my jacket on.

After a month or so of this, I began to think maybe I could go it one better, so I tried, alternately, jogging fifty paces, then walking fifty paces. I soon found it didn't work. Brisk walking into the wind was one thing—I would get a little breathless, but the exertional angina would not clamp down. Launching into a jog for even twenty-

---

* Not that she gave up walking, which she continued doing for her own benefit; she simply took her own walks each day in her own direction at her own time. To this day our neighbors may think we're awfully antisocial because each of us walks alone.

five paces, I found, brought me right up against the brick wall. After trying it off and on for about a week, I discarded even intermittent jogging as a thoroughly bad scene.

Of course, there is more than one way to skin a cat. Up until March or so I had confined my walking to the relatively level stretches of the Taneum Canyon county road. But as the snow melted in March, it became possible to travel secondary roads and logging roads, or just to take off cross-country. At the edge of Knudson's field, for example, there was a service road for the irrigation ditch that led up a dry hill at a moderate incline, then, two or three hundred feet above, leveled out to follow the irrigation ditch back around the hillside for a mile or two. I began climbing that hill on some of my walks—not rushing up it, by any means, just taking it as slowly as necessary, stopping to catch my breath now and then, but working my way up to the top and then taking the level walk along the ditch at the top. On the other side of the canyon was another farm road going up into the hills. Up the canyon beyond Brain's farm, there was an old logging road that started slowly into the hills, then forked, with a very steep climb up toward forested hills on the right and a less steep road to the left that made its way up into the wooded area known as Cobain's Pocket. From time to time I would explore one or the other of these roads, taking as much time as necessary, pausing whenever I got slightly short of breath, but climbing just the same.

These treks, for the most part, didn't bring on angina as long as I didn't try to hurry. They made a very refreshing change of scenery from time to time. They also brought me into areas frequented by a great many deer that came out as the snow receded. They would appear in groups of three or four, up to two or three dozen, and would stand staring at me with their heads up and their big muley ears out, watching as I approached as close as forty or fifty yards before bouncing away. I had explored Cobain's Pocket from above during hunting seasons in the past but hadn't fully understood how it lay or where the road down led to, so on these walks I kept making hunting-season notes in my mind.

As this sort of recovery program got underway, yet another goal, or benchmark, began to emerge: a more careful assessment of coronary artery disease *risk factors* as they applied to me, and an attempt to do something about them. At that time, a number of such risk factors—just plain elements of everyday living—were coming to be recognized as very strongly associated with coronary artery disease and myocardial infarctions. These were life-style risk factors, of course: high-fat, high-cholesterol diets, cigarette smoking, high-tension, high-anxiety type-A personality behavior, and so forth. It seemed to me worthwhile to start actively working to reduce some of those risk factors in my own life while still maintaining a life-style that I could live with.

In a sense, trying to reduce risk factors at that stage of the game was really like locking the barn door after the horse was gone: Nothing was going to restore what had already been lost. But, more and more, things I read in the medical literature were suggesting that reduction or elimination of some risk factors in the very midst of severe coronary artery disease might at least have some beneficial effect in *slowing the progress of the disease*. There was even some speculation among doctors that eliminating some risk factors might conceivably help reverse the ongoing disease process to some degree. Nobody was making any promises, and everybody agreed that the ones who might benefit the most would be the ones who had early, mild coronary artery disease that had not yet reached the point of catastrophe. But it seemed to me, more and more, that if risk factors really did contribute to worsening of the disease, and some of them could be reduced, it might make sense for me to pay attention to reducing them.

A Look at the Risk Factors

As we saw earlier, nobody knows precisely why atherosclerosis occurs or why it seems to pick coronary arteries as a favorite target. Certainly there is no simple cause; it comes about as an accumulation of numerous different influences. The disease seems to be a wide-spread affliction among Americans, Englishmen, Germans, and other European populations, yet the distribution is uneven. Certain things seem to place some people at greater risk than others in the same populations.

What's more, the distribution of the disease is by no means universal worldwide. Although Americans, Canadians, and northern Europeans seem highly prone to trouble, it is much less common in such southern European countries as Italy or Greece. The highest incidence anywhere in the world is among the people of Finland, whereas, until very recently, the condition was extremely rare among the people of Japan. Oddly enough, this "relative immunity" enjoyed by native Japanese did not seem to extend to Americans of Japanese extraction living in America, and, indeed, following World War II the incidence of atherosclerosis rose markedly among the affluent Japanese living in Japan. Coronary artery disease remains relatively rare in China and such underdeveloped countries as India and the central African nations, and among Arabian peasants, although it is very common among the Israelis living right next door. We might argue, of course, that many poverty-stricken people in underdeveloped nations simply don't live long enough to develop coronary artery disease, but this alone doesn't seem to explain the overall low incidence—even those third world people who live long enough don't get coronary artery disease very often.

Obviously there must be some significant variables at work to explain this spotty and uneven incidence. Whatever they are, each of these variables present in a given person's life might act to increase that person's individual risk of developing coronary artery disease, or developing it more rapidly than might otherwise be expected. These speculative variables came to be known as "risk factors."

Emerging with this concept were a couple of rather obvious corollaries. First, it seemed that if these risk factors could be identified, then it might be possible to match individuals with risk factors and identify which individuals might be more or less likely to develop coronary artery disease than others. If that were possible, it might also be possible for those individuals who seemed to be at high risk to reduce their risk by making changes in the way they lived. And, in fact, if truly valid risk factors could be identified and acted upon by changes in the way a person lived, then it seemed possible that widespread, lifelong attention to reducing or eliminating risk factors might very substantially reduce the overall incidence or frequency of coronary artery disease in whole populations.

The trouble with that was that possible risk factors appeared to be quite numerous, and anything but simple and straightforward, and first of all they had to be identified. Bit by bit over the past twenty years, a number of these factors *have* been identified. It would be worthwhile at this point to look in more detail at some of them that seem to be very clear cut:

1. *Heredity.* Atherosclerosis is basically a generalized disorder of the body's metabolic and physiological function. As such, its development is influenced by a person's genes, since both metabolism and physiological function are strongly directed and guided by those genes. This is one part of the reason that two virtually identical persons with identical environmental backgrounds may have widely differing degrees of atherosclerosis. Thus, one of the major risk factors for coronary artery disease, as we understand it today, is a *family history of coronary artery disease.*

This is not to say that CAD is a hereditary disease, passed directly from parent to children according to clear-cut principles of Mendelian genetics, like Tay-Sachs disease, Huntington's chorea (Woody Guthrie's disease), or certain kinds of hemophilia. CAD does not have any known hereditary links in this direct sense. Neither does this mean that an individual with no immediate family history of CAD won't get it. I came from a family of long-lived progenitors with no history whatever of CAD, yet I certainly developed the condition. When I did so, however, I instantly *created* a strong family history of CAD for my daughter and my three sons, who had previously had only their maternal grandfather known to be afflicted with the disease. Finally, this is not to say that a person whose family tree is studded with CAD on both sides necessarily *has* to fall victim to the disease.

In short, heredity is not in most cases a direct, identified cause of CAD. It is merely a risk factor—one variable that, when present, suggests that a person is more likely to fall victim to coronary atherosclerosis sometime during life than another person without a record of the disease in his or her family tree. We could say that person is *more prone* to the disease, more *predisposed* than others. There are many other diseases and disorders that have similar patterns of hereditary predisposition—diabetes, for example, or breast cancer in women, or perhaps endogenous depression. Even vulnerability to addiction may have some hereditary predisposition.

Oddly enough, there is one small group of people who have a much more direct genetic vulnerability to CAD than normal. These are people who carry genes that cause them to accumulate extraordinarily high levels of cholesterol or other lipids known as triglycerides in the bloodstream. In this hereditary condition, known as *familial hypercholesterolemia*, individuals have serum cholesterol levels in the range of 400 or 500 milligrams per deciliter, compared to the normal range of 150 to 220. Other people have a *familial hyperlipidemia*, with triglyceride levels that regularly range five or six times higher than normal. People with this type of hereditary affliction (fortunately relatively few) tend to develop generalized and coronary atherosclerosis very frequently, quite early in life and in a markedly severe degree.

Unfortunately, nobody can choose his ancestors; you're born with what you're born with. What you *can* do, if it applies to you, is recognize a family history of CAD as one black mark on your chart, so to speak, so that it becomes all the more important to reduce or eliminate any other risk factors that you *can* influence. No single risk factor necessarily condemns anyone to coronary artery disease, but risk factors piled upon other risk factors compound the risk.

2. *Gender.* Coronary artery disease, historically, has been preponderantly a disease of males. True, some women developed the disease, but comparatively few—until quite recently, only something

like 1 woman for every 30 or 40 men. In addition, when it did appear in women, it seemed to appear later than in men, progress less rapidly, and, generally, prove to be less severe.

Why this difference? The main reason, as we understand it today, is that there are distinct physiological and psychological differences between men and women, and that these differences distinctly tend to favor females as far as coronary artery disease is concerned.

Take hormone differences, for instance. From puberty through menopause, a woman's body generates markedly higher levels of estrogens and progestogens, the main female hormones, than a man's. These hormones not only regulate ovulation and sustain pregnancy; they also seem to exert a distinct protective effect on the woman's cardiovascular system. Historically, most women who develop severe coronary artery disease seem to manifest the disease some years after menopause, the point at which female hormone levels drop markedly, or else they also have diabetes, another independent and powerful risk factor for CAD.

Of course, there have been other considerations, too. Until recently most women spent their lives in the home and were less likely than men to be subjected to the tensions and pressures of the workplace. Women were less subject to such pressures as territorialism, aggressiveness, or fierce competition for position, wealth, rank. They were—perhaps—less subject to driving pressures and ambitions, less likely to generate huge quantities of adrenal hormones in response to anger or fear. In addition, for years fewer women than men indulged in heavy cigarette smoking or heavy alcohol use. As a result, many were largely sheltered from some of the more devastating risk factors for CAD and thus enjoyed relative freedom from the disease.

In the last thirty or forty years much of this has changed. Incidence of the disease is still predominantly male, but far less so than previously. More and more women *are* developing coronary artery disease in their forties and fifties. In many of them today the disease is progressing just as rapidly and becoming just as severe as in men. It is not that their bodies are producing any less of the protective female hormones; rather, more of them are becoming more vulnerable to other risk factors. More women in the current "coronary generation" have been lifelong heavy cigarette smokers than previously. Many have moved into the formerly male workplace, taking on the tensions and pressures of careers and competing with men for position and income. More and more are functioning on higher adrenaline levels than ever before. All these newly assumed risk factors tend to reduce the protective benefits of *nonrisk* factors such as plenty of estrogen; and as a result, the male-to-female ratio of coronary artery disease has become much closer to 3 or 4 to 1 than the previous 30 or 40 to 1. In the words of the familiar cigarette ad, women have come a long way, baby, in terms of rapidly increasing incidence of lung cancer and coronary artery disease.

Of course, gender is another risk factor that nobody can do anything about. The male is automatically at higher risk for the disease than the female, if not so much so as thirty or forty years ago. For a woman, CAD is no longer a threat you can afford to ignore simply because you're a woman. It is a real threat, it is increasing in incidence among women and it is just as pernicious a threat to women as to men. Neither men nor women can alter their gender (ordinarily); but as with heredity, they *can* recognize the risk and seek to reduce other risk factors that *can* be altered.

3. *Race.* Coronary artery disease is relatively uncommon among black people in underprivileged nations in central Africa, but in America blacks are at significantly higher risk than their white counterparts, whether male or female. Some of this difference may be due to other risk factors that go along with being black—increased vulnerability to hypertension, for example, or diets more rich in cholesterol and animal fats, with heavy reliance upon fried foods and refined carbohydrates. There may also be plain genetic racial predispositions for increased atherosclerosis and increased CAD among blacks that simply have never yet been defined or identified. Needless to say, nobody can do anything to alter the burden of race, but there is good reason to believe that blacks, by paying increased attention to factors such as diet, physical conditioning, and other risk factors, may largely be able to counteract the risk factor of race and at least achieve a par with whites.

4. *Hypertension.* Of all disorders that human beings are subject to, high blood pressure is perhaps the most widespread and pernicious. It is estimated that some 40 million people in America have blood pressure elevated above healthy norms, and half of those people don't even know it. What *is* known is that high blood pressure is a major physiological risk factor for development of atherosclerosis and CAD. The hypertensive person not only has that disorder whittling away at the functional vitality of his cardiovascular system, particularly the arteries supplying the heart, the brain, and the kidneys, but is also more vulnerable to early progressive atherosclerosis. There is no question that many people who develop severe CAD have either suffered from long-standing uncontrolled hypertension or else have had their hypertension controlled only by a lick and a promise, sporadically, which amounts to the same thing.

Here at last is a risk factor that really *can* be reduced or eliminated, because hypertension is easily detected and in most cases can be effectively and permanently controlled. Our high intake of dietary sodium contributes to high blood pressure. We are also a nation of overeaters, with large numbers of us carrying 10 to 20 percent more avoirdupois—plain fat—than normal or necessary. Although no studies that I know of have actually demonstrated this, it is highly likely that if everyone with measured hypertension were to reduce his or her weight by 10 percent and reduce sodium intake by 50 percent, one-quarter of the hypertension in this country could be controlled by those two measures alone. Medical treatment could effectively deal with the rest.

Effective medical treatment of hypertension, unfortunately, involves some difficult problems. For one thing, the condition doesn't go away: Continued medication can bring the pressure down, and keep it there, but it will pop right back up again when the medication is terminated. This means that to eliminate hypertension as a risk factor for CAD by medical treatment, that treatment must be continuous lifelong and involves eating a lot of very expensive pills. What's more, the medicines themselves may have undesirable side effects, such as lethargy, lack of energy, lightheadedness, or—especially notable in males (as discussed earlier)—loss of libido or relative impotence.

On the other hand, the kind of damage that high blood pressure can do to the body, over the long run, is not particularly appealing, either. In addition to speeding the development of coronary artery disease, hypertension can lead to long-term kidney damage, cause visual disturbances, and make one increasingly vulnerable to strokes. On balance, *anyone* with high blood pressure needs to be diagnosed and treated, and hypertension is one active risk factor for coronary artery disease that can be eliminated, not just reduced, through continuing treatment by whatever means are necessary.

5. *Diabetes mellitus.* Here is another diagnosable and treatable disorder that greatly increases a person's risk of coronary artery disease and accelerates the CAD's progress and severity unless it is discovered and controlled. There are some 5 million known diabetics in the United States today; experts estimate that another 2 to 3 million people already have undiagnosed diabetes.

Two types of the disease are recognized. Type 1, sometimes called *juvenile onset diabetes*, often severe, tends to appear during childhood or adolescence. Type 2, or *adult onset diabetes*, a milder form of the disease, appears during the decades of the thirties, forties, or fifties. Both types are influenced by heredity, although the exact genetic pattern of transmission of the disease has never been thoroughly identified and understood. What is most important in terms of coronary artery disease is the fact that either type of diabetes, if not carefully and continually treated and controlled, causes greatly accelerated development of atherosclerosis. The atherosclerotic changes can affect arteries in the kidneys, eyes, and brain, as well as the coronary arteries. Thus, diabetics who are undiagnosed or treated inadequately are vulnerable to a whole host of accelerating problems, one of which is rapidly progressing and unusually severe coronary artery disease.

Since *any* individual with diabetes has a built-in risk factor for coronary artery disease that can at least be reduced with treatment, whether by diet, oral medication, or insulin injections, early diagnosis is critically important. Diabetes is usually first suspected when sugar is found in the urine on routine urinalysis exam, or an abnormally high level of sugar is found in a blood sugar examination. These are laboratory tests that ought to be done at appropriate intervals throughout a person's life in the course of routine physical examinations. In addition, everyone should be aware of the three so-called *cardinal signs*, or flagrant symptoms, of developing diabetes: abnormally frequent urination, abnormal thirst, and abnormal and unexplained increase in appetite. These cardinal signs are sometimes spoken of as the three polys—*polyuria, polydipsia,* and *polyphagia.* Any such symptom deserves immediate investigation, for it may be the first sign of developing diabetes.

6. *Plain obesity.* There has been so much nonsense written about obesity and coronary artery disease that perhaps we should just stick to the facts here. There is no direct cause-and-effect relationship between obesity—generally defined as being 10 or more percent over the actuarial "ideal weight" for one's height and body build—and coronary artery disease, but it is a plain statistical fact that the person who is persistently overweight is more at risk of developing coronary artery disease than is the individual whose weight is in the normal range.

This is not quite the simple, straightforward risk factor you might think at a glance. It may actually represent a number of risk factors at work, all with one outward manifestation. The trouble is that overweight people may be overweight for a multitude of reasons, and their obesity may be all scrambled up with other risk factors.

Most overweight people are overweight because they eat too much, and because they eat too much of the wrong foods. These are often people whose daily diets are loaded with animal fats from red meats, dairy products, and eggs, high in cholesterol, high in saturated fats. Many of them don't engage in *any* physical exercise to speak of, often because they're so fat that physical exercise is uncomfortable for them. Many also are hypertensive; others have diabetes, with their obesity directly related, in part, to the disturbance in their carbohydrate metabolism. And obesity often is related to emotional pressures and tensions that encourage the person to overeat or make it difficult not to eat.

Obviously, sorting out all these possible causes for obesity can be a tough job, even with the help of a perceptive physician. But it isn't all that difficult for a person to determine whether he or she is actually overweight. Men, for example, can use a simple formula: The ideal weight for a male is approximately 110 pounds plus five additional pounds for each inch of height over five feet. (This formula, of course, doesn't account for such things as differing bone structure, body build, or habitus—mesomorphic, endomorphic, or ectomorphic, but this doesn't really matter. The formula is not intended for fine tuning, but it will work perfectly well to suggest whether one is even within striking distance of ideal weight or not). The ideal weight formula for a woman is approximately one hundred pounds plus five pounds for each inch over five feet. Probably the person very close to ideal weight, according to these formulas, can disregard obesity as a risk factor for CAD; the person who overshoots by very much should recognize that he or she, indeed, does have a risk factor for CAD and that this risk factor can be reduced or even eliminated, regardless of cause, *simply by losing weight.*

Easier said than done? Yes, indeed. Multitudes of people, both men and women, exert enormous effort trying to lose weight and either fail completely or lose it only to pile it back on again almost immediately. What's the problem? Certainly there are metabolic differences that allow one person to eat apparently unlimited quantities of food and never gain an ounce, while others have to reduce their food intake almost to starvation levels in order to lose any weight at all. Certainly psychological or social factors may be at work. But a major reason so many have difficulty losing weight is sheer lack of any significant, recognized motivation. Many people think they'd like to lose weight in a vague sort of way but don't have any clear, specific reason. Fancied improvement in physical appearance, the possibility of wearing more attractive clothing or some indefinite perception that thinner is healthier just won't do it. But a clear recognition that whatever its cause, obesity is a major risk factor for a thoroughly unpleasant, lifelong debilitating disease can be a powerful motivation.

There is immense value in controlling or eliminating that risk factor. True enough, for a person who is not immediately threatened, controlling obesity as a risk factor may seem like buying a hundred shares of Apple Computer stock today in the vague hope that it may be worth a million dollars in twenty years. But if a person reviews *all* the risk factors that may be at work in his own life, each one compounding the others and clearly pointing to trouble down the line, recognizing obesity as a real future threat can provide the motivation for prolonged, determined effort to modify it.

This becomes even more imperative in the individual whose coronary artery disease has already been demonstrated in one way or another. People who just couldn't or wouldn't control their obesity before catastrophe struck may find it far easier to control after. As a large-boned, six-foot male individual, I spent most of my adult life ranging in weight from 210 pounds to 235, despite numerous desultory attempts to knock off weight. After my hospitalization with my acute MI, I came out with a weight of 195 pounds, naked, still some 15 pounds above my ideal weight, but not totally out of reason. Subsequently my weight began creeping up toward 210 pounds again at one point, but it yielded quickly to attention and has remained comfortably stable at about 200 pounds ever since. Before my MI, the motivation was not there; afterward it was. This obviously is not the ideal scenario, and for people seeking to *avoid* coronary artery disease, a search for valid motivations for controlling weight could prove far more fruitful than a search for quick and easy diets.

7. *Physical indolence.* What an unpleasant term to apply to oneself! Most of us don't regard ourselves as indolent, yet many people are just that. They come equipped with bodies that can tolerate and, in fact, require a certain amount of physical exercise on a regular daily basis, yet they never seriously think about obtaining it, and the body slowly deteriorates. Until the last ten or fifteen years, many people regarded vigorous physical exercise as something reserved for nuts and athletes. Physical laborers or migrant farm workers may obtain plenty of such exercise, but a great many blue-collar workers—factory workers, assembly-line workers, deliverymen, repairmen, and the like—obtain practically none whatever. White-collar workers have to seek exercise to find it, and all too often they choose not to. Professional people, business people of all sorts, multitudes of housewives—all build their lives around laborsaving devices to spare themselves any physical effort at all.

For many years, first as a practicing physician, then as a freelance writer, I had no more physical exercise in my life than was required to walk out to the car, make hospital rounds, and then sit in my consulting room, or, later, at the typewriter desk. Ann and I did some intermittent backpack hiking in the summer, and we got quite a bit of exercise for about two months during hunting season each year, but from late November through May or June we engaged in no exercise much more strenuous than lifting our forks to our mouths. Ann, with her physical therapy work, got somewhat more exercise than I did, but not very much.

For me, part of the problem was that I had no real interest in physical exercise, never had. I *hated* exercise just for its own sake. For one thing it bored me; for another, I spent my school days as an uncoordinated 98-pound weakling who despised physical education and sports and never got over it. As a result, it became normal for me to be "busy" and begrudge the time that exercise would take out of a "busy" day. Even on backpacking trips I found no particular exhilaration in carrying a forty-pound pack two miles up and nine miles in during the course of a day. I enjoyed the wilderness, the fishing, the peace and quiet, the relaxation *when we got there*; but getting there, to me, was just a form of forced labor.

Perhaps now, six years after my MI, I have begun to reach a state of grace in which I find that modest physical exercise is reasonably pleasant and rewarding in itself. Perhaps. I may never be entirely certain about this, since I feel that I have no choice about it anyway, at this point. To sit around in my former degree of total physical indolence would now, I think, be suicidal. I suspect that if somehow I were suddenly dropped into an alternate world in which my MI had never occurred, even bearing all the memories of what had occurred, in this world, it would be exceedingly difficult for me to continue an exercise program of any serious dimension. And certainly it would not be honest for me to try to contend that *you* will necessarily find physical exercise pleasant, rewarding, exhilarating, or any of the other things that physical exercise is supposed to be.

All this notwithstanding, the fact is that physical indolence is a very major and deadly risk factor for coronary artery disease. The reverse is also true: a life-style that involves regular physical exercise not only reduces or eliminates a risk factor but has a very positive effect as a *negative* risk factor, actively protecting against the development and danger of coronary artery disease.

Exercise builds and develops muscles, and muscle activity requires a good blood supply. The heart must pump the blood; when it is forced to exceed a bare physically indolent level of activity for periods of time each day, the heart itself develops good muscle strength and good myocardial circulation. Atherosclerosis may still progress, and the machine may still suffer catastrophes—but the machine is in far better condition to absorb an insult and adjust to it.

What's more, exercise has been found, in carefully controlled scientific studies, to have a positive or beneficial effect on the metabolism of fats and carbohydrates in the body. Among the various fatty materials in the blood that we know are related to atherosclerosis, cholesterol is a bad actor. Too much cholesterol in the blood serum seems to increase and accelerate the development of atherosclerosis. In addition, certain lipoproteins—metabolic by-products of the fats and carbohydrates we eat—also seem to have an effect. One class of lipoproteins with very low density in terms of molecular size and weight are now clearly associated with accelerated development of atherosclerosis. Other lipoproteins with much higher density tend to slow the progress of this condition.

These fatty materials can easily be measured by simple laboratory blood tests, and their effects have been outlined statistically. We now know that people who carry constant high blood levels of cholesterol and low-density lipoproteins are prone to coronary artery disease; they develop it more frequently and more rapidly than those with lower levels. On the other hand, people who have larger quantities of high-density lipoproteins seem to be protected against atherosclerosis and CAD. At least in theory, anything that increases the level of high-density lipoproteins in a person's bloodstream and lowers the level of low-density lipoproteins is beneficial. There is a great deal of evidence today that regular, vigorous daily exercise does just that. To be effective, the daily exercise periods should last for thirty minutes to an hour at a time and should be vigorous enough to give the heart a workout—brisk walking, jogging, swimming, bicycling, tennis, that sort of thing.

Fortunately, during the last fifteen years we have seen widespread public recognition of the protective value of physical exercise as part of the life-style among many people. Young people in particular have recognized the value of such exercise, and of course it is in young people especially that establishing such a lifelong habit is of the greatest benefit as a continuing protection against atherosclerosis. Exercise also helps combat two other risk factors: obesity and hypertension.

What about people in their middle or older years? They, too, can benefit from exercise, but should consult a physician before shifting abruptly into a vigorous exercise program to avoid precipitating trouble that may already be present. This is especially important for anyone who already has symptoms that might be related to coronary artery impairment—angina on exertion, for example, or cardiac arrhythmias and irregularities, or shortness of breath. People in this age group may also want to select the kind of exercise they undertake on a rational basis. A vigorous round of tennis every day may not be a rational choice for a sixty-five-year-old man with some shortness of breath. An overweight person might choose swimming for exercise while simultaneously endeavoring to reduce his weight. In fact, for a great many such people, the best and most sane form of exercise may be brisk walking a couple of miles or more a day.

I have been dwelling on this subject simply because exercise is one positive, protective venture that anyone can undertake and maintain at some level or another. The only way you can "fail" at physical exercise is not to take it.

8. *Cigarette smoking.* Although this risk factor appears far down on this particular list, it really belongs at the very top since it is more heavily loaded with direct danger than any of the others. Cigarette smoking is damaging to health in many ways, some direct, some indirect, but its relationship to coronary artery disease is direct and specific.

Nobody has yet defined precisely *how* cigarette smoking accelerates coronary artery atherosclerosis, but the evidence that it does so is overwhelming. Certainly a number of a specific damaging effects can be clearly defined. We know that the nicotine in cigarette smoke is a violent poison, even in very small amounts, and that even a small amount serves as a powerful cardiac stimulant, whipping the heart rate up far above normal levels. At the same time, nicotine causes small arteries supplying the heart muscle to pinch down, to constrict. Thus, the overall nicotine effect of cigarette smoking is to increase the heart's work load while simultaneously restricting its blood flow, so that the whole myocardium suffers a relative degree of ischemia.

This wave of ischemia is imposed on the myocardium repeatedly with each dose of nicotine from each cigarette, hour after hour, day after day. A person with a healthy heart and no coronary artery disease may not notice this relative ischemia in terms of any obvious symptoms or limitations. For a person with any degree of coronary atherosclerosis, however, introducing this relative ischemia is simply adding insult to injury. An already impaired heart circulation is made worse, and in many cases the nicotine effect of smoking may actually help precipitate such symptoms as acute angina.

There are other effects of smoking, too. The tars and other by-products inhaled in tobacco smoke actively irritate the mucosal lining of the bronchial airway in the lungs, causing a continuous outpouring of mucus that has to be cleared up, and a certain amount of airway obstruction. This repeated irritation eventually can lead to physical changes in the walls of the bronchioles; these tiny air tubes lose their normal elasticity as fibrous tissue forms in their walls. Ultimately, anyone who smokes cigarettes regularly, and especially the heavy cigarette smoker (a pack a day or more), develops *some* degree of chronic obstructive pulmonary disease, a condition that may eventually become severe enough to cause death from *pulmonary emphysema*, but long before that extreme level of damage is reached, there is a chronic, continuous impairment of air movement into the lungs, so that the oxygen available to the bloodstream becomes limited to some degree or another. Thus, in addition to suffering repeated episodes of increased heart rate and restricted coronary artery flow due to smoking, the blood reaching the smoker's myocardium is just not as well oxygenated as it should be, which naturally increases the relative ischemia of the myocardium.

The carbon monoxide in cigarette smoke presents a third danger. The trouble with carbon monoxide is that it successfully competes with oxygen for positions in the oxygen-carrying hemoglobin molecules. When carbon monoxide is present in the bloodstream, the hemoglobin, which ordinarily takes up oxygen in great quantities for transport throughout the body, will pick up the carbon monoxide some *245 times more easily* than the oxygen, and then cannot carry oxygen in addition. What's more, once carbon monoxide is picked up and bound to the hemoglobin, it doesn't let go readily, so a quantity of totally useless hemoglobin remains in the bloodstream for prolonged periods, during which time it cannot transport any oxygen. The heavy smoker, as a result, is constantly carrying a *lower* concentration of oxygen in the blood than normal, and this inevitably robs the myocardium of some of the oxygen that it ought to be getting. This development alone forces the myocardium to work harder, forces the heart to beat faster, just to stay ahead of its constant need for oxygen. The more carbon monoxide in the blood, the tougher it is for the myocardium.

Obviously, all of these heart-damaging effects of cigarette smoking tend to compound each other, and the effects get worse the more one smokes. The one-pack smoker is subjecting his heart to twenty 10-minute periods of induced overwork and artery constriction each day—over three hours a day of active torment. The two-pack smoker is achieving almost seven hours a day of self-damage. At the same time, at each level of cigarette consumption there is a progressively higher load of carbon monoxide continuously present in the blood—so much, in fact, that it may not even be completely cleared out of the blood in the course of a normal sleeping period.

The person who has never smoked cigarettes or used other forms of tobacco has simply lived his life free of these damaging effects, and thus has always been free of one major risk factor for coronary artery disease. For those who have smoked, or who continue to smoke, the beauty of stopping is that these heart-damaging effects all come to a halt immediately as soon as cigarette smoking is discontinued. Even a person who is already in serious potential trouble with coronary atherosclerosis can sharply reduce the risk of eventual catastrophe within a matter of days or weeks after smoking has ceased. In short, terminating smoking is one of the most immediately and massively beneficial things a person can do to protect against a CAD catastrophe, whether that person has mild trouble or very severe trouble. To continue cigarette smoking in the face of known or demonstrated CAD simply doesn't make sense.

This is not to say that cessation of smoking is any ironbound guarantee that a catastrophe will be averted—cigarette smoking is only one of many risk factors involved. But it is such a very important risk factor that for anyone who really seeks to evade a coronary catastrophe or to prolong survival after one has occurred, cessation of smoking is an obvious and necessary first step.

Having delivered myself of that little screed, I now have to add that it may not necessarily be easy to do, no matter how firmly you're convinced that you absolutely must. I found it frustratingly and infuriatingly difficult. I mentioned earlier that I did not quit smoking immediately after my heart attack. I cut way down, but I did not cut *out*, and that was no good. It was not until the summer of 1982 that I finally, in desperation, found a way to quit, through an outside agency.* Since then I have fallen off the wagon, briefly, a number of times, but so far have always slapped the addiction down. To this day I find it extremely difficult to be in the presence of smokers, not because their smoking is distasteful, but because I want to join them. Neither do I pretend to think that this personal fight is over. When I recently signed an insurance application declaring myself to be a nonsmoker, my hand trembled.

9. *Alcohol.* The question of alcohol consumption as a risk factor for CAD is considerably more muddy than the question of smoking. It has long been known that alcohol and its main metabolic breakdown product, acetaldehyde, are cellular poisons. When they are present in the blood in continuing, large quantities, these chemicals damage the function of cells all over the body, including the muscle cells of the myocardium. The exact nature of the damage done to heart muscle is not clearly understood—it's a long-term thing that occurs in people who consume large amounts of alcohol regularly over a prolonged period of time—but, among other things, it has been documented that drinking large quantities of alcohol in a brief period of time can be irritating enough to the heart to trigger various kinds of arrhythmias in some people. It's also not clear to what

* Smoke-Enders, one of many available, and helpful, commercial stop-smoking programs.

degree chronic heavy drinking may contribute to the development of atherosclerosis; it upsets the carbohydrate metabolism in the body, certainly, and may influence cholesterol levels and triglyceride levels as well.

Of course, we are speaking here of possible heart damage from heavy, prolonged alcohol consumption. But a number of careful scientific studies have indicated that a *small* amount of alcohol taken daily actually may have some protective effect against coronary atherosclerosis and heart attacks. For one thing, a small amount of alcohol causes dilation of the smaller arteries and arterioles, as evidenced by the sense of flushing and warmth one feels from a cocktail or two, so that coronary blood flow may actually be increased temporarily. In addition, some studies have indicated that small amounts of alcohol tend to increase the level of protective high-density lipoproteins in the blood and reduce the level of the low-density lipoproteins, which are known to contribute to atherosclerosis.

Clearly, a moderate alcohol intake at least is not a terrible threat, in terms of coronary artery disease. The problem is to define precisely what we mean by "small amounts" of alcohol. All the studies reporting beneficial effects speak of a daily alcohol intake limited to approximately one beer a day, or a glass of wine daily, or a cocktail. Quantities above these very modest levels do not *increase* the beneficial effects, and quantities very much above these levels begin to be counterproductive because of cardiac toxicity. Most doctors I know would agree that no nondrinker should go out of his way to ingest alcohol in order to obtain the beneficial effects. The person who drinks at the modest level mentioned here can probably disregard his alcohol intake as any kind of risk factor, but the person who drinks significantly more than that on a daily basis may indeed be increasing his risk, even though the nature of the risk is not nearly as clearly defined as that of cigarette smoking.

10. *Age.* In most cases, coronary atherosclerosis does not tend to claim its victims until the middle decades of life. Catastrophe occurs most often during the decades from age forty through age seventy, with the peak incidence probably appearing at age fifty to sixty, slightly later in the case of women. As a general rule, the earlier a myocardial infarction occurs, the more likely it is to be severe. The individual who has an MI in his early forties is likely to have a severe, rapidly progressing degree of coronary atherosclerosis; the myocardial infarction that occurs is likely to be massive and the likelihood of death during the initial episode very high. By the same token, the individual who first develops evidence of CAD after age sixty is likely, in general, to have more slowly progressing disease,

with better collateral circulation already established, so that the MI, when it occurs, is likely to be less severe, its damage more limited in scope and the chances of survival far better. A woman is more likely to enjoy the protection of her estrogens during her forties, so that early severe MIs in women of that age are less common; but then, women become more vulnerable to more rapidly progressing disease after menopause, during their fifties and early sixties.

11. *Diet.* So many different things have been written about diet as a risk factor for coronary artery disease that many people are totally confused, and well they might be. The trouble is that nobody yet knows all the answers here, and patients may encounter as many different recommendations as there are doctors—or writers of special-diet books.

Many of the scientific studies, until recently, have been contradictory, but in spite of the confusion, certain facts seem to emerge as overall guidelines. Usually—not always, but usually—people who develop coronary atherosclerosis and later have myocardial infarctions are found to have high levels of both cholesterol and other blood lipids known as *triglycerides* in their blood. Although the body actually manufactures cholesterol out of other materials continually, most people with abnormally high cholesterol levels also eat large amounts of cholesterol-containing foods: whole eggs, cured fatty breakfast meats, fat-marbled beef, such seafoods as shrimp, clams, oysters, and anchovies, as well as organ meats, such as liver, sweetbreads, or kidneys, to name just a few foods that are extraordinarily high in cholesterol. In addition, these people also tend to eat large amounts of butter, cheese, whole milk, pork, lamb, and other foods loaded with saturated animal or vegetable fats. For example, almost all classical cheese (except a few skim milk cheeses) are high in butter fat; so are whipping cream, sour cream, and half-and-half. Saturated vegetable fats are found in the "old-fashioned" cooking oils and margarines made of cottonseed, coconut, or soybean oil, and to a lesser extent in peanut oil and olive oil as well. To make matters worse, recent studies suggest that many people may be genetically predisposed to manufacture more cholesterol than normal from such fatty foods—their genes may actually force their metabolisms to do this.

Other recent research also suggests that it may be the *total quantity* of fat in the diet that matters just as much as the *kind* of fat as far as elevated cholesterol and triglyceride levels are concerned. The average American diet may be composed of as much as 40 percent fat, but studies have indicated that if total fat intake is reduced to

30 percent or even 20 percent of the daily diet, cholesterol and triglyceride levels will usually decline.

What can a person do to reduce this dietary risk factor enough to do some good and still end up with a diet one can live with? The problem may not be as difficult as it would seem if you consider that many of the "dangerous" foods do not necessarily have to be totally eliminated—merely sharply reduced. The "typical American breakfast" of two fried eggs, three slices of bacon, hash brown potatoes, and toast slathered with butter offers a number of opportunities for reasonable and livable substitutions. Butter can be eliminated totally by substituting unsaturated margarine made from safflower or corn oil for frying and for toast. Nobody *has* to have two eggs when one will do just as well, and additional fat can be eliminated by boiling or poaching that egg rather than frying it. In addition, there are a number of very palatable cholesterol-free egg substitutes on the market, made largely of egg white and flavorings. These products, suitable for scrambling or omelets, may not taste exactly like real fresh eggs, but one can, with a little effort, suspend disbelief and use them at least part of the time. By reducing the breakfast eggs from two to one per day, then substituting a cholesterol-free egg substitute two mornings out of seven, a person can reduce his average weekly intake of cholesterol by 30 to 40 percent right there. If that same person substitutes medium-size eggs (which weigh about 50 grams each) for extralarge eggs (which weigh 70 grams apiece, with proportionately more cholesterol-laden yolk), the weekly cholesterol intake can be lowered even more without any terrible sacrifice in the quality of one's breakfast. Further reductions can be achieved by substituting a whole-grain cereal and toast for breakfast once or twice a week, and by substituting 1 percent or skim milk for half-and-half on the cereal and in the coffee.

You can take the same approach to reducing the saturated fats in your diet. As an example, a person can institute a rotation schedule for the dinner meals, serving fish one evening, poultry the next, a pasta meal the third evening, and a red meat—beef, pork, lamb—only every fourth dinner meal. To the person long accustomed to red meat and potatoes six days out of seven, this may seem like a radical shift in diet, yet it is perfectly workable and actually offers a pleasant variety that may have been absent before. Further, the person who uses classic cheeses—Cheddars, jack, bleu, or ripened cheeses—in some quantity almost daily, can easily reduce the use of cheese to once every three or four days, perhaps in association with a pasta meal. Butter use can be eliminated almost completely by substituting polyunsaturated margarine as a spread. The new butter-and-magarine mixes containing from 15 to 40 percent butter, depending on the brand, don't do the job as well as unsaturated margarine, but they are better physiologically than pure butter and tend to *taste* more like butter than plain margarine.

People could argue that this kind of approach to more healthful eating habits is merely hedging. I disagree. I think, on the contrary, that it is a pattern of eating that could be started early in life, and, if pursued as a matter of habit, would substantially reduce cholesterol and triglyceride levels on a lifelong basis, thus largely eliminating the dietary risk factor and very probably helping to control the obesity risk factor as well. The person who *must* change his eating habits following an MI might find this kind of program permanently tolerable, practical, and *achievable*. Bear in mind that we are talking about altering a slow, progressive disease process, and any changes directed at that goal, to help significantly, must be undertaken over the long term. Two or three months, then back to the old routine, just won't do. But widespread, long-term control of the dietary risk factor could make a very substantial difference in the incidence of coronary artery disease in the whole population.

12. *Tension, apprehension, and dissension.* Hardly anyone acquainted with cardiovascular disease seriously questions that such factors as anxiety, tension, or emotional conflict play a role in the development and progress of CAD, yet nobody yet has defined clearly what that role is, or, for that matter, clearly demonstrated that modifying these factors in one's life will necessarily reduce one's risk significantly. All we have is some reasonable speculation that reducing these factors may well be beneficial for some people.

Back in 1959, a cardiologist named Meyer Friedman, and his associate, R.H. Rosenman, in a now-classic article in the *Journal of the American Medical Association*, introduced the idea that so-called type A and type B personalities might respectively contribute to CAD or protect against it. People with type A or type 1 personalities, as described by Friedman, are all too common in our American society. These are the people with tense, anxious, hard-driving personalities, with obsessive-compulsive elements in their makeup— the ambitious, rarely satisfied workaholics who devote their lives to "achievement" on their own terms. These are the people who drive themselves constantly, work obsessively, and forever punish themselves for underachievement. They tend to eat irregularly and all the wrong foods. They often tend to drink too much, have never learned to let themselves relax, and are never satisfied with less than the most they can achieve (or more), at all times.

Type B or type 2 people are in sharp contrast. These people tend to be less tense, more easygoing or laid-back in their attitudes toward work and the world. They tend to do as little as necessary to get by, are not driven by ambition and are perfectly happy being relaxed. Type B personalities aren't entranced with work for its own sake; they suffer very little anxiety and tend to have more placid, accepting emotional responses to everything that happens to them. From his studies of people in these differing personality groups, Friedman concluded that people with the type A personality were markedly more vulnerable to coronary atherosclerosis and coronary artery disease developing earlier, and far more severely, than were their counterparts, the type Bs.

From the beginning many cardiologists disagreed with Friedman, but his ideas had a certain fascination, seeming to embody a certain amount of scientific common sense as well. It seemed reasonable that type A personalities would constantly be operating at higher adrenaline levels than their B counterparts, constantly living in states of fright, flight or siege, so to speak, with adrenergic hormonal factors constantly pounding away at their blood pressures, their hearts, and their coronary arteries. Maybe some people couldn't be clearly distinguished as A or B, but it did seem clear that many of the people, particularly the males, who were dropping dead of heart attacks in squadrons in their early forties, or were suffereing massive MIs in their early fifties, tended to have far more type A in their personalities than type B.

However a given type A personality may exert its influence, one thing seems clear: Once atherosclerosis is present in the coronary arteries, so that the myocardium is vulnerable to ischmia, there is no question that anger, anxiety, interpersonal conflicts, or obsessive-compulsive behavior can indeed trigger angina attacks just as effectively as hard physical exertion. It would follow that to whatever degree a person could reduce these emotional influences the better, as far as the health of the heart is concerned. Precisely how to go about altering these personality factors is beyond the scope of this book, but recognizing that such a risk factor exists is obviously a necessary first step in doing anything about it. For some people, just a careful, thoughtful, private reappraisal of relative values in one's life may reveal positive steps that could be taken to reduce levels of tension, apprehension, and dissension. For others, a perceptive physician might provide guidance, while in still other cases psychological or psychiatric counseling might help root out underlying reasons causing one to be driven to living a life in the fast track. But clearly the hard way to deal with the problem is to have your myocardial infarction first.

Assessing Your Risk Factors

It is clear from what we've just seen that practically everyone has at least *some* risk factors for coronary artery disease. But in order for you to do anything effective about reducing your risk, you need some way to assess which specific factors apply to *you*, and some scale on which to judge how minor or how grave your own individual risk may be.

The risk factors we have been discussing fall into three general groups, which can be listed as follows:

1. *Uncontrollable risk factors:*
    a. Age.
    b. Heredity.
    c. Sex.
2. *Controllable risk factors that must be discovered by medical examination:*
    a. Hypertension.
    b. Diabetes.
    c. Elevated blood lipids.
3. *Obvious and reducible or controllable risk factors:*
    a. Cigarette smoking.
    b. Obesity.
    c. Physical inactivity.
    d. Dietary habits.
    e. Tension, apprehension, and dissension.

This breakdown of risk factors is important if you are to make a sane assessment of the ones that affect *you*. Obviously you can't do anything about your age no matter how much you'd like to, and if you are in your late forties, fifties, or sixties, you are more vulnerable than if you are in your twenties. Equally obviously, you can't pick your parents, and, at least in most cases, you can't do anything about your gender. Nevertheless, these are factors that bear upon your risk and, therefore, need to be considered.

It's also obvious that you can't do anything about controlling the second group of factors if you don't know they're there. There are probably as many people with high blood pressure who just don't know it as there are who do. There are also multitudes of undiagnosed diabetics wandering around, and many people have no idea what their blood lipids are. These things, however, are all easily discoverable; a routine physical examination and a few simple, inexpensive laboratory tests will tell the story.

As for the self-evident risk factors in the third group, these obviously *can* be controlled or altered when they are present. But how can a person put all these things together and come up with an individual overall risk factor rating on some kind of meaningful scale?

It's not all that hard. What is needed is some kind of self-applicable test or individual risk factor examination. Recently, the Arizona Heart Institute, an outpatient facility for the diagnosis, treatment, and prevention of cardiovascular disease, based in Phoenix, Arizona, has come up with just such a self-applicable test that can be of immense value to virtually anyone who wants to assess his CAD risk factors as a baseline and guide for doing something about them. This simple, do-it-yourself test lists twelve basic risk factors and allows a person to score himself on each factor in order to come up with an individual risk factor score. The test not only checks for each risk factor but also assesses its relative importance, weighing the more dangerous or influential risk factors more heavily, the less dangerous ones more lightly. With the permission of the Institute, I have reprinted this cardiovascular risk factor analysis on page 182 in such a form that any reader can score himself to obtain a numerical risk factor rating. Immediately following the test is an analysis of the scoring provided by the Arizona Heart Institute.*

Dealing with Your Risk Factors

By using the previous test, you can obtain a remarkably accurate idea of precisely where you stand with regard to risk factors. But what can you actually *do* in terms of modifying or eliminating risk factors in your life? I can give you a living example from my own experience, simply by analyzing the risk factor score that applied to me before my heart attack five years ago and comparing it to my score today.

Before my heart attack, my risk factor score would have been 43 points. Now, five years later, on the program that I am currently pursuing, my risk factor points add up to only 26—and I could trim another 7 points off that score if I could bring my weight down another twenty pounds and reduce my cholesterol level just a few milligrams below its current level.

The message is clear: Coronary artery disease risk factors *can* be

---

* A similar risk factor self-appraisal test, called RISKO: A Heart Hazard Appraisal, has been developed by the American Heart Association. RISKO appraises most of the same factors as the Arizona test, but in a somewhat different way, and also produces an individual numerical risk-factor score, with an analysis of what the score means. If you want to compare results, you can obtain a copy of the RISKO test by writing: The American Heart Association, National Center, 7320 Greenville Avenue, Dallas, Texas 73231, or by telephoning the American Heart Association state office nearest you (telephone numbers listed in most major city directories).

Arizona Heart Institute
Cardiovascular Risk Factor Analysis

score

1. Age	Age 56 or over..	1
	Age 55 or under	0
2. Sex	Male...	1
	Female	0
3. Family History	If you have:	
	Blood relatives who have had a heart attack or stroke at or before age 60...........	12
	Blood relatives who have had a heart attack or stroke after age 60...............	6
	No blood relatives who have had a heart attack or stroke...................	0
5. Personal History	50 or under: If you had either a heart attack, a stroke, heart or blood vessel surgery..	20
	51 or over: If you had any of the above....................................	10
	None of the above...	0
5. Diabetes	Diabetes before age 40 and now on insulin....................	10
	Diabetes at or after age 40 and now on insulin or pills.........................	5
	Diabetes controlled by diet, or diabetes after age 55..........................	3
	No diabetes...	0
6. Smoking	Two packs per day..	10
	Between one and two packs per day or quit smoking less than a year ago...........	6
	If you smoke 6 or more cigars a day or inhale a pipe regularly.....................	6
	Less than one pack per day or quit smoking more than one year ago..............	3
	Never smoked..	0
7. Cholesterol (If cholesterol count is not known answer 8.)	Cholesterol level—276 or above................................	10
	Cholesterol level—between 225 and 275..........................	5
	Cholesterol level—224 or below................................	0
8. Diet (If you have answered 7, do not answer 8.)	Does your normal eating pattern include:	
	One serving of red meat daily, more than seven eggs a week, and	
	daily consumption of butter, whole milk, and cheese..........................	8
	Red meat 4-6 times a week, 4-7 eggs a week, margarine, low fat dairy	
	products and some cheese...................................	4
	Poultry, fish, little or no red meat, three or less eggs a week,	
	some margarine, skim milk, and skim milk products.........................	0
9. High Blood Pressure	If either number is:	
	160 over 100 (160/100) or higher..............................	10
	140 over 90 (140/90) but less than 160 over 100 (160/100)......................	5
	If both numbers are less than 140 over 90 (140/90)............................	0
10. Weight	Ideal Weight Formula:	
	Men = 110 lbs. plus 5 lbs. for each inch over 5 feet	
	Women = 100 lbs. plus 5 lbs. for each inch over 5 feet	
	25 pounds overweight..	4
	10 to 24 pounds overweight...................................	2
	Less than 10 pounds overweight...............................	0
11. Exercise	Do you engage in any aerobic exercise (brisk walking, jogging, bicycling,	
	racketball, swimming) for more than 15 minutes:	
	Less than once a week.......................................	4
	1 to 2 times a week..	2
	3 or more times a week.......................................	0
12. Stress	Are you:	
	Frustrated when waiting in line, often in a hurry to complete work	
	or keep appointments, easily angered, irritable..............................	4
	Impatient when waiting, occasionally hurried, or occasionally moody................	2
	Comfortable when waiting, seldom rushed, and easygoing.......................	0

SEX: _____ AGE: _____ STATE: _____ TOTAL POINTS: _____

Score Results

Tabulate your points. Compare with the charts below.

Please note: A high score does not mean you will develop heart disease. It is merely a guide to make you aware of a **potential risk.** Since no two people are alike, an exact prediction is impossible without further individualized testing.

With Answer to Question 9		**Without Answer to Question 9**	
High Risk............................40 and above		High Risk...........................36 and above	
Medium Risk...............................20-39		Medium Risk..............................19-35	
Low Risk.............................19 and below		Low Risk.............................18 and below	

identified and quantified, at least roughly, as low, medium, or high for each individual, using such a self-evaluation test. Once identified and quantified, many of these risk factors *can* either be eliminated or sharply modified without reducing the overall quality of life to any serious degree. This can be done even in the face of established coronary artery disease, with the overall effect of reducing the risk, reducing or slowing the progress of the disease, and, very possibly, evading or postponing catastrophe.

For young people the message is especially appropriate—and exciting. Without any question, modifying or controlling CAD risk factors is the wave of the future. If present or potential risk factors can be identified at the age of twenty or thirty and can be eliminated or at least modified on a lifelong basis, the likelihood of future trouble with CAD can be reduced very substantially for multitudes of people. For a great many the future risk can be virtually *eliminated*. It is not at all inconceivable that such programs, applied widely throughout society, promoted by public awareness and supported as a commonsense life-style in all age groups, could reduce the incidence of acute myocardial infarction by as much as 60 percent from the current level. And we are not talking about marginal numbers here, either. We are talking now about 300,000 *deaths* per year that could be prevented or postponed.

— 10 —

Autumn 1981 on the eastern slopes of the Cascade mountains was singularly beautiful. The summer had been long, warm, and dry, although not by any means warm enough for me. There were only a few summer days warm enough to drive me into our swimming hole in the chilly Taneum Creek, even though I tolerated the swimming perfectly well. By September the undergrowth on the hills and in the woods had turned a crisp, crackly brown, in contrast to the deep green of the firs and pines. The weather was sunny, the sky intensely blue, the nights becoming nippy. By deer hunting season in mid-October, the tamaracks were already turning their bright yellow, in contrast to the other conifers, and filling the air and covering the ground with thin yellow needles. From high points on Taneum Ridge or Cle Elum Ridge, one could look down into the

Taneum Canyon to see the glorious autumn display of cottonwoods on the creek bottom—huge, magnificent trees, turned flaming orange-yellow with the chilly nights.

That hunting season held particular significance for me, since I had made it a major first goal in my first year of recovery. The first anniversary of my heart attack was approaching, and I was determined to be on my feet and in the field again throughout the hunting season. In this respect the exercise program seemed to be paying off well. I was walking three miles every day on the level at a brisk pace, or else climbing up the irrigation ditch road or the old logging roads on either side of the canyon and finding that if I went slowly enough, I could evade the ill effects both of angina and shortness of breath. Of course, these exercise periods were confined to about an hour at a stretch, a far cry from the 5 to 10 miles of walking spread out over ten hours in a day that was our usual custom during hunting season, but I was determined to manage and was infuriated with Ann when I found her poring over our hunting maps planning easy hikes and undemanding downhill hunts for me to take.

As it turned out, Ann was right—I could not handle the physical exertion of "hunting as usual" nearly as well as I had hoped. We did have a hunting season, but it was severely limited. With the continuing use of the beta-blocker medication and judicious use of additional nitroglycerin to combat angina, I was able to travel the woods and game trails reasonably well, but found that exhaustion caught up with me after two or three hours. As it also happened, our deer season turned out to be sharply abbreviated when Ann bagged a small spike buck on our first morning out and I encountered a two-point buck with a crumpled horn up near the Gypsy Camp meadows above our house two days later, thus filling our deer cards in the first four days of a three-week season.

The elk hunt that year was not as generous. Our actual encounters with elk, male or female, always infrequent at best, were especially infrequent during that particular season. Neither of us saw a sign of a bull elk from the beginning of the season to the end. Many of our favorite hunting areas were slowly being destroyed by logging. On the one day that we made our way along the trail on the south Cle Elum Ridge to the Elk Tuileries—a hunt I insisted upon making—we not only saw no elk at all but found that loggers had clearcut over half of that beautiful area in the course of the summer. Thus our season that year was mostly devoted to seeking out new places to hunt, and I was able to take it in shorter, less vigorous spurts than usual. We searched out hunting spots where I could be deposited at the top and could then hunt downhill through an area to a prearranged place down below where Ann would leave the car.

Again, my fatigue determined the length of the hunt on any given day, and for the first time in years we did not attempt to cut up windfalls and load the Bronco full to build up our winter firewood supply. The gasoline-powered chainsaw we owned was more than I dared try to struggle with, too heavy and too awkward. We confined ourselves to scavenging cut-up pieces and small chunks of scrap wood we picked up along the road's edge and could take back home to cut up with a small, lightweight electric chainsaw we had there.

Thus as the elk season ended, my feelings were very mixed. I was grateful that I'd been able to get out in the field as much as I did, but I was bitterly disappointed that I couldn't really get out and *hunt*. It was like trying to hunt on crutches—the brick wall of physical limitation was always there. This was not only disappointing but depressing as well. It began to occur to me that maybe my recovery—my cardiac rehabilitation—was never going to be as complete as I had imagined it might be, no matter what I did to help it along. No matter how uncrippled I might feel from time to time, I was still crippled in a very basic way, and maybe the crippling wasn't going to get a lot better.

These feelings were borne out as that fall of 1981 moved into the winter months. My recovery seemed to have reached a plateau. Although things did not in any way seem to be deteriorating, they weren't perceptibly improving either. I was not quite sure at that point exactly what further improvement I expected or looked for, but it seemed to me there ought to be *some*. Meanwhile the fall had had other excitements than just the hunting season. After a careful assessment of all factors, Ann and I had decided to proceed with our original plans to enlarge our house at Thorp. The basically one-room kitchen–dining room–living room–bedroom with a tiny little study isolated by partitions in a corner was clearly not suitable for continued full-time living. Even though Ann was now gone for most of three or four days per week seeing her physical therapy patients, we were constantly tripping over each other, our household effects, and any guests we might happen to have. With the aid of Wayne White, the Ellensburg architect who had originally designed the cabin, breezeway and bunkrooms of the existing house, we designed a large additional wing, connected at an angle to the original building, two stories high, with a solarium at the same floor level as the original cabin, a large "sunken study" half a flight down, and an equally large master bedroom and balcony two-thirds of a flight up. Thus all autumn long, straight on through to the end of November, we had daily visitations of carpenters, electricians, plumbers, and sundry other artisans building on the new wing. It was finished and ready for us to occupy just before Thanksgiving.

Having this done just at the beginning of winter season went a long way toward relieving many sources of pressure and tension in our lives. It gave us our first real opportunity to spread out and find individual privacy since we had moved to Thorp full-time the year before. Throughout the turmoil and dust and dirt and noise of building, I had gone on with the intensive job of revising and finishing *The Fourth Horseman*, a task that extended well into February and March of 1982. This was the first "sustained drive" of intensive writing work that I had done since the heart attack, and I found that it came along very well—not as fast as before, perhaps, but fast enough, and most important of all, ultimately bringing in a satisfactory and publishable novel.

In short, the work level, the energy level, the basic physical capacity to do my writing seemed largely restored. Fred Cleveland's repeated question during my visits with him involved how I felt about the "quality of my life" and my "capacity to do what I wanted to do," and I always answered that I couldn't complain. In this respect I was getting along well on the medical program. He agreed, upon reviewing a repeat electrocardiogram, chest X ray, lab tests, and physical examination in March, that I was coming along swimmingly from his viewpoint. My blood pressure, which had fallen from borderline high levels before the heart attack to a stable 132/80, had never risen higher than that during this period, partly, no doubt, because the Inderal I was taking as an antianginal medicine also served as an antihypertensive medicine as well.

But if the medical program seemed to have established at least livable control of most symptoms of my coronary artery disease, it was not at any time providing complete control. Angina was still the major limitation. Medicine or no medicine, I still had episodes almost daily, sometimes on exertion, sometimes on exposure to cold, sometimes totally at rest, and sometimes waking me up in the middle of the night. I had long since learned to be very crafty about when to take additional nitroglycerin prophylactically before I intended any period of physical exertion in order to minimize or avoid the angina, yet it crept up on me every day in one way or another. It was a cold and unpleasant continuing companion that winter of 1981 to '82. I certainly did not care to have it with me as constantly as it was, yet at least I became used to it to the point that it didn't frighten me or distress me unduly.

It did distress Fred Cleveland, and he began talking hopefully of the new calcium slow-channel blocking agents that were being used in Europe quite successfully to control angina, especially angina at rest, or variant angina, and that were coming up for FDA approval during the spring and summer of 1982. Fred thought that I might well get a lot of help from one of these new medicines, and his enthusiasm at the prospect was contagious—I, too, began to look forward impatiently to the FDA approval of nifedipine, one of the calcium slow-channel blockers that could be taken orally.

When it finally did become available, however, it turned out to be a very bizarre drug indeed, at least in my case.

There were two of these drugs that came into use at that time: *nifedipine*, later marketed under the trade name Procardia, and *verapimil*, marketed under the trade names Isoptin and Calan. Verapimil got FDA approval first, but only for intravenous or intramuscular injection, and then only for specialized emergency use.

These drugs' supposed activity was very interesting. Evidence had been growing that so-called variant angina, or Prinzmetal's angina, or angina at rest, often resulted not so much from atherosclerotic plugging of coronary arteries as due to irritation and spasm of the smaller branch arteries, which could happen at any time, even when the heart was relatively at rest. Such spasm was thought to be triggered, at least in part, by perfusion of calcium ions into the muscle cells lining these arteries. The theory was that these new drugs could block perfusion of calcium into the artery walls and, thus, reduce muscle spasm that could bring on angina. In addition, these drugs could reduce the irritability and contractility of injured myocardial cells, thus reducing the work load on the heart and, perhaps, reducing the irritation that might trigger dangerous cardiac arrhythmias.

These drugs had been used in Europe on patients with coronary artery disease for several years prior to FDA approval in the United States. The European reports had all indicated that they did indeed work as anti-angina medications, but that their effect was erratic and could vary a great deal from patient to patient. It was as though part of the true picture of how these drugs acted was known but another part remained unknown or undemonstrated. Some cardiologists, therefore, regarded them pretty much as wild cards in dealing with angina, but because the drugs didn't seem to do any active harm to the people who used them, their use had been explored. Such questions had led the Food and Drug Administration to be very cautious about approving these drugs, to the intense frustration of cardiologists like Fred Cleveland, who believed that their usefulness far outweighed any possible hazards and who were agitating vigorously for their approval.

As soon as Procardia became available, Fred had me start using it in very small doses. The drug, which came in 10-mg capsules, was ordinarily supposed to be used in doses of up to three capsules four times a day, or 120 mg per day, but Fred started me off with one 10-mg capsule four times a day, with instructions to observe and report carefully what changes in my own anginal pattern I observed on that low dosage.

From the first it was apparent to me that this was a potent medicine indeed. During my first three or four days on the drug, it seemed to me that the amount of resting angina, far from decreasing, actually increased significantly, I began having episodes during the day when I had practically never had them before, and the episodes seemed to be prolonged and quite refractory to the nitroglycerin I usually took to relieve them. In addition, during that first week, I was awakened from sleep at one or two in the morning with angina attacks, for two or three nights in a row. Since Fred had said that I might experience some curiosities the first few days on the medication, I didn't report this to him, but after the third or fourth day I simply reduced my own dosage to one capsule three times a day, omitting the bedtime dose. On doing this, almost like magic, virtually all the resting angina that I had seemed to disappear. I had just as much angina on exertion as before, but far fewer attacks when I was sitting at rest, and, for a week or two, none at all at night. Since I had been bothered at least one or two nights a week with some degree of resting angina before, I regarded this as a great step forward.

The problem with this medicine was that this pattern seemed slowly to revert back to the original pattern after a week or two, so Fred recommended that I increase the dose again to four times a day, and if that seemed to stabilize, then go to two tablets three times a day. Thus, we started a period of dose-juggling with this medication, using my response as a kind of litmus-paper indicator of how much or how little I should be taking. Oddly enough, I found that virtually every *change* in daily dosage, whether a small increase or a small decrease, seemed to bring about a day or two of increased angina at rest, which would then settle down. Fred finally had me settle on two capsules three times a day, and in the long run, once the ups and downs were stabilized, I felt that the Procardia had brought about some degree of overall improvement in the resting angina, even if not a great deal.

I spent much of the summer and fall of 1982 playing with dosages of this new medication and staying more or less on an anginal plateau. Some weeks seemed a little better, some a little worse. I still managed to maintain my level of physical activity without increased discomfort, but once again I became aware of the brick wall that guarded its periphery. Push it a little too much, the angina was always there. What's more, it became obvious to me that my level of "permissible" physical activity was not increasing anymore: It remained flat, without any of the slow, gradual improvement in physical capacity that I had enjoyed before. In particular, I was bothered by muscular use of my upper torso—my arms, shoulders, pectorals, or upper back muscles. Sexual relations didn't seem to cause any trouble, but during that winter such activities as chopping kindling, carrying logs in for the fireplace, or anything else involving upper torso muscles seemed to bring on more angina, so I resigned myself to back away from these kinds of activities.

In addition, during that fall and winter I encountered an emotional reaction that rather surprised me in its intensity. During a visit with Fred in September (I was seeing him at about three-month intervals at this time), he informed me that he was reaching mandatory retirement age and that my December visit would be the last time that I would be seeing him. He intended to turn my care over to Dr. Robin Johnston, the cardiologist who had done my catheterization and angiograms.

When I heard this news, I was absolutely appalled. I knew, of course, that Fred was a few years my senior, but I had unthinkingly assumed that he would just go on forever as my doctor. I also knew that the Mason Clinic had definite retirement rules so that the "old boys" would not just hang around indefinitely, so it was not any choice of Fred's. But I was totally shaken at the prospect of suddenly shifting my care into the hands of someone I didn't really know. What I had never realized fully was how very much I had come to depend on Fred Cleveland as my doctor; to count on his wisdom, his quiet unflappability, his unerring good judgment, and the depth of his experience. From the first, to me he had seemed like a citadel of protection in the midst of a disastrous and frightening illness. But appalled or not, I made my last appointment with Fred for early December, after which I'd move down the hall to Dr. Johnston's office for care and advice.*

At the appointed time in early February I went in to see Robin Johnston. I knew him by reputation as a thoroughly competent cardiologist, and had encountered him very briefly at the time of the cardiac cath and angiography, but this was really the first time

---

* Fate plays bizarre tricks where coronary artery disease is concerned. I did see Fred in early December; he made some final adjustments in my medications; we spent some time talking about what he felt the future might hold for me at that stage in my recovery from catastrophe. We didn't talk much about what fate might hold for him; he said only that he and his wife had often wished that his work would allow them to travel more, and that they were contemplating a trip to Paris or some place like that come springtime. Fred's retirement date was December 31, 1982, but just a few days before that, I learned later, he himself suffered a severe myocardial ischemic attack, in the middle of his office schedule, and Dr. Richard Anderson and Dr. Wei-i Li performed coronary artery bypass surgery as an emergency procedure. He recovered and was doing well when last I talked to him in early 1986.

I had seen him as his patient. Whatever else might be said, it was immediately apparent that Robin Johnston was not Fred Cleveland. From the beginning he seemed a little more detached, a little more brusque, a little more hurried, and a little less interested overall in my unique problems than Fred had ever allowed himself to appear. At that visit, Robin reviewed the medication program that I was on, then began outlining some changes. First, he wanted me to stop taking the Norpace—I had had no trouble with arrhythmia for over a year now. No, it didn't have to be tapered off, just stop it abruptly, he said. He also wanted me to double the dosage of the calcium blocker, Procardia, that I was taking at that time, from one capsule four times a day to two, immediately, since, in his experience, it was only fully effective at the higher dosage level. Finally, as soon as that was accomplished, he wanted me to taper off the Inderal, if I found that I could do so without too much anginal distress. It was his feeling, he said, that it would be most ideal if my angina could be controlled by the nifedipine together with the Isordil and supplementary nitroglycerin, in order to dispense with the beta-blocker altogether.

I didn't argue, but I found the whole idea thoroughly alarming. The medical program I had been on wasn't doing the job completely, by any means, but at least things had been reasonably stable and predictable, and the thought of making sudden, abrupt changes was downright frightening. I thought of Fred's concern earlier about rocking the boat. Wasn't that what this amounted to? I wondered to myself if maybe Dr. Johnston was just indulging in the "new guy routine"—when the new guy takes over he's got to change everything right away to show that he's the boss.*

I expressed my concern about the changes to Dr. Johnston. He did seem to understand my apprehension and suggested that I might be more comfortable making the changes serially, one at a time, rather than all at once. This seemed sensible, especially if I could let him know of anything that seemed to be happening, and I agreed.

There was no problem discontinuing the Norpace. I stopped taking it that very afternoon and found no evidence of any recurrence of the arrhythmia. This was pleasing, because that drug alone was costing me around $45 a month to take. Changing the other two

---

* In all fairness to Dr. Johnston, I learned later, when I reviewed my medical records, that Fred Cleveland had written an extensive note in my chart after my December meeting with him, recommending almost all the changes that Dr. Johnston had mentioned. Among other things, Fred was apprehensive that the Inderal, the beta-blocker I was taking, might eventually bog me down into heart failure (something those drugs sometimes do), and he wanted me off it very soon, if at all possible.

medicines, however, seemed to lead to nothing but trouble. When I increased the nifedipine from one to two capsules four times a day, doubling the dose, a few days after dropping off the Norpace I found exactly the same thing happening as before when I increased the nifedipine dosage—the amount and duration of the resting angina sharply increased, exactly the opposite of the effect that was desired. These changes disappeared when I reverted back to the dosage I had been taking. Then, instead of trying to increase it all at one time, I tried increasing it just one capsule a day, and found myself faced with a changing pattern of angina with each small, incremental increase. After a couple of weeks, I managed to get the dosage of that drug up to two capsules three times a day, but not the four times daily that Robin Johnston had recommended, because those two extra capsules seemed to *cause* angina at rest every night that I took the bedtime dose.

Cutting down on the beta-blocker was even more disastrous. With the previous dosages, I had gotten used to having relatively little angina on exertion, just one or two brief episodes a day, especially in the morning, easily eradicated with nitroglycerin. When I started tapering back the Inderal, however, I immediately discovered just how much antianginal protection it really was providing. I dropped the four doses down to three, taking one in the morning, one at about three in the afternoon, the third at bedtime, and within a day I was having markedly more angina on my afternoon walk. When I tried discontinuing the bedtime dose, too, reducing the effective dose by half over a period of a week, I was faced with three or four quite severe angina attacks every day, and I found it extremely difficult to complete my hour-long walk without having two or three attacks before I got home. Within a week I found that I was eating nitroglycerin tablets like popcorn and still not achieving even halfway acceptable control of the angina. I went back to the original dose of the Inderal and found that all this trouble cleared up immediately. Then I tried reducing the dosage by just a half-tablet every other day. That time, it took four or five days before I began noticing the recurring severe angina, but there still seemed to be a limit to how little I could take without running into severe trouble.

I fiddled around with this for about two bad weeks, with much more angina on exertion than I cared to put up with, before I called Robin on the phone and reported what was happening. "Well," he said, "it was worth trying, but some people's angina won't let them get off the stuff. Cut the dose down as low as you can, and then don't worry about it."

Ultimately, I found that I could cut the total daily dosage down from 160 mg a day to about 140, and that was the lowest limit I could tolerate. Without the protection of the beta-blocker, I was having lots of severe angina. I found this very depressing, since I had always more or less anticipated that as my recovery continued, the angina would improve so that I ultimately might get off some of these exceedingly expensive medicines. (My bill for medicine alone was running about $1,600 a year.) Now it seemed that I was really going to have to take relatively large doses of this antiangina medicine forever.

It may seem, with all this medication-adjusting done largely on my own, that I was just playing doctor again, exactly what Fred Cleveland had urged me not to do. Maybe Dr. Johnston was a little disgusted at this, too, although he never said so. But the fact was, *I* was the one who was having the angina. With these medicine changes, I was having a lot of it, and it *hurt*, and I was very sensitive to it, and by that time very, very tired of it. It was extremely depressing to know that it was constantly waiting just around the corner, ready to slug me any moment that I got to feeling too smart or self-satisfied. There were times, during a two-hour seige in the middle of the night, when the thought would come to me that I'd just about had it, that it might not be all that bad if I just shuffled off in the middle of a siege and had it over with, instead of having to live with it, forever. There was absolutely nothing even remotely suicidal about this thinking, it was far more a matter of anger and frustration than hopelessness, a matter of sitting in recurrent agony waiting for the other shoe to drop, and thinking that, if it *did* drop, it might not be as bad as not having it drop.

Ann, of course, was aware of the trouble, and she coped as best she could, but there was very little she could do. There was the unspoken understanding between us that she would ignore my angina attacks, or pretend to, because I couldn't bear to feel that she was being upset by them. Her job, it seemed, was to go along as if everything were going reasonably well, and not make waves. The problem was that she couldn't keep herself from sometimes making waves, and I couldn't keep myself from resenting it.

There was an additional depressing element that Ann and I both came to recognize during this period: the plain fact that our sexual relationship was slowly but steadily deteriorating. I haven't said much about our sex life so far in this account, largely because there hadn't been anything particularly remarkable to say about it. Neither of us had ever been wary or scared of sex since the heart attack, as many coronary patients are. A particularly vigorous session could trigger a little angina, but this seemed easy enough to prevent with an extra dose of nitroglycerin or two taken in advance. What was happening now was something different: An odd degree of emotional alienation seemed to be setting in, together with a decline on my part both in interest and in performance.

Unquestionably, a lot of the problem had to do with medicines. Beta-blockers are notorious for knocking down the libido, although doctors and drug manufacturers alike seem reluctant to mention this to patients. Antidepressant drugs, including lithium, can do the same thing, and I was taking both beta-blockers and lithium. But much of the trouble lay in the emotional relationship that had evolved between Ann and me. I was certainly excessively irritable and self-preoccupied during those days. Ann kept doing little things that angered or irritated me, often to an irrational degree. I would irritate Ann back; then she would get mulish, plant her heels in the ground, and refuse to budge, no matter how ridiculous the point might be. Often, the irritating things were completely petty: her calling up-stairs in the morning with her imperative, three-minute warning for breakfast, when I didn't feel like rushing to get dressed; bringing home packages of fake bacon for me to eat that were low in salt, low in cholesterol, and low in flavor as well; forgetting to stockpile an extra jar of freeze-dried coffee, so that I would run out in the middle of the day; that sort of thing. Probably an element of cabin fever was at work too: I didn't get out much or see too many people, often by choice, yet I resented Ann's gallivanting around seeing her patients.

Whatever the causes, the problem was real, and it certainly didn't help during a very troublesome time. We didn't hide from it; we tried to deal with it the best we could, which wasn't very well. It was just one more headache we didn't really know how to handle.

Eventually, of course, the long period of juggling medication came to an end, with at least temporarily "ideal" dosages of everything established once again, and the angina once again reasonably under control, but on a somewhat poorer plateau than before. Unfortunately, however, during that winter and spring of 1983 I began to notice the appearance of some other problems, problems that I hadn't really noticed before to speak of. Occasionally I would awaken at night and find myself having some slight difficulty breathing, a fullness in the chest, as though I had some phlegm or mucus in my bronchi that I couldn't quite clear out. This was not painful in any way, merely annoying, enough of an irritant to keep me just dozing for a couple of hours instead of really getting back to sleep again. While I *was* asleep, Ann began to notice that I had occasional episodes of Cheyne-Stokes breathing—seconds-long periods of not breathing at all, followed by periods of deep, rapid breathing, to catch up, so to speak. At the same time, I noticed a little bit of edema or puffiness of the ankles occasionally, present one day, gone the next. Finally,

I found that the shortness of breath would appear much more markedly on my vigorous walking expeditions than ever before. Bit by bit, on occasion, I would have more trouble in the morning on awakening and getting showered and dressed than I had before. I would have spells of angina in the process of dressing, accompanied by shortness of breath brought on with as little exertion as just bending over to tie my shoes.

All this came into particular focus during a visit we made in late February 1983, when we spent a week at a friend's condominium at Lake Tahoe. We had been invited repeatedly to use the place on a moment's notice, and an opportunity presented itself when a cardiology conference was scheduled at a Lake Tahoe hotel, offering me a chance to earn some of the necessary Continuing Medical Education credits required annually for me to maintain my state medical license.

Lake Tahoe, of course, is located at an elevation of six thousand feet, four thousand higher than our home in Thorp. It was a nasty February in Nevada, cold and sloppy, with intermittent snow, and it was necessary to keep hopping in and out of our rented car to put on or take off chains driving to and from the hotel where the meetings were held. In addition, the condo was a two-story apartment in a two-story building, with our bedroom on the ground floor, the kitchen and living room up a steep stairway on the second floor.

During the five-day visit, I began having very noticeable problems with dyspnea—shortness of breath—getting up, showering, dressing on the bedroom level, then walking upstairs for breakfast on the second level. I could *do* it, all right; I just had to do it very, very slowly, stopping to rest, for example, between putting on one shoe and putting on the other. At the same time I noticed that the ankle swelling was more marked than it had been before, and this continued all the time we stayed at Lake Tahoe. I also seemed to have more trouble with angina here than before, with a couple of bad nights: awakening with angina, taking as much nitroglycerin as I dared, and still having the angina persist for a couple of hours before it passed.

Probably this was a perfect example of a doctor-patient knowing too much for his own good. None of these new symptoms or changes was particularly dramatic or sudden, or, for that matter, even physically demonstrable, except for the ankle edema. What I was feeling were some subtle internal, visceral sensations indicating that something was different, that something was changing. But these changes seemed to strike a chord from my years of practice. They were very much the sort of symptoms that I had always associated with borderline heart failure—a slow weakening of overall heart function, with the heart slowly failing to keep up with the pumping job demanded of it. As soon as I realized that, I immediately recalled Fred Cleveland's remark, two or three years before, that the real galloping threat to my life was not so much a recurrent myocardial infarction as plain old heart failure. And I had quite enough medical awareness to do a thoroughgoing job of worrying about these changes.

On returning from Lake Tahoe, I saw Robin Johnston at my next scheduled appointment and reported these things to him. At that precise moment I didn't actually have any ankle swelling to speak of. He listened to my heart and listened to my lungs, ordered a new chest X ray, and then sort of spread his hands. "I don't see any sign whatever of heart failure," he told me. "Your lungs are perfectly clear, your heart sounds fine, you have no edema, your liver isn't tender—don't worry about it."

I suggested that maybe this was something that was beginning to turn up on a very borderline level, that perhaps I was aware of subtle indications of trouble that he couldn't detect or confirm because he couldn't feel the sensations himself, and could find no physical evidence to support them. "Maybe so," he said, "but frankly, I just don't see anything to treat. I don't think anything bad is going on, except that your weight isn't down any since last time. Why don't you work on that a little harder?"

And, in fact, these problems did seem to quiet down during the rest of that summer and fall. I was still having too much angina on exertion during my afternoon walks, yet even this varied from day to day. One day I would have to stop two or three times to take nitroglycerin and allow the angina to quiet, whereas another day it would hardly appear at all. The "borderline heart failure," as I came to think of it, did recur now and then, perhaps once a month, for a couple of days; then it would seem to settle down again. I continued to report this to Robin at my quarterly checkups, and he continued to pronounce me completely free of any evidence of heart failure and suggest that I was worrying too much. And, indeed, we went into the hunting season that autumn of 1983 and moved through it with relatively little trouble. Here, during my season of highest-level physical exertion, I found myself with very little angina, except when I tried to speed things up too much. By hunting very slowly, and selecting downhill hunts, I got along without any more problem than I had had the season before.

In fact, one episode toward the end of the elk hunt that year suggested that I was really doing much better than I thought. Deer season had been dull—we hardly even saw a doe—and elk season was much the same, until one afternoon two days before the season ended. During that last week, Ann and I had been hunting an area of middle elevation, a partly logged, part heavily wooded foothill area surrounding an old abandoned homestead cabin, known as the Cummins place. We had explored and found a "northwest passage" up into this plateau area from the Taneum Creek road at the bottom, and there was an old logging road that led down into the area from above. On this particular day, Ann dropped me off at the road up above so that I could make my way slowly down to the Cummins place. She was then to drive down to the bottom, take the northwest passage road and trail up to meet me in the middle, a hunt that we knew would take approximately three hours, with both of us hunting toward each other through an extremely promising elk area.

The night before, two or three inches of fresh snow fell on top of three or four that had already fallen, and the weather had been quite cold, so the new snow was fluffy. I made my way slowly down the main logging road through some cut-over areas, then into a patch of woodland that gently sloped down a series of benches, from left to right. Farther right, the land fell steeply through dense woods toward a camping place called "Josh's" on Taneum Creek. I was going slowly and quietly, not really expecting anything much to happen, since we had seen so little evidence of animals this season. At one point I jumped a large doe out of the woods to the left of the road; she crossed the road, and, in a series of enormous bounds, went down the steep slope to the right before stopping a hundred yards away to look back up at me through the trees. Since her tracks were immediately in front of me on the road, I paced them off, marveling that she had been clearing fifteen to twenty feet with each bound.

As I worked my way on down the road, about one o'clock in the afternoon I stopped and ate my lunchtime sandwich. I was coming to a point where several small logging spurs cut up to the left from this main road, curving around a shoulder of a logged-off hill that had a little timber and lots of tall buckbrush standing on it. On a whim I started walking up one of these little spurs, glancing up the hill, and then, quite suddenly, I saw a large cow elk standing in a tiny clearing about seventy-five yards above me, staring down at me. When I stopped and froze, she moved into a dense clump of saplings and buckbrush, but then I saw movement farther up the slope, and three more cows came down out of a clump of woods into the little clearing behind the first one. They were followed by a small, spike-horned bull that crossed the clearing in the course of a couple of seconds. He was followed by yet another cow, then a larger spike bull.

These animals had appeared suddenly, almost magically, as though they had just materialized right there on the hillside, their black heads and tawny bodies in sharp contrast to the snow-covered hillside and the dark blue-green of the firs. I had simply glanced up the hill and there they were. I was so startled that I didn't even bring my rifle up until I saw the first bull. They were not running, but covered the ground very swiftly with their long-legged walking gait. I got the second bull into my sights for a split second and fired a single shot just as he disappeared into the buckbrush. The shot startled the elk, and I heard them crashing through the thick patch of woods, around the shoulder of the hill, to my left.

I ran down the little spur to the main road, hoping that they might drop down the hillside and cross the road in the open, but I saw nothing. Then I went back to where I had fired the shot. My heart was pounding with excitement, and the angina moved in; I stuck an Isordil tablet under my tongue, along with the usual nitroglycerin, and waited for the pain to pass. I felt sure that I'd missed my shot; there had been no sign or suggestion of any animal going down up there. But as soon as the angina passed, I began climbing up the steep, snowy slope some seventy-five yards toward where I'd seen the animals. At least they would have left tracks in the snow, and tracks could be followed.

I had to stop three or four times on the climb up, slipping in the snow, grabbing buckbrush to keep from sliding down, the slope was so steep. Each time I stopped I had to wait until I got my breath back. I began grasping at straws: Maybe I would get up there and find that second bull lying dead on the ground—it was conceivable that I might have hit him; you never knew until you looked. Finally, after ten or fifteen minutes of very hard work, I reached the point where the tracks went across. There was no dead bull there, but there was a small sprinkling of blood in the snow.

I followed the tracks through the woods, around the shoulder of the hill. There was not much blood, only a drop or two here and there, but obviously I had at least nicked the animal. According to the rules of hunting, when you know you've hit an animal, you follow it and find it if you possibly can. I traced the tracks for another two hundred yards in the snow, through dense brush and small firs. Then, quite some distance around a bend in the main road, the animals' tracks turned straight downhill, indeed crossing the road up above a curve that I could not have seen from below. They went straight across the road, then down, down, down an almost-vertical slope to another bench some five hundred feet below.

I knew that beyond that lower bench the land dropped precipitously another five hundred feet, through dense woods, to a large, flat area, before descending to Josh's camp and Taneum Creek at the bottom of the canyon. I also knew that going after that elk was obligatory—but starting off on a rugged, three-hour chase all by myself just didn't make sense. I was already short of breath and waiting for the lingering edges of the angina to subside. Since it was common hunting lore that following hard and fast on the trail of a wounded elk in the snow was not necessarily the most fruitful tactic— many hunters would deliberately delay for half an hour or so in order to allow the animal to find a bed somewhere where he might be surprised later—I decided to go on down the road to meet Ann first, then come back with her to pick up the trail. She was longer than I had expected, partly because she was having trouble with a knee that she had twisted earlier in the season, so it was a good hour before we returned to the trail crossing the road and started down the steep slope to the first bench, beginning at about two-thirty in the afternoon.

It was clearly evident before we had gone very far that I could only have nicked the bull in the flank with my single shot, since there was no evidence whatever that he had been badly wounded. There were occasional blood drops every twenty or thirty feet, but there was no place where the animal had crept into a thicket to lie down, as almost certainly would have happened if he had been seriously wounded at all. What's more, the group of elk had all stayed together, whereas a badly wounded bull almost certainly would have soon broken away from the rest. We followed the tracks down the five-hundred-foot slope, out on the bench, meandering back and forth around on the bench, then starting down through the deep woods to the other bench below. No sight or sound of any elk. At one point, the blood trail did break away momentarily from the rest of the elk and pass into an extremely thick area of brush, but then immediately backtracked and rejoined the group.

At the bottom of this second slope, which was extremely steep and difficult to negotiate, there was a large area of flat land that had recently been logged over and then abandoned, because, according to rumor, the gyppo doing the job had run out of money. For an area of about ten acres trees had been fallen in a jackstraw jumble, lying on the ground, criss-crossing each other, an almost impenetrable thicket of two-foot tree trunks covered with big heaps of limbs and needles. The elk had come into this area and apparently had just as much trouble getting through it as us; time and again, tracks indicated starting off in one direction, running into a blockade, turning around and heading another direction, only to run into another block. At the bottom of this logged area was a fresh skid road, which Ann thought would lead down to the creek and Taneum Road, and she decided to leave me to wander through the tangle while she went to retrieve the car and bring it back to Josh's. The plan was for me to go on down and come out at Josh's by dark, which meant around four-thirty at that time of year, whether I had found the elk or not.

I spent a good hour climbing up and over logs and brush, following those elk tracks with the encouragement of a little drop of blood in the snow here and there, indicating that I was still on the right trail. Two or three times I stopped for nitroglycerin, expecting to jump the elk beyond the next tree trunk at almost any moment. No such thing happened. Finally, I followed the trail out of the logged-over bramble, around the side of a little knob hill, and into the undisturbed deep woods above Josh's. Just when it became dark, I came on a very old road that I knew worked its way down to the creek, but at this lower elevation the snow had disappeared and the elk trail vanished into the thick ponderosa pine duff lying on the bare ground. At one point, making my way slowly down the road, I saw an animal out of the corner of my eye crash through the brush, away from me, at the noisy dead run so characteristic of a spooked elk, but all I saw really was a flash of tawny hide, black legs, and it was gone.

I never did see that elk again. The three-hour chase was exhausting, but we were back at dawn with our neighbors, Bob and Wilma Dlouhy, to comb the area once again, with no result. Once again the quarry had proved incredibly elusive. Later that morning, we encountered a hunter who said that he had come up from the bottom at Josh's at dawn, much as we had, and had jumped two or three cows and a spike bull out of the dense brush near the creek, but they had vanished before he could get a shot off, leaving no trail in the pine duff. He said that he had hunted them down there all morning without ever seeing or hearing them again.

That experience at the very end of the elk season demonstrated two things to me with equal clarity: first, that I could, indeed, still hunt effectively, since I don't think I would have done anything any different had I been in tip-top condition; but second, that there were clear limitations on what I could do, and that probably on that day I had pushed myself about to the limit that I could tolerate. Progressive recovery, and good control of the angina and the shortness of breath, were just as elusive as that bull elk had been. During the December and January that followed, Ann and I made one or two trips over to the Columbia Basin for an undemanding look for ducks and geese, but, for the most part, that winter I stuck close to my desk, maintaining my regular walking program but recognizing that the angina was gradually, almost imperceptibly, closing in, and that the "borderline congestive failure" episodes were occurring more frequently, particularly in the mornings, and becoming more bothersome.

There were days during that winter and spring of 1984 when I just didn't feel good, in a vague sort of way, until nine-thirty or ten in the morning, and the nocturnal angina was becoming a more frequent visitor. But the next time I saw Robin, in March or so, he again insisted that there was no evidence that he could see of any congestive heart failure. He fiddled with my medications, again urging me to increase the Procardia and try to cut back on the Inderal, both of which I tried, both of which I could not succeed in doing. More and more during that spring I began to feel that there was a gulf of communication—or at least a gulf of comprehension—between what I was experiencing and feeling going on inside me and what Robin Johnston was able to determine objectively from physical examination, and it seemed to me, more and more, that he wasn't really crediting my perception that something new and different was going on.

When the time came for my next visit with him in early June, a turning point was finally reached. This time, unlike other times, I asked Ann to come in to Robin's office with me. When Robin came in, I confronted him with the fact that I was very certain something untoward and undesirable was going on, whether he could find any evidence of it or not. I told him my angina on exertion was growing slowly but perceptibly worse. I hadn't had any recurrence of the arrhythmia, but I was bothered more and more by the nocturnal angina episodes, which tended to hang on for two or three hours when they came, regardless of any nitroglycerin that I took. I told him that the sense of terrible fullness in my chest and shortness of breath that came on so many mornings was becoming debilitating. I said I clearly did not feel that things were getting better or even remaining stable, despite his physical findings on my visits. Things were getting progressively worse, and it seemed to me that this worsening was beginning to accelerate.

At that visit I had the feeling that Robin was finally really listening to me. "Of course, you could be right and I could be wrong," he said when I had finished. "Maybe I've just been hoping too much that things were happening that aren't actually happening at all, or trying too hard *not* to see things that really are happening. Whatever is going on, you're obviously unhappy, and that's no good at all. Maybe it's time for a complete reevaluation, time to take a fresh look at the whole picture."

With that, he then suggested a plan of attack that seemed eminently sensible to me. Then and there, he did a complete and exhaustive physical examination; then he asked me to stay in Seattle until the next day in order to get a new chest X ray, an electrocardiogram, and a variety of lab studies. "Let's get a baseline of where you are as far as we can see right now," he said. "Meanwhile, I will pull out all the old records of your cardiac cath and angiograms and look at them again, take another look at all the opinions that led to the course of treatment we're following. Then when all this is together, let me take the whole current picture back to the cardiac conference and see if there's any consensus that we ought to be considering something different." I agreed to come back for an appointment with him a month later for a review of this new workup and of any new cardiac conference assessment.

When that time came, in July 1984, Robin Johnston went over his findings in detail. The physical and laboratory findings, as far as he could see, were unchanged from a year before, even two years before. My blood pressure was staying down to a safe 130/80. The chest X ray was clear, and there was no sign of any heart enlargement that would suggest any progressive heart failure. The EKG was unchanged, with no evidence of new infarction or damage, no evidence of ventricular hypertrophy that might be consistent with approaching or progressive heart failure. "Frankly, I *still* don't see any evidence that you have any degree of heart failure," Robin told me. "But I have to believe that you really are feeling something going on. Your blood cholesterol level is down to 240, which is about the lowest we've ever measured it. All your other laboratory studies are fine. Basically, all the evidence that I have before me suggests that your recovery is on a stable plateau, and staying there."

"And the cardiac conference assessment?" I asked.

"They aren't quite so sure that things are really all that stable," he admitted. "The general consensus was that there is nothing going on that should stampede us into reconsidering our treatment, no reason suddenly to rush in to do bypass surgery, because you really have been doing at least adequately well on the medical program. On the other hand, the consensus is that your recovery reached a plateau maybe a year or a year and a half ago, and that now maybe you are gradually beginning to lose ground. Maybe you're going to have more and more angina. Maybe you are indeed going to get into some overt trouble with congestive heart failure. Bypass surgery won't help congestive heart failure a bit, but it might help relieve the angina."

"So what does this add up to?" I asked.

"The others think, and I agree, that this decision has really got to be up to you," Robin said. "Let's go along for a while longer just as we are but pay more attention to these internal feelings of yours. Even if you're having more angina, you're generally able to do most of the things that you want to do without a really distressing amount of discomfort. If the angina gets worse, you'll know it. If in the next few months or the next year, you reach a point that the angina is bothering you more than you want to put up with, then we have to consider acting. You'd be a higher-risk patient for coronary bypass surgery than any of us would like, particularly the surgeons, but if you reach a point that you're having angina every time you get out of your chair, or even to the point that it's an active daily distress and you don't want to live with it anymore, then maybe the benefit could outweigh the risk." He looked at me. "Put it this way, Alan: If *you* decide that *you* think the time has come to consider a bypass, the cardiac conference would not be opposed to the idea. But in a very real sense, you've got to be the doctor now, because you know what's going on better than I do. In fact, *any* patient in this situation has to be the doctor."

We went along through that summer and fall as Robin had suggested. Certainly, this reevaluation presented me with a totally different way of looking at what was going on. There were suddenly options that could be based on circumstances and events. The very thought that there *might* be options when no options whatsoever had been available before seemed to me both uplifting and exhilarating. Before this reevaluation it had seemed to me that I was looking forward to a steadily descending spiral of capacity and capability, with no ultimate hope for relief in sight—a matter, in a way, of "dying inside," as Bob Silverberg had put it so beautifully in one of his novels. At the same time, the sudden appearance of possible options was startling and frightening. I was by no means ready to rush into the surgeon's office the next day. Although I had complained about it a lot, I knew that I really was not yet in all that much desperate trouble with the angina. Perhaps it was just the terribly depressing aspect of having no options that had worried me the most, and if the options were now there—if the possibility of corrective surgery at some later stage was now there—I could ride with what was going on. If the time came that I really wanted to act, as Robin had expressed it, I would jolly well know it. So ride I did.

During that summer and fall, two experiences helped define what was happening and mold the direction in which it would be necessary to go. Since early spring, my son, Jon, and I had been planning a fishing trip to the high Cascades, in the Pasayten wilderness area, when he came home for a short vacation from his graduate studies at Cal Tech. I knew that I was not about to carry a forty-pound backpack twelve miles in and five thousand feet up to the high fishing lakes in that wild area, but there was an alternative: to make it a pack trip, with horses to ride and mules to carry our gear. We made our plans for a six-day trip to some highland lakes at about the six thousand-foot level and arranged with a wrangler to pack us in and out. We started off on the trip during the third week in August.

I will not dwell upon the delights of that trip into the wilderness, other than to say that if riding a horse miles and miles up a mountainside is better than walking up with a heavy backpack, it isn't a whole lot better. Neither of us were riders, the horses were uncooperative, the mode of travel incredibly uncomfortable. But finally, at the end of a seemingly endless day, we were deposited, with far more gear than we ever could have backpacked, on the shores of a lake, twelve miles into the Pasayten wilderness, for a five-day fishing trip.

Nothing exactly disastrous happened during those five days, and yet I seemed to have a bad time of it. We made a snug camp with separate tents near a fine large fire pit, and it didn't rain, but the weather was cold at that elevation, especially for mid-August. And although we had plenty of warm clothes with us, I never really got thoroughly warmed up from the time we arrived to the time we left. The sun was out only intermittently during the day, accompanied by a chilly wind, and at night it became downright frosty. I had some angina on the trip up, wrestling with the horse, and, once there, I seemed to have increased amounts of angina on very little exertion, turning up far more frequently than at home. In addition, the first two nights I had severe and prolonged trouble with nocturnal angina at one-thirty in the morning, and lasting almost until four, even though I ate so much nitroglycerin that it gave me a headache— something that rarely happens. The only way I could seem to get it to quiet would be to sit up in my tent, with it recurring as soon as I lay down again. So I spent two or three hours each of the first two nights sitting up in my sleeping bag, wishing the pain would go away. The third day and night it seemed much better, but the fourth night it was right back again.

On top of all this—or, perhaps, because of it—I found that I just didn't feel very well, and that I had very little energy to do anything but putter around camp or read a paperback novel, while Jon went gallivanting off in his hiking boots up over rocky ridges and down into neighboring lakes to fish. I did some desultory fishing in the lake where we were camped, and on the outlet stream that ran down a hill into a series of meadow pools, but even though the fishing was reasonably good and we had a couple of nice trout dinners, I couldn't seem to get enthusiastic about it. Jon noticed that I wasn't at my best and undertook most of the heavy work around camp— going out to forage for firewood, for example, and breaking it up for burning. It irritated me that I had to flop around like an invalid at a time when I had planned to join him in activities, but there seemed to be an activity stone wall that I just couldn't scale. I tried to explain it to myself, saying that it was just a matter of altitude sickness, that I was trying to do too much with too little oxygen in the air, but then I realized that this was really just another name, in my circumstances, for "borderline heart failure." When I tried to define the difference, I found that I couldn't find any clear distinction. Certainly, the altitude had something to do with it, since it all seemed to settle down immediately on returning home—at least to the level it had been before.

All in all, not such a good trip for me, or for Jon, either. At home, before we left, he had sensed that things were not totally placid between his mother and me; he had noticed that I seemed hyper-irritable, shorter with her than he remembered, and we talked about this a little during the trip, about some of the frustrations and irritations that both Ann and I were increasingly experiencing—the sort of things I had never talked about with any of our children in my life. He was distressed about this, but he was *really* taken aback at the amount of physical distress and debility I was experiencing. I realized later that I had never really indicated to any of the kids how much the continuing angina and other physical problems were bothering me. Jon had assumed, once the immediate crisis of the heart attack was over, that I had really fully recovered, and "just had to take it a little easy," as he put it. Thanks to my lack of communication and sense of secretiveness about this, it was not until now that he realized how far off the mark that assumption was.

The second experience, far more alarming, occurred about two months later in the fall, at about the beginning of the second week of deer season. The opening of every hunting season necessarily marked a radical change in Ann's and my pattern of daily activities. Each morning that one or both of us intended to hunt, we would shift our alarm clock awakening back to five A.M. then galvanize ourselves into vigorous action: an abbreviated sip of coffee, dressing as fast as we could in the layer upon layer of hunting clothes that we had laid out the night before, preparing and eating enough of a breakfast to sustain us for several hours' hunting, fixing a Thermos of coffee and sandwiches for lunch,* then climbing into our hunting boots, lacing them up, all accomplished in the space of an hour in order to get into the car and on our way to wherever we were going

---

* Neither Ann nor I ordinarily drank enough coffee to amount to a hill of beans, certainly not so much as to threaten my heart in any way or interact with any of my medicines, but on bitter cold hunting days we *did* like to have a cup of coffee after our first morning hunt, and again at lunchtime.

to hunt, all before daybreak, which came at around a quarter of seven at that time of year.

This year, I found this unaccustomed rush in the early morning was noticeably more distressing than it had ever been before. I would start out short of breath, stop to combat angina two or three times in the middle of things, stop to rest in the midst of dressing, take ten minutes to get into my boots and get them laced up, because leaning over to tie them was such an effort, then remain short of breath until we got out into the car on the road. It was not always the same every day, nor was it always consistent. One morning I would have relatively little trouble, the next a great deal, without any rhyme or reason to it.

At the particular time in question Ann and I had been hunting in an area quite close to home, really just up at the top of the ridge across the creek from us, but accessible by road only by driving five or six miles out into the valley, then cutting back up a logging road that went up on the top. It was not a singularly good area for elk during the season, but earlier, during deer season, we would almost always encounter deer in this area.

This year, we had worked out a new scheme for hunting the region: Ann would drop me off at the top of the area, so that I could hunt through a series of meadows and woods, then down an old abandoned logging spur, while she would take the car around and down below me a couple of miles, then still-hunt very quietly at the bottom of the region, in hopes of seeing animals that I might spook out from above. We would take about two and a half or three hours for this particular hunt, and I would end up meeting her at the car down below.

The particular morning in question, in mid-October, was only a little worse than usual. We had slightly overslept, and, consequently, felt somewhat more hurried than usual that morning. Once we were ready to leave, the car didn't want to start (it was cold and frosty), and we had to fiddle with that for a while. After we had driven out to the end of the Hutchins road and started up it, still in darkness, another hunter's rig planted in the middle of the road with its lights out suddenly started up, turned on its lights, and raced on up ahead of us, a commonplace little trick that some hunters will pull that invariably infuriated me. As a consequence, I remained short of breath all the way up into the hunting area, even when the other rig turned off to the left to go up the old road into Rattlesnake Canyon, an area that we were not interested in hunting. We arrived at my drop-off point in good time, still quite dark, so that I would have the time needed to make my way across a small, open meadow and over a fence and gate to a posting place, where I ordinarily would stand and watch for movement until it became light enough to make out animals at greater distance. This would give Ann enough time to get down and reach her starting place.

As I stepped out of the car and Ann took the wheel, we reaffirmed our plan. She would drive down and start slowly out along the bottom of the area while I came down slowly from the top. If we didn't meet somewhere in the middle, she would return to the car in time to meet me there in two and a half hours. If either of us got anything, we would use our usual "come quickly" signal—two quick shots, followed by two more five minutes later—and, in the event that we somehow didn't meet at the appointed time where she'd parked the car, she would come up and wait where she had dropped me off; she had to come back that way anyway in order to go see patients later in the morning.

As she drove on up the road, I could hear the car clanking away in the ruts. It was still quite dark, but I wanted to get across the little meadow, over the fence, and into the woods before more cars came up the road, since I didn't particularly want to advertise that I was hunting in this area or attract other hunters to follow me. I loaded my customary four shells into my rifle—a very accurate .270-caliber Browning that I had used for years, with 120-grain shells for deer. I closed the bolt with a shell in the chamber, set the safety, slung the rifle over the shoulder of the heavy red-and-black-checked woolen lumberman's jacket that I was wearing, and started walking briskly across the meadow toward the gate.

I got about halfway there, when suddenly I realized that something was going on that was very different and very wrong. Quite abruptly, I couldn't breathe. The slight shortness of breath I still had when I got out of the car suddenly magnified itself a hundredfold and I was literally gasping for air, while a deep underlying surge of angina began welling up.

I stopped stock-still in the middle of the meadow and got a nitroglycerin tablet under my tongue, but I knew that this was not just another ordinary attack of angina. I definitely was not breathing right. I was so obviously not breathing right that I couldn't seem to get any air into my lungs at all, and I could actually *hear*, deep in my chest, a crescendo of bubbling and gurgling sounds, as though my whole bronchial tree suddenly were full of water.

I knew exactly what was happening. I had observed it many, many times in my medical practice. I'd heard that same bubbling, gurgling sound coming from other people's chests—in people suffering acute attacks of pulmonary edema, a form of acute heart failure in which the lungs suddenly become permeated with fluid forced out into the air spaces.

The moment I stopped moving, this attack at least stopped getting worse, but I was desperate for air, gasping as rapidly, as deeply as I could. I simply couldn't seem to get any air in. I dropped the rifle off my shoulder and leaned on it, fighting down panic. I knew that an attack of pulmonary edema could get worse and worse, and my mind raced through the succession of things that might help slow it and relieve it. The nitroglycerin was no help, since this was not an ischemic event but simply a matter of a heart suddenly failing to do its job of pumping blood adequately. In an emergency room or hospital, an injection of morphine would be a powerful weapon to fight an attack of this sort, but, of course, I had no morphine with me, or anything to inject it with. Sometimes, it could help to put a tourniquet on a leg to try to reduce the return of venous blood to the heart, temporarily, and give it a moment's respite, but the thought of shucking all those clothes in order to get at a shirt that I might use as a tourniquet seemed absolutely beyond my physical means at the moment. For a while, I kneeled, holding onto the rifle and squeezing my knees in flexion, thinking that that might slow venous return somewhat, but the acute dyspnea and the gurgling sound of fluid in my chest continued.

I remember thinking other things, half-irrational. I said aloud to myself. "Alan, this is ridiculous, you can't just stand here and suffocate in the middle of a meadow—what if somebody drives by and sees you?" That might, in fact, have been a good thing, but it didn't seem like a good thing to me at the moment. Above all, I was determined to get myself across the rest of that meadow and into the edge of the woods, so I got to my feet, used the rifle for support, and worked my way along one slow step at a time across the rest of the meadow, then laboriously climbed over the gate into the edge of the woods.

Once there, I simply stood and waited, gasping like a fish out of water. Very, very slowly the attack seemed to begin easing. I still could not get in *enough* air, but I was getting more than before. I waited some more, checking my pulse, and was amazed that my heart rate was quite slow, perhaps 65 or 70 beats per minute. Then I remembered that that was the action of the beta-blocker, the Inderal, and I realized, with a blinding flash of insight, that that was exactly why beta-blockers were contraindicated in people suffering heart failure—it prevented the heart rate from speeding up to compensate. If my heart were able to beat 90 or 100 beats per minute at that moment, I thought, this effusion of fluid into my lungs might clear up very quickly, but as it was, it was clearing up very slowly.

Thirty minutes later, I was still standing there. Daylight had come, but the attack was still not over. I considered several alternatives. I didn't think it was going to be possible for me to hunt my way down to meet Ann—at least, I didn't dare try. Much as I wanted to hunt, the obvious wisdom was to find a tree stump close by, sit down on it, and not go anywhere. I thought of firing our "come quickly" signal, but that might, ultimately, simply bring Ann up looking for me on foot in the wrong place, leaving the car down below, which would do nobody any good. I realized that when I did not arrive at the car, sooner or later she would come back up to the drop-off point, and that was my decision—simply to wait near the drop-off point until she turned up.

An hour later, the attack had almost completely subsided, and, aside from the fact that I was feeling totally exhausted, I was at least breathing again. Taking it very slowly and easily, I climbed back over the gate, and walked slowly back across the meadow to find a windfall log near the road to plant myself on, and plant myself I did.

Finally, at about a quarter of ten, I heard the car clanking down the road and Ann appeared, not knowing whether to be alarmed or disgusted to see me sitting on a log exactly where she had left me. I told her what had happened and we debated what we should do. I felt like nothing so much as going straight home to bed, but obvious wisdom dictated that I should have Ann drive me into Ellensburg to consult with young Dr. Horsley, to see what ought to be done— I did not want another attack of this sort occurring again.

I was feeling much better, breathing quite freely, by the time we got to Ellensburg, but I was scared enough by the experience that I didn't even object when Horsley threw me into a hospital bed, took an EKG and chest X rays, drew blood for enzyme levels, and decided to keep me incarcerated for twenty-four hours for observation. When he examined me, he found no physical signs of pulmonary edema whatever. He said that my lungs were perfectly clear—but at least he believed me when I told him exactly what had happened. With his finest bedside manner, he wanted to know what the hell I was doing up in the woods hunting, anyway, when all this was going on, so I patiently explained to him that all this *hadn't* been going on until I got halfway across that meadow. His main concern, and mine as well, was what might have transpired to trigger this sudden episode, since it seemed highly suspicious that it might have been another myocardial infarction. But there was no current of injury on the electrocardiogram, and the first enzyme tests came back negative. Horsley insisted that they be rechecked twelve hours later, but those repeat tests were negative also, so he released me, reluctantly, about midday the following day. While I was still in the hospital, he gave me a couple of doses of a powerful diuretic, and I lost ten pounds of water in twelve hours. He also put me on a small loading dose of digitoxin, a medicine specific for combating heart failure. While I was under his care, he had contacted Robin Johnston by telephone, and when I got home I called Robin's office to make an appointment for the following week.

When I saw Robin, I told him straight out that I'd had an episode of acute pulmonary edema, that I *knew* it was pulmonary edema, and nothing else. After he examined me, he said, "Okay, I believe you. I still don't see any objective evidence of heart failure, but I have to believe that history and agree that it was probably acute pulmonary edema. I don't know why it turned up that way, and I don't know why it cleared up so quickly, but I don't think I like it very much."

"I don't like it either," I told him.

He looked at me through his glasses, with his head tipped to one side. "I think maybe it's time we quit fooling around," he said.

"I'm afraid I think so too."

After a moment, he nodded his head, as if he had made a decision. "Okay, let's keep you on the digitoxin and have you take the Lasix diuretic morning and evening. At least that will help prevent any more heart failure. Then, let's have you come in to the short-stay receiving ward next Wednesday morning, for a repeat angiogram. And then, when we have that in hand, we'll have you see the surgeons. I think the ball is in their court now."

IV

THE CUTTING EDGE

— 11 —

We did not know then, and we still do not know, precisely what it was that triggered that episode of acute pulmonary edema in the mountain meadow that October morning. I had clearly not suffered another infarction catastrophe—there was no sign of it on repeated electrocardiograms, no evidence of it in the enzyme studies, and no hint of it in my general condition during the following days. The only residual I had from that morning's experience, aside from a few more gray hairs, was another small quantum jump of increased angina—not a large jump, no sharp or severe change for the worse, just a little more trouble a little more often than before. Clinically, we had no explanation for what had happened, but very clearly some change had occurred internally; some watershed point had been reached and things were not the same afterward as they had been before.

Clinical evidence or no clinical evidence, I *knew* what I had experienced. Looking at a patient sitting on his examining table, no doctor has any way of seeing *inside*, seeing the minutiae of changes that may be taking place in the patient's coronary circulatory patterns or in the responses of the living myocardial cells under constant attack from ischemia. In a very real sense, the doctor, like the blind man examining the elephant, can detect a trunk here, an ear there, a leg somewhere else, a tail another place, yet never once see the elephant.

Looking at it from the inside out, however, I had the additional data of subtle but clear-cut visceral perceptions of things happening— very minute things, perhaps, that I could perceive as happening only by subtle changes in the way I felt inside. It was these visceral perceptions that led me to an insight into what was going on and to an insight into a basic difference between any patient with coronary artery disease and any doctor attempting to treat him.

At that time, I was approaching the fourth anniversary of a catastrophic myocardial infarction. I had spent a period of more than three years apparently on a generally stable, relatively unchanging plateau of recovery—at least as far as my doctors could determine, to the best of their ability, from examining me. But throughout that time, I was growing more and more certain that my coronary artery disease—and, probably, anybody's coronary artery disease—was not, and never had been, a condition that sat there like a toad on a rock, solid, stable, and unchanging. Rather, I was convinced, that underlying disease was an extremely dynamic, constantly changing condition, a give-and-take of healing and breakdown, of bettering and worsening.

That this should be so is hardly surprising, considering that coronary artery disease involves the most dynamic multiplex of organ systems in the body: the heart, the lungs, and the vascular system. No matter what damage or insult may occur, whether it be a catastrophic MI at one extreme, or, at the other, merely a steadily progressing limitation of heart circulation followed by ischemia and angina, the heart must continue to pump blood as long as it can. The blood continues to circulate throughout both the lungs and the rest of the body, and the lungs continue to take in air and oxygenate the blood. It seemed logical to me, therefore, that when there was an injury or insult to the heart, changes would take place not merely at the time of the insult but over a prolonged period of time thereafter; sometimes swift, dramatic changes, sometimes changes so slowly as to be almost imperceptible, sometimes sporadic changes— but all of them changes that the patient can be very much aware of simply through a certain deep-seated, dynamic perception of the way he feels from moment to moment, or day to day. The patient can know for certain that these changes are occurring because he *feels* them—yet they may be totally imperceptible to the patient's doctor, to any examining technique, or to any laboratory study.

Perhaps the most obvious and simple example of this can be seen in the waxing and waning of angina. When an attack of angina begins, it means that some segment of myocardium somewhere is starving for oxygen. When the angina begins to ease up, this means that that portion of myocardium that had been starving for oxygen a few moments before is once again getting oxygen because an artery is relaxing and opening, allowing more blood to flow through, or because overactivity has stopped, reducing the amount of oxygen the myocardium needs, or because the patient has taken nitroglycerin, which has begun to help dilate arterioles supplying the myocardium, or even because an area of arterial spasm somewhere in the coronary tree has relaxed for some other reason. There is no way in the world that any doctor can tell that patient *when* he should take nitroglycerin to combat his angina, because the doctor can't know what the angina is doing at any given moment. Even if the patient is hooked up to an electrocardiograph, and a running tracing is registering an S-T segment depression, this may only be a present-moment reflection of an episode of ischemia that happened some seconds or minutes earlier. The only one who has any way of telling when to take the nitroglycerin is *the patient himself*, and he has to rely on how he feels at the moment, what his symptoms are, or what his own visceral perception dictates to him.

In my own experience, I always knew up to thirty seconds before the pain began when I was going to have an attack of angina, not from any actual, perceptible pain, but from a peculiar, probably very individual feeling of fullness and coldness in my chest—a visceral perception I learned to recognize instantly when it began, and knew precisely what it was going to evolve into. Fright, panic, cold, or severe pain can all affect both the patient's physical dynamic process—the starving of the myocardium for oxygen—and his own internal perception of this dynamic process going on, but only the patient can tell. The physician could examine that patient ten minutes after the angina passed, or two minutes after, or even while it was going on, and might find absolutely no physical evidence that it was present.

It seemed to me that exactly the same thing might apply to a very early low level of congestive heart failure. After I saw Robin Johnston that October day, I realized that I was quite certain I had been having episodes, or periods, of borderline congestive heart failure, on and off, for months, maybe even for a couple of years, sporadically, before I had finally suffered this frank episode of pulmonary edema that I knew couldn't possibly be anything else. I had no way to *know* that this had been happening, exactly; I merely *suspected* it had been happening, to the point of near-certainty, on the basis of my own internal feeling of *something different going on*—sudden, unexpected episodes of shortness of breath, for example, without any particular reason for them; sudden episodes of a sense of fullness in the left chest that was uncomfortable but wasn't exactly angina, and that didn't really seem to clear up completely with nitroglycerin; changes in the pattern of the variant or nocturnal resting angina that I had, with increasingly poor response to medication, and the discovery that, more and more commonly, it would begin to quiet down if I sat up in bed, but would immediately recur as soon as I lay down again.

As this account indicates, I had told Robin Johnston about these episodes on more than one occasion and asked him if I might be in borderline congestive heart failure. Each time he examined me *when I told him*—not, of course, in the midst of an episode, since I never had an episode like that while I was in his office—and he had assured me each time that there was no sign of congestive heart failure. I'm certain that he was telling me exactly what he believed to be true— there *wasn't* any objective sign that he could detect of congestive heart failure. *I* was the one who said I was having borderline congestive heart failure, based on internal feelings that he could not possibly detect to ratify. If he made any mistake at all, it was a perfectly understandable and, maybe, inevitable mistake: He didn't believe or credit with validity my visceral perceptions that something different was going on. It was a case in which the doctor was perfectly right, and the patient was perfectly right, also, and, in this case, the patient was quite considerably more right than the doctor was.

Was this situation entirely unique to *me*, perhaps, because as a physician, I was more alert to my deep-seated feelings of things changing inside than some untrained patient would be? I wonder— but I don't really believe this is true. I suspect that every person with coronary artery disease develops similar visceral perceptions and simply *must* believe what he feels and tell his doctor about it, again and again, until his doctor believes it, too. I think any person with angina, or shortness of breath, or beginning heart failure, becomes "trained" in recognizing his internal sensations in very short order indeed; he becomes a veritable expert in perceiving such sensations in himself. He may not know how to interpret them, but he knows they're there when they're there, and he knows that something different is going on. But the doctor is trained to believe only what he or she can see, or feel, or hear, or measure. And this means, through nobody's fault at all, that it can be the doctor who is the blind man.

In my case, I am sure that Robin Johnston was quite genuinely startled and surprised when I had a sudden, unexpected episode of acute pulmonary edema that nearly suffocated me in that mountain meadow one morning. He was surprised, but *I* wasn't surprised; I could only say to myself, "I kept *telling* you, man, and you didn't believe me." Today, I think I find this more amusing than distressing, but there is still a remnant of regret in my mind. Possibly Dr. Johnston and I, between us, should have had enough sense to have figured out what was actually happening two years earlier, when my own internal feelings first began to flag me that something was different, something was changing. Perhaps I lost two years that I need not have lost, because we might have started reevaluating things that much sooner.

Certainly, I welcomed the decision to repeat the angiograms and at least consult with the surgeons. It seemed to me that there was a certain inevitability to all of this, and that something had been necessary to get both me and my doctor off the stump. As it turned out, just performing that repeat angiography demonstrated to Robin that something different was indeed going on, very clearly and convincingly: I developed another attack of acute pulmonary edema, just as severe as the first one, right under his nose in the cath lab, just as he was finishing the angiograms. There was, once again, the acute dyspnea, the gurgling noise in my chest (which the doctor listened to while it was going on), and the severe chest pain, just after the last coronary artery pictures had been taken. Nitroglycerin was administered then and there, and, demonstrably, did not turn the attack. Morphine was administered, and that helped. An abrupt sag in blood pressure was noted, measured, and documented. This attack, probably brought on during the injection of the contrast agent into my coronary artery, passed more quickly than the first, and I was considerably more happy to be having it there in Virginia Mason Hospital than out in a mountain meadow at dawn, but I felt that now, at least, Dr. Johnston knew beyond doubt what had happened up there.

My appointments a few days later were scheduled first with Dr. Johnston, then with Dr. Richard Anderson, a Mason Clinic cardiovascular surgeon who did bypass operations at the hospital in teamwork with Dr. Wei-i Li. Ann was along for the meetings. Presumably, both Dr. Johnston and Dr. Anderson had had a chance, by the time of my appointment, to study the new angiograms and consult between themselves as to what course of action should be recommended. Ann and I presented ourselves at Dr. Johnston's office at the appointed time but found that he was tied up in the operating room performing an angioplasty (about which more later) and that he would be delayed for a bit. While we waited in his examining room, however, Dr. Anderson walked in.

I had met him a number of times before at Virginia Mason Research Foundation board meetings and other hospital functions, and I was well aware of his fine reputation as a cardiovascular surgeon. He was young—maybe in his early fifties—tall, slender, a quiet-spoken man with very level gray eyes and a slightly turned-up nose on which he wore a pair of very thick-lensed half-glasses, which I assumed to be magnifying lenses that he used during surgery. Weighing heavily in his favor was my impression that Dr. Anderson was not any surgical prima donna; his manner was quietly unassuming, and he wasn't afraid of eye contact—he looked you straight in the eye when you talked with him. I knew that he had been operating at Virginia Mason for over ten years, and was now chief of surgery there, the position once occupied by Dr. Joel Baker, the "quick brown fox" of my *Intern* narrative. I also knew that Dr. Anderson had performed over two thousand coronary artery bypass operations, with an overall operative mortality rate of less than 1 percent.

Coming into the examining room, he greeted us both and perched on the end of Robin's examining table. "I'm supposed to see you later this afternoon, but since you're waiting right now, I thought I'd look in. Robin thinks you're ready for surgery, but actually I can't make a decision to move in any direction at all until you give me the answer to one very critical question. I can see by your record and from what Robin tells me that you've been having a lot of trouble in the last six months, especially the last month or two. What I need to know is very simple: What single thing is bothering you the most? Is it the angina, or is it these episodes of heart failure?"

"The angina," I said, without the slightest hestitation. "There's no question about that. It's bothering me a lot, it's getting progressively and rapidly worse, and it's reaching a point that it's disabling me. The heart failure business is more *scary* than the angina, but from where I stand, the heart failure is not the most desperate problem, at least not yet. The angina's at the top of my list."

Dr. Anderson smiled. "Well," he said, "you've just said the magic words. Now I've got to check my operative schedule. That really wasn't a trick question, it was very important and very real. We don't do coronary artery bypass operations to treat congestive heart failure. The record shows that the operation doesn't seem to help heart failure very much, and there are far, far more effective ways to treat that problem medically. But if angina is really driving you to the wall, I am almost certain that we can do a bypass that will help a lot. It may not wipe it out completely, but at the very least it should help it. Now you go ahead and see Dr. Johnston for his reports, and then come back to my office up the hall and we'll go over some things you'll need to know."

When Robin finally came back to his office, he went over the results of the angiography with us, using a diagram of the coronary circulation that had been marked to correspond with my own cine–X-ray films. Johnston pointed out that there was no gross evidence of any progressive obstruction in any of the coronary arteries over the four-year interval since the first angiogram, "but we have to realize that the technique is just not detailed enough that we would be able to distinguish as little as a five or ten percent increase in obstruction of one vessel or another." The films again had shown the right coronary completely obstructed and an unusually short and narrow circumflex artery, with much of the usual blood supply, in my case, supplied by the left anterior descending (LAD) artery. This simply meant that there might be only a limited additional blood supply to one part of the left ventricle, even if a bypass graft were to run to the circumflex artery. The new angiograms, however, did show that my regular walking had paid off: There seemed to be new collateral arteries that had developed from the lower branches of the right coronary artery connecting with the lower distribution of the left anterior descending coronary artery branches, providing additional circulation to the tip of the heart and the lower end of the interventricular septum.

"When Dick Anderson looked at your films," said Dr. Johnston, "he felt that he might get one good graft from the aorta to the left anterior descending artery below the obstruction, and a not-so-good graft perhaps from the aorta to the circumflex. In addition, he thinks that if he's lucky he might possibly be able to get a graft down to those right coronary collaterals, if any of them turn out to be big enough to accept a graft. He thinks that this will help the angina to some degree, but he can't be sure just how much until he's actually in there and can see what can be done. But he's worried about the heart failure. Experience with bypass surgury shows that bypassing those arteries won't do anything to change or improve or reverse the heart failure."

I couldn't understand why not, and I told Robin Johnston so. The bypass operation couldn't possibly relieve angina unless the grafts allowed a better and richer supply of oxygenated blood to reach areas of the myocardium that were ischemic, areas where the myocardial cells were sick, or, perhaps, just barely hanging on at all, or, in some cases, progressively dying from oxygen starvation—wasn't that so? Yes, that was the idea, Robin agreed. But if borderline heart failure was developing that hadn't been present before, wouldn't this be occurring because of a weakening of portions of injured or ischemic heart muscle that were slowly losing their capacity to do an adequate job? Yes, Robin said, that was probably why the heart failure was developing to whatever degree it was developing. But if this were true, and if the bypass operation were to suddenly supply that sick ischemic area of myocardium that was beginning to fail with a fresh, copious supply of oxygenated blood, wouldn't that help support and heal the failing myocardium and lead to a reversal of the heart failure?

Robin looked startled. "It would make sense, wouldn't it?" he said. "Maybe you're right; maybe this *would* happen. But the general experience of cardiovascular surgeons and cardiologists is that bypass surgery is not a good treatment for heart failure; it doesn't seem to accomplish a lot to reverse it. The two major things that bypass surgery *can* accomplish are to relieve severe angina—we *know* it can do that—and, in cases in which there is severe obstruction of a coronary artery branch—a myocardial infarction just waiting for a chance to happen—a bypass graft can prevent damage, if we can get it in there first. In fact, with the right patient, we now think this operation can turn the clock back about ten years in the progress of coronary artery disease. Of course that doesn't happen with every patient, and we only have about twenty years' experience doing these operations at all, so we can't be too certain, but we think that many patients can gain as much as ten years' ground."

I later saw figures from the ongoing Coronary Artery Surgery Study that placed the magic number at about seven years, rather than ten, but the study did confirm that the operation could help individuals, anywhere from six months to ten years or longer. And, indeed, I knew enough about the nature of the coronary artery bypass graft surgery or CABG (sometimes irreverently called the cabbage operation), to be comfortable enough with these statistics regarding results.

Exactly what does coronary artery bypass graft surgery involve? The procedure, I knew, was time consuming and a technically difficult surgery to perform. Once the patient is anesthetized, a midline incision is made down the front of the chest, and the breastbone, or sternum, is split down the middle with the refined equivalent of a buzzsaw. Then a retractor with opposing flanges is placed in the cut, which divides the sternum in half from top to bottom. A ratchet mechanism is turned (actually, a rack-and-pinion gear), and the divided sternum is forced apart, exposing the front surface of the pericardium and the heart. The exposure is very good, the procedure smooth and efficient. The patient's shoulders are then thrust back, pushing the chest forward to provide even better exposure.

While one part of the surgical team is busy "cracking the patient's chest" in this manner, another part of the team is involved in a more delicate dissection: making incisions on the inside or middle surfaces of both the patient's legs, from knee to ankle, then carefully dissecting out undisturbed lengths of the patient's greater saphenous veins. In order to provide a natural physiological vessel, or channel, to use as a bypass shunt to carry blood from the aorta to a portion of a coronary artery below an obstruction, some kind of blood vessel must be provided from some other part of the body. The greater saphenous veins in the legs are the most frequently used source of graft material. Normally, these rather small, thin-walled vessels lie just under the surface on the inner side of the lower and upper legs, and carry blood from the skin and subcutaneous tissue of the feet and legs, up into the femoral veins and thence into the abdominal vena cava and on to the heart.

In spite of their size and normally assigned job, these veins are really somewhat superfluous to normal venous return from the lower extremities. Thus, surgeons have found that the greater saphenous veins can be removed and used for graft material without causing any serious disruption in blood return from the patient's lower extremities. Since nerves that normally carry pain, touch, heat, and cold sensations in the inside of the lower legs must be injured in order to remove these veins, however, the patient may have a persisting area of numbness along the whole inner surface of the calf as a long-term, sometimes permanent result of this part of the operation. In addition, because the return of venous blood from the feet and lower legs is diminished, at least temporarily, the patient will usually have a certain amount of lower extremity edema following the operation, but neither of these effects disturbs normal function of the legs very much.

From the beginning of bypass grafting, the greater saphenous veins were most frequently employed as graft material, partly because they were easily removed in most patients, partly because they seemed to function very satisfactorily as bypass conduits for the blood from the aorta to the lower segments of the coronary arteries, once grafted into place. But other potential graft materials that could be "spared" by the body were also explored in the early days of bypass surgery. The artery in the abdomen that supplied the spleen, for example, was large enough to use, and it had the advantage of being closer to the natural arterial anatomy of the coronary arteries than the saphenous veins—but the spleen had to be removed to make the splenic artery available, and this involved a difficult, potentially dangerous abdominal operation in addition to the chest operation. Another, more or less superfluous artery that was easier to obtain was the internal mammary artery, which runs down the inside of the front of the chest wall on either side, and some surgeons prefer to use these vessels for grafts. So far, no kind of artificial arterial graft material has been found successful enough in preliminary studies in laboratory animals to qualify for use in human beings. (I will have more to say about the search for artificial graft materials a bit later.) Mostly, however, surgeons today continue to favor the saphenous veins for graft material simply because they seem to work so well.

Once removed, the saphenous vein graft material is kept in a saline solution, ready for use as soon as the patient's chest has been opened and the heart prepared. The actual implanting of a graft is a fairly simple, straightforward maneuver, at least on the surface. An incision is made into the side of a coronary artery, below the level of disease and obstruction, and one end of the saphenous vein graft is sewn into place there in a delicate microsurgical operation. The graft is then laid on the outer surface of the heart extending up to the point that it can be sewn into an opening made in the ascending aorta, another delicate operation. This is not easy work: The surgeon must make watertight connections of these small blood vessels, using sutures finer than a human hair and requiring 4x magnifying glasses even to see. Obviously, the skill of the surgeon comes very much under the gun. In competent hands it has been possible to attach such grafts to coronary artery branches as narrow as 1 millimeter in diameter (3/32 inch, a bit larger than 1/16 inch). The diagrams that follow show in sketch form how these grafts are placed, and what they look like once the grafting is completed. (See Figure 9.)

Before the actual grafting process can begin, however, there is one further crucial step that has to be taken. Obviously, if an incision is made into the bulb of the aorta while the heart is beating and blood is being forced into the aorta from the left ventricle, the surgeon would not only have to work on a moving target (which would render microsurgery virtually impossible) but would also have arterial blood squirting all over the operating room. In order to perform the graft, it is first necessary literally to disconnect the heart, the pulmonary arteries carrying the blood to the lungs, the pulmonary veins carrying the blood back to the heart, and the ascending aorta completely from the patient's circulation, and channel the flow of his blood temporarily through a heart-lung machine. This massive temporary bypass of the whole cardiopulmonary system accomplishes two things: It provides the surgeon with a "dry" (bloodless) field on which to operate, and it enables him to stop the heartbeat temporarily so that he also has a quiet, nonmoving operative field on which to work.

Unfortunately, bypassing the patient's entire circulation through a heart-lung machine is not good for any prolonged period of time. Surgeons have found that, ideally, a patient should not be left on the heart-lung machine much more than one to three hours before he or she is "weaned off," his blood circulation reestablished through the heart, and the heart restarted again. Indeed, the use of a heart-lung machine for *any* length of time during cardiac surgery carries the risk of such serious, possibly permanent complications as stroke, brain damage, damage to the myocardial cells of the heart, or problems getting the heart restarted once the patient is off the machine,

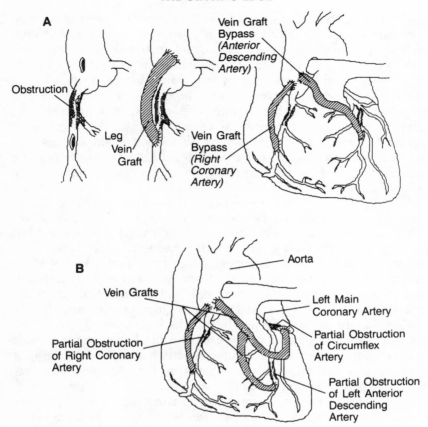

Figure 9 (A) A double bypass to bridge obstructions in the right coronary and left anterior descending arteries.
(B) A triple bypass to bridge obstructions in the right coronary, left anterior descending, and circumflex arteries.

and these risks increase, minute by minute, from the moment the heart-lung machine is started. This means from the moment the heart and lungs are bypassed, the surgeon is under a countdown of steadily mounting risk to get the bypass grafts installed as quickly and skillfully as possible in order to get the patient off the bypass machine and functioning on his own again.

Implanting the graft or grafts obviously involves the highest degree of experienced clinical judgment on the part of the surgeon, since it is then and there, actually looking at the heart, that he must finally decide which bypasses are technically possible and which are most likely to serve a useful purpose. Once the grafts are implanted, the bypass machine is removed, and the patient's heart is shocked back into a normal rhythm again and again begins to circulate blood, including through the bypass grafts, and an actual measurement of the amount of blood flowing through each graft is made. Interestingly enough, the *number* of bypass grafts that are installed may not be nearly as important as most people assume. It is the *end result* of the grafts, whether one, five, or six, that matters. The overriding purpose of grafting is what the surgeon calls complete revascularization, that is, bypassing *all* the important arteries that are seriously narrowed. If that is done, the surgery has done the best that could be done, whether one graft or seven grafts were involved.

In my particular case, in advance of the operation, Dr. Anderson suspected (but could not be certain) that there might be only two grafts possible that would benefit my angina, with a possible but very questionable third graft left to be considered at the time of the surgery. In other words, it appeared that he had only two or three targets. Once in the midst of the operation, however, he actually saw by direct examination a much different picture of my coronary arterial tree than was revealed in my angiograms. In fact, the situation was much more favorable than he had expected, so that he was able to place four good grafts, each of which he felt would provide real benefit, instead of the minimum of two and the maximum of three that he had originally anticipated for complete revascularization (but this is getting ahead of the story).

Once the bypasses are completed, and the patient's heart is restarted, what remains of the operation is the necessary but tedious reclosure of the patient's chest. This means controlling any bleeding from small vessels that may be going on inside the chest, then firmly wiring the two halves of the sternum, or breastbone, back together again, to hold the divided bone as motionless as possible, before closing the subcutaneous tissue and skin. Because the surgeon must be certain that the patient is going to be able to breathe by himself when disconnected from the respirator, he is delivered back to the recovery room with an endotracheal tube still in place in his trachea and connected to a functioning respirator, which is used to assist breathing for an indefinite period of time during early recovery. In order to be sure that the chest remains dry inside, free of any blood or serum that may seep into it, and to be sure the lungs (which partially collapse during the operation) fully reinflate, two drain tubes are inserted in the lower end of the chest cavity and run to underwater seals below the patient's bed level so that fluid can be drained out but air from the outside atmosphere can't inadvertently be sucked in to prevent the lungs from inflating. Finally, the patient's dressed leg wounds must be firmly wrapped to prevent swelling or bleeding in the immediate postop period.

Obviously, this kind of operation is no casual undertaking. In the best of hands it will take anywhere from four to six hours, and it may take longer than that in some cases. It will require not only expert anesthesia administration and an expert, experienced, skillful team of surgeons, assistants, and nurses in the operating room, but also the services of an expertly trained medical and nursing staff in the Intensive Care Unit in which the patient is placed immediately after recovery from anesthesia. This is not a matter of some lonely GP taking out a child's appendix by himself on some farmer's kitchen table at two in the morning and expecting a good result. A group of ten to twelve highly trained, competent people must work as an efficient team in order to reduce the overall risk to a patient to the lowest level possible. It is also not the sort of operation for which such a team, from the chief surgeon down to the circulating nurse, can maintain their competence if they only do two or three such operations a year. Although there was a great deal of pressure, in the early days of bypass surgery, for relatively small, inexperienced, low-volume institutions to try to undertake this kind of work, it soon became evident that by far the best results were obtained by highly skilled and experienced teams performing many bypass operations—several a week, even more—so that all the necessary medical skills were kept constantly honed to a razor-sharp edge. Such high-volume, intensive teams in large medical centers were able to reduce risks to the point that a really competent team would not have more than 1 or 2 percent serious complications or operating room deaths out of hundreds of cases done each year, whereas less experienced, low-volume teams, by comparison, might have 5 or 6 percent major complications/mortality with a much lower volume of patients. Clearly, the large-volume medical centers were—and still are—the way to go in selecting where to have bypass surgery done.

Even under the best of circumstances, the whole procedure is fraught with hazards that the OR team or the Intensive Care Unit team must be prepared to detect and deal with on the spot. The anesthesia for such an operation, for example, can be extremely tricky. Anesthesia, obviously, must be profound and prolonged, yet the inhalation anesthesia commonly used for, say, abdominal operations has the effect not only of depressing brain and nervous system function but of depressing myocardial function and irritating the lungs as well, with the ill effects becoming more pronounced the longer the anesthesia must be maintained. Consequently, for bypass surgery the anesthesiologist may choose a different sort of anesthetic, including one of the very fast-acting, fast-clearing narcotic agents, which will produce the depth of anesthesia needed, with very little depressing effect on the heart, while maintaining just the right degree of anesthesia, no lighter or deeper than necessary, throughout the operation. This, of course, requires constant monitoring of the patient's respiration and blood pressure, and the pressure of blood in different parts of the heart throughout the operation. Many of the monitoring lines and tubes that have to be placed in the patient before or during the operation are important in order to permit the anesthesiologist to keep second-by-second control of what is actually happening inside the patient during the operation.

Other hazards must also be faced. Since there may be bleeding, and since transfusion blood is needed to operate the heart-lung machine, there must be an adequate supply of cross-matched transfusion blood available; the patient may receive up to three or four units of blood in the course of the operation. Preparing and maintaining this blood leads to additional expenses, which might seem superfluous if the patient didn't really need all the blood that was prepared, but there is no alternative but to have it ready in the event that it is needed.

Probably the trickiest part of the operation comes after the graft or grafts have been implanted and the patient is disconnected from the heart-lung machine, when the patient's heart must be restarted to resume its usual work of regular beating and pumping blood. In most cases, a simple electric shock is all that is needed to restore normal heartbeat, but occasionally there is a patient whose heart simply will not start beating again on its own, despite repeated efforts to restore it to normal activity. This should not be surprising when you consider how many patients go into coronary artery bypass surgery with very sick hearts, hearts that have been virtually beaten to death by myocardial infarction, coronary artery obstruction, or prolonged repeated episodes of ischemia, hearts that are just hanging on by a thread already, without the additional insult of the ischemia period when the heart is bypassed by a heart-lung machine and the critical part of the operation is performed. What's really amazing, in fact, is how very seldom this kind of disaster occurs. When it does, a variety of heroic measures can and must be taken, then and there, and in most cases the heart *can* ultimately be restarted, but there are those rare tragic cases when it simply cannot.

Even when the heart has been restarted successfully, the patient still may not be out of the woods. In many cases there are situations in which the heart resumes its beating but then slips into failure, sick enough to begin with and/or traumatized enough by the surgery that it cannot immediately resume efficient enough contractions to maintain the circulation properly—in short, *failing* to do its job. In some such cases drugs such as digitalis or other heart-stabilizing medications can help the patient over the critical hours after the surgery. In other cases a cleverly devised balloonlike pump on the end of a catheter can be inserted into a femoral artery and advanced up into the aorta. This "balloon pump," the so-called Left Ventricular Assist Device, or LVAD, can be used in its temporary location in the aorta to help pump blood along, relieving the failing left ventricle of some of its work load—literally *assisting* it—for a period of time, perhaps hours or even days, until it has time enough to recover its strength and resume its normal activity. This device, which is then simply withdrawn with the catheter when it's no longer needed, is one of the simplest forms of "partial artificial heart" in regular use today, employed temporarily to help bridge a crisis that might otherwise be fatal. Still other patients may have trouble resuming normal respiration naturally, needing to remain longer than normal on the respirator, so that the job of clearing the lungs of secretions, and allowing them fully to expand and take over their job, has to be postponed awhile.

Coronary artery bypass surgery was first performed in human patients in the mid-1960s. By the early 1970s, it had become a widely used, vastly popular, and extremely expensive procedure. In those early days, a great deal of criticism was leveled at surgeons and hospitals for the frequent, heavy use of the procedure, and some of that criticism persists today. Having once proved that the procedure could be done, it was widely espoused by a whole generation of enthusiastic surgeons and it soon became part of a certain euphoric mythology among patients. It seemed that almost everyone who suffered a twinge of angina was being subjected to the operation, willy-nilly. The operation became so popular in patients' minds that it became sort of a status symbol. A great many patients actively demanded it, as though anybody with heart trouble who had not had a bypass operation was somehow declassé. Meanwhile, surgeons and hospitals were getting rich offering the procedure so widely and freely, often at very high and uncontrolled cost to the patients and the patients' insurers.

Clearly, this was not a good situation, considering the very real risks and hazards of the operation. Critics claimed that surgeons and institutions were actively merchandising the procedure to patients, like peddling automobiles, whether it was needed or not. Arguments arose in those days that there weren't any clear-cut indications to determine which patients might benefit from bypass surgery or which might not, or when the surgery ought to be performed in a given case. There were complaints that nobody could even tell for sure whether a given operation was successful or not, that there was absolutely no evidence that bypass grafting increased a patient's prospects for longevity to any degree, and that considerable question existed as to what other benefits it might offer. And, in the meantime, costs were skyrocketing, with total-cost figures ranging from $25,000 to $50,000 per operation at many institutions.

Some of those arguments and criticisms may have been justified, at the time. Perhaps the CABG operation was overused, and abused to some degree, in the early 1970s. Patients were encouraged to submit to it without any clear understanding of potential benefits or proper indications. I question whether this was entirely a matter of greedy surgeons latching onto a popular operation in order to make themselves and their hospital institutions rich. There was a widespread perception among cardiovascular surgeons and cardiologists at the time that here, at last, was something active and specific that could be done for patients with severe coronary artery disease; that instead of the pills, promises, prayers, and postmortems—long the most that cardiologists could offer—here was something positive and exciting. Much of the aggressive use of this operation arose from the sense of impotence and frustration that had prevailed before.

But what about today? I think the physicians and other critics who are still complaining about overuse and abuse of the operation, or about surgery for remuneration only, or about lack of indications for the operation and lack of evidence of results, are simply talking ancient history. Things have changed since the early 1970s. The surgical techniques of the bypass operation have been steadily honed. The incidence of operative morbidity and mortality has steadily dropped—there is now far less risk involved. At the same time, indications for the operation have become more clearly defined, and the selection of patients more discriminating, as surgeons and cardiologists have learned more and more about the results that can be achieved. Large-scale, carefully controlled scientific studies have been carried out—and still continue—to help determine more clearly exactly which patients will or will not benefit from surgery, to clarify exactly what indications for the surgery are really valid, and to determine which benefits various patients may actually enjoy and which are likely to be illusory. Responsible medical institutions now have cardiac conferences in which many cardiologists and surgeons pool their knowledge and experience to help determine which patients might benefit the most with the least risk, and which might best be left untouched by the surgeon's knife. And individual surgeons or surgical teams keep careful tabulation of specific indications for surgery on their patients and publish careful, objectively honest assessments of all aspects of their surgery, including complications, failures, degrees of success, and so forth.

In 1976, one especially important controlled multicenter prospective study drew the attention of everyone concerned: the so-called Coronary Artery Surgery Study, or CASS. This study was *prospective* ("looking ahead") in that patients with ongoing disease were entered into the study and followed, over a period of years, to see what happened to them with various forms of treatment. It was a *multicenter* study, meaning that patients were enlisted in the study from a large number of major medical centers specializing in medical and surgical treatment of heart disease, including some of the finest, most prestigious medical centers in the world. It was *controlled*, meaning simply that it was set up in such a way that individual patients with closely comparable degrees of coronary artery disease could be assigned at random—with fully informed consent and permission—to one of two or more different methods of treatment so that the overall results of those methods of treatment could validly be compared.

In the CASS study, prospective patients were divided into categories according to the history of their illness. In one grouping, for example, people were classified according to myocardial infarction in their history. One class included only patients who had never had an infarction, another included those who had had a mild MI, a third included those with a history of a very severe MI. Similarly, patients could be classified according to no history of angina at all, or a history of mild exertional angina, severe exertional angina, variant angina, and so forth. Patients also were classified according to the findings on their angiograms—that is, according to the degree of obstruction demonstrated in the main and branch coronary arteries.

Then, among those patients who were so classified, those who agreed to enter the study were "randomized," that is, placed at random into either a medically treated group or a coronary artery bypass group. The progress of these patients was then closely followed, whichever approach to treatment was selected, and the results over a period of five years were analyzed statistically to determine, if possible, which patients from which classes seemed to benefit more from one approach to treatment than another.

It might seem at first glance that such an approach to treatment was terribly hard-eyed and coldblooded for the unfortunate fellow with coronary artery disease, but actually it was not. The only patients who were considered eligible at all were those for whom there was, by current knowledge, *no* clear-cut known advantage of one method of treatment over another. In the course of the study, any patient whose circumstances changed, so that one method of treatment was clearly more desirable than another, was immediately dropped from the study and placed on the form of treatment considered most beneficial.

The results of this multicenter CASS study were tabulated in 1981, and published and intensively reviewed in 1982. In the analysis of results it appeared clear that coronary artery bypass surgery did not offer any clear-cut advantage over conservative medical treatment in vast numbers of patients. There was, for example, no overall increase in longevity or any overall decrease in mortality in bypass patients, except for one specific class: Among those patients who had severe left main coronary artery obstruction demonstrated on angiogram, those who had bypass surgery had a significantly lower mortality rate—fewer of them died during the five-year period of the study—than did those with the same lesion who underwent medical treatment. People in this group who had the bypass also suffered fewer new myocardial infarctions than occurred among those on conservative medical treatment during the same time period.

But perhaps equally important, one other group was found to clearly benefit from surgical treatment as compared to medical treatment: patients with severe and debilitating angina pectoris. Here, the difference was not a matter of living longer or having fewer new infarctions; it was simply that the bypass patients almost uniformly had significantly more relief of their angina than was possible to achieve by medical treatment. Thus, two clear-cut criteria for bypass surgery emerged: Patients with debilitating angina that was poorly controlled by medication could be helped; and those with severe left main coronary artery lesions could be offered hope of greater longevity and less risk of recurrent infarction catastrophe after bypass.

Similar studies continue to this day, and, bit by bit, the benefits and drawbacks of CABG surgery are becoming more and more clearly defined. The timing of the operation—whether in the midst of a myocardial infarction, or six weeks later, or four years later—is being investigated to identify when is the best time for eligible patients in each classification of coronary artery disease to have the surgery. And, as time goes on, more and more statistics are being gathered regarding how those earlier bypass patients have fared.

Certain problems seem to plague all such patients. Once bypasses are installed around partially obstructed coronary arteries, the natural coronary arteries tend to close, so that the patient must depend more and more on the flow of blood through the bypass channels. In the vast majority of patients, over a period of time, those bypass channels also tend to plug up slowly, so that reoperation becomes necessary in some to maintain coronary artery circulation. In recent studies, there is some evidence that bypass channels made from internal mammary arteries may not plug up as quickly as those made from saphenous vein segments. Yet many surgeons still choose saphenous vein grafts, perhaps with the idea of preserving the internal mammary arteries for later use if and when repeat bypass surgery becomes necessary. In addition, internal mammary artery grafts are technically much more difficult for the surgeon to perform. These arteries are not cut out and used as separate grafts, as with saphenous vein grafts; they are left attached to the arterial circulation at one end, and the free end must be tunneled through to the heart and won't even reach the back of the heart. Operating time—and, thus, time the patient must remain on the heart-lung machine—is often much longer, and the risks are higher. Thus, the question of which graft material is better remains unresolved, at least in early 1986.

How does all this add up, as far as is known today? Beyond any question, in some patients who are carefully selected according to the indications and criteria now being developed—patients with severe left main coronary artery obstruction or severe triple-vessel disease, for example—CABG surgery can indeed be lifesaving or life prolonging. For a vastly greater number of patients, relief of angina achieved by the surgery can bring about a striking improvement in the quality of life. Further progress in the use of this operation is certain to depend upon these criteria and new criteria that may be discovered from ongoing studies, as well as the success or failure of still newer alternative procedures being developed today, procedures that we will discuss later.

In my individual case, the degree of obstruction of my left main coronary artery was not, in itself, sufficient enough to provide a clear-cut indication for bypass surgery, and my particular coronary artery anatomy, as seen on the angiograms, seemed to militate against the operation. But the progressive development of debilitating angina tipped the scale, in the minds of my cardiologist and the cardiovascular surgeons—and in my mind as well. By the time Ann and I waited for our appointment with Dr. Richard Anderson, I had reached a point that I was willing to accept the necessary risk if it in any way seemed to be reasonable.

— 12 —

The risk of surgery was just one of the things that Dr. Anderson discussed and explored with us in his office that afternoon in early November. In view of the severity of my original MI and in view of the history of what had happened since, particularly the progressive angina and the appearance of borderline heart failure, he felt that my potential risk from the operation was substantially higher than usual. According to his own statistics from the operations he had performed during the last two years, he said that fewer than 1 percent of his patients, overall, had actually died or suffered severe life-threatening complications during or following their surgery—but, in my case, he assessed the potential risk as being closer to 7 percent.

He then discussed the nature of the complications that might occur and the measures that were always on hand to help deal with them. He explained that the most critical period, once the operation was completed, was the first twenty-four to forty-eight hours postoperatively, during which time the patient is in the Intensive Care Unit under continuous observation by specially trained nurses and physicians. He anticipated a hospital stay of eight to ten days.

Dr. Anderson also discussed with us some of the details about how the surgery was performed and what one might expect in the hospital following the operation and during the recovery period. He pointed out that perhaps the hardest part, from the patient's standpoint, has to do with the endotracheal tube—a tube inserted through the patient's mouth, then passed down through the larynx, or voice box, into the treachea, to permit administration of oxygen by the anesthesiologist during the operation, and later to permit the respirator to be used until it is felt that the patient can breathe on his own. Insertion of the endotracheal tube is no problem, Dr. Anderson pointed out, because it isn't done until the patient is already partially anesthetized. But once the patient recovers from anesthesia, the tube can be an enormous trial. It tends to be highly irritating, stimulating both the gag reflex and the choke reflex. These problems can be controlled to a large degree by the use of various sedatives and antianxiety medications, but the patient still experiences periods of acute discomfort until the endotracheal tube can be taken out. In addition, there is a problem with the tube that medications cannot solve: Because it passes down through the voice box and separates the vocal cords, the patient cannot talk—not even a squeak—as long as the tube is in place.

Dr. Anderson detailed these and other things that I should anticipate—the need to force myself to breathe deeply and cough up mucus, for example, in spite of the fact that coughing with a freshly closed chest incision, involving separated bone, is very painful, one of the things that the patient is inclined to want to do least of all. There is also the need to get up and move about as early as possible postoperatively in order to avoid the threat of venous stasis—the pooling of blood in the veins in the legs and other large veins, and the threat of developing venous thrombi—blood clots in the veins. Both can be avoided by movement of the legs. There is the need to use physical therapy measures to keep parts of the body, particularly the upper extremities, limber despite the fact that the patient isn't likely to be eager to move a great deal. And so forth.

Dr. Anderson went through these things patiently, making each point clear, without any sign of hurry. When my turn came to ask questions, I brought out a little list of things I wondered about, and he carefully fielded all those that had not been covered already. No, in the course of studying the films of my new angiograms, he had not been able to see any perceptible change in the arteries—at least no evidence of additional obstruction—compared to the angiograms taken four years before, but he repeated what Robin had said: There seemed to be somewhat better collateral circulation at the base of the right coronary artery distribution than before, so at least religious attention to the exercise program may have paid off to a degree. Since I didn't actually understand the hand-sketched angiogram road map that Robin Johnston had shown me in my chart, I wasn't exactly sure what could be told from it; I asked if there was any possibility that the surgeon might get in there with my chest open in the operating room, only to discover that he couldn't really do anything at all. No, that wasn't likely, Anderson said, because he knew from studying the actual angiograms that there were at least two bypasses that he was dead certain he could complete that ought to help to some degree. The only question in his mind was how feasible the third bypass graft might be. I asked him if there were any of the serious complications that might turn up about which nothing could be done. "Well, aside from the extremely rare eventuality of a stroke during the surgery or the immediate postop period," he said, "which occurs very seldom but can sometimes come out of left field without any apparent reason or warning, all the other complications are at least deal-with-able—they usually can be countered quickly and effectively. Unfortunately, however, once in a rare while there will be a patient who for one reason or another will present complications far over and above anything we expect, and sometimes these patients are ones who have very serious, permanent problems or may even die." He cited as an example a patient who might develop heart failure during surgery, and continue to remain in heart failure in spite of the use of an aortic assist pump, so that the temporary use of the pump might have to be extended far too long. In such a case there could be the additional problem of having to wean the patient from the pump. Usually, a patient's failure will be temporary, and with a few hours' "rest" provided by the assist pump, will recover itself, but if the myocardium isn't there to recover from the failure, it isn't there, and this is why there are people who die of congestive heart failure during or soon after surgery.

I asked him if there were any common or likely postoperative problems other than cardiovascular problems. This he thought over for a while, then said, yes, there were some, the sorts of things that might complicate any major surgical procedure—unexpected kidney failure, for example, or unexpected liver damage, or the exceedingly rare patient who suffered a new myocardial infarct in the midst of the operation, or the development of a clot in a deep vein that then moved to the lungs as a so-called pulmonary embolus, or the threat of wound infection—"So far, I haven't had any infections, but someday a patient is going to come along and break my record"—things of this sort, that might complicate any major surgery. In addition, he said, many postop coronary bypass patients at one point or another in the course of their recovery suffer some degree of depression, and in some cases this can be bothersome. "We don't know why this happens, but it does seem to happen in enough people that we have to be aware of it as a real concern. Maybe it has to do with some degree of cerebral anoxia during the procedure. Maybe it has to do with the long slow recovery period. Nobody has defined it, but occasionally there it is."

Then I asked him how much total down time I could expect from the operation—not just hospital time but at home as well, either in bed or housebound. "Well, we don't want you in bed or housebound any more than you have to be," he said. "In fact, we will hoist you unto your feet with a derrick if necessary to get you moving, like it or not. So there won't be that much down time in the sense you're speaking of, of being completely laid out. But overall, you should expect a period of about two months before you're feeling up to assuming full, normal activities, moving around freely, driving, going shopping, et cetera, and three months before your energy level begins to pick up again. Maybe six months before you really get into the full swing of things in terms of energy and activity—but it varies a great deal from patient to patient."

Finally, I asked him a question that was very much on my mind. His presentation had been a matter of providing me with information on which a go/no-go decision could be made. He was prepared to authorize the surgery and prepared to do it. It was his professional opinion that the surgery would be beneficial. But he had in no way urged me to decide in favor of it. I had to make that decision on my own. From my point of view, my situation had changed quite radically for the worse in the course of the past two or three months, but now we were going into a holiday season, with plans already made with family members for Thanksgiving and Christmas. For this reason I asked him how he would feel, in the event I decided for the surgery, about delaying it until after the holiday season was over; that is, lying low and not rocking the boat until family and kids had come and gone.

He gave me an odd look. "I think that if your decision is to go ahead, it would not be wise to delay any longer than necessary. If we're going to jump, I think we'd better jump." He then consulted his schedule and indicated that he had two dates close at hand that he could commit—either Monday the twenty-sixth of November, the day after Thanksgiving weekend, or Wednesday, December 5, nine days later. He indicated that if we decided to proceed, I should contact his office as quickly as possible and set one of those dates. Then he smiled. "I do think, however, that the idea of lying low and not rocking the boat between now and the target date is an extremely good idea. Between you and me, I wouldn't go hunting."

It was quite late by the time we left his office. Dr. Anderson had been tied up in an obligatory hospital staff meeting until almost six o'clock and had spent over an hour with us discussing options and prospects. The weather in the pass was not good, and we debated whether to try to go home that night with the risk of a snowstorm in the pass or stay in the Busbys' apartment and cook up something for supper. I vetoed both these plans, saying that I felt like nothing more than going out for a couple of drinks and a steak dinner.

As we left the clinic building in the November dark and rain and drove out of the parking garage across the street, I found myself thinking of the old apocryphal gladiators' salute: "Hail Caesar, and farewell; we who are about to die salute thee." Actually I was not feeling anything as fatalistic as that would imply. More than anything else, I felt a sense of immense relief and guarded optimism as a result of that long interview with Dr. Anderson, an immense release of tension I had felt building all summer that had reached a climax that morning in the mountain meadow. Here, at last, after four long years, a solid, firm, plausible alternative had been placed within my reach, a real and rational option that I could now accept or reject. Although I had not been able to address the idea consciously before, I realized then that the one thing I had dreaded most before this afternoon's interviews with Robin Johnston and Richard Anderson was the possibility that I would hear that nothing whatever could be done, that I would have no alternative, no option but to continue in the deteriorating spiral of the past nine months, which had seemed to me to be reaching the point of the intolerable in the past six weeks. I had feared that the new electrocardiograms might have shown evidence of new myocardial damage, so that there was too little myocardium left to operate on; that the drift into congestive heart failure might have been interpreted as so great as to completely outweigh any possible benefits that the surgery might offer; or that the surgeon himself might have rejected the project as merely begging for trouble or presenting too ridiculous a risk for him to be willing to lay his good operative record on the line. Now that none of these things had happened—now that the option *was* available in formalized terms—"I have authorized the surgery"—I found that my sense of relief and release, and the attendant euphoria, made it very difficult to consider the dark side of the picture at all.

I was quite sure that evening as we drove away from there that I was going to opt for the surgery, dark side or not. In a sense, I felt that I didn't really have any rational choice—that to reject it now would be virtually suicidal. True enough, I was not yet driven to the point of desperation. No doubt I could continue to limp along as I had been for some period of time longer, but only at the cost of progressively more discomfort and limitation, and I felt very strongly that the inevitable end of that road was disaster. The question was not whether I needed the surgery but merely when, how soon; and passing the option by now or temporizing, even for a few weeks, could all too easily mean losing the option forever. On the dark side, there was a very real risk that I might agree to this elective surgical procedure and not survive it—a 7 percent risk of mortality or of disastrous irreparable complications was, by any manner of figuring, an extremely high risk factor for any elective surgical procedure—but even that seemed to me to be a more favorable prospect than I had imagined. I had thought the surgeon might have been anticipating a 10, 15, even 25 percent risk—and I learned that Ann had been worried about exactly the same thing. The other part of the dark side was that having gone through the operation, and surviving it, I might find that it actually did very little good and that, ultimately, I would end up in essentially the same boat I had started out in, with the trial and trauma of recovery from massive surgery piled on top.

We drove over the Evergreen Point bridge, across Lake Washington, to Bellevue and went to a restaurant appropriately named The Butcher, a crowded steak house, where we found seats at the bar, had a couple of drinks apiece, then ordered steak dinners. I do not recall precisely what our conversation was that evening, but I realize, in retrospect, that at least in this instance Ann kept her hands off, and we left the restaurant with the decision made—that I would accept the option—and expressed in words. By that time we both realized that we did not want to spend the night in the apartment; more than anything else, we wanted to be home. So, we made a late-evening, two-hour drive, through the pass and down to Thorp, in a teeming rainstorm.

— 13 —

The meeting with the doctors had been on a Friday afternoon and evening. On the following Monday, I called Janice, Dr. Anderson's office nurse, schedule keeper, and general organizer, and told her of my decision to go ahead. She confirmed the two dates Dr. Anderson had mentioned, the Monday, November 26, just after Thanksgiving, or December 5, and I told her I thought the sooner the better. She said that she would make the necessary prearrangements with the hospital, and that I should plan to appear there for admission at about two o'clock in the afternoon on Sunday, November 25. She also reiterated something that Dr. Anderson had told me on Friday— that if anything should happen in the meantime to distress me in any way, to come directly to the hospital for admission without bothering to call. "They'll know why you're there, and Dr. Anderson is ready to move anytime he has to."

I didn't completely adhere to Anderson's admonition against hunting, but the hunting during that elk season had been severely limited anyway. Since the episode of pulmonary edema in the meadow, there had been no more early rising and scrambling to get out in the field. The few days we went out at all, we went out at a leisurely pace at ten in the morning, for an hour or two, or an hour or two late in the afternoon, when Ann got home from work. I had not gone out alone at all, and on the few occasions when I went out with Ann, my hunting consisted largely of posting an area, sitting quietly on a stump somewhere while she hunted toward me. In fairly typical fashion, we saw a number of elk during deer season and multitudes of deer during elk season. It was almost a parody of a pattern we had seen over the years: An area that was totally bereft of any deer throughout deer season was suddenly teeming with deer during elk season, bucks and does alike, sticking their heads out from behind trees and waggling their ears at us. On one two-hour hunt, in a beautifully wooded area above the Cummins place the morning after a fresh four-inch snowfall, Ann and I, between us, saw no fewer than eight deer in groups of two or three, including two spike bucks and one beautiful, large four-point buck. We had not seen so much as the tail end of a doe in that area during deer season. As for elk, one afternooon, on an old logging spur at the base of the woods on the hill above our house, I stood and watched a herd of twenty or more cow elk come down a draw out into the open, swoop in an enormous curve over toward the promontory above the Brains' farm, run into Ann, who was hunting in that area, and turn back to pass within twenty-five yards of me as they went back up the gully into the woods again, not running, merely walking fast, and starting away when they were spooked. They were fascinating to watch in their preambulations, but there was not a horn in the crowd.

It would have been nice to have gone back home and done nothing whatsoever during that last ten days before the surgery was scheduled, but we already had plans made and we decided to proceed with them; perhaps just as well. I was not feeling particularly well; both the angina and shortness of breath were there, repeated reminders of continuing trouble. Having decided on the surgery, I was eager to have it over with, and the waiting was difficult. Having house guests added to the pressure but it also provided something to occupy the mind. During the last week of elk season, our lifelong friends Jack and Phyll Martin came down from Sammish Island to spend a few days with us. Ann would take Jack out hunting for a couple of hours in the morning, while I stayed home and helped Phyll make bread. After the Martins had left, Bill and Mo came over from Spokane to spend Thanksgiving with us, an extremely quiet and sedate one. Becky was there for two days, but none of the other kids, for one reason or another. We visited, listened to music, played bridge; exciting things like that.

Earlier that week, I had called each of the kids to let them know about the impending surgery and reaffirm what I strongly felt—that there was no point or reason for them to come home, since there was nothing that any of them would be able to do. I told Bill and

Mo much the same thing. On Thanksgiving night, and again on Saturday night that weekend, I had severe and prolonged episodes of angina in the middle of the night, and I remember thinking how great it would be if just possibly this kind of recurring torment would soon be over, one way or another.

On Sunday morning, Ann and I left Bill and Mo to close up the house at Thorp and we headed back to Seattle to meet the two o'clock admission time at Virginia Mason Hospital. As Ann remarked, it seemed as if we had done all this before, but, of course, we hadn't— not precisely. While Ann remained downstairs in the admission office, filling out the inevitable forms, I was trundled up to a room on the surgical floor of the hospital, and the usual parade of activities began—the interns' visits, the resident's admission visit, the inevitable repetition of medical history, the succession of laboratory people drawing their tubes full of blood, the EKG technician trundling up the EKG machine for a fresh go at me. I found that I was unable really to get into the spirit of things, since I knew that the people that mattered already had all the information they needed, and that all this repetition for the sake of formality was ridiculous— necessary, maybe, for one obscure reason or another, but still ridiculous.

Ridiculous or not, necessary things were done. At one point a second wave of lab technicians came in to take a second wave of blood, carefully explaining (as though I were going to refuse to donate) that my blood gases—the amounts of oxygen and CO_2 in my arterial blood—had been far lower than they had expected, and they wanted to repeat the tests. Precisely what they were going to do with this information when they had it was left unexplained. At another point a respiratory therapist came in with a portable respiratory tank, a plastic-and-cellophane cylinder, about a foot tall and eight inches in diameter, with a breathing tube attached to the bottom. I was supposed to exhale as completely as possible, then suck through the breathing tube to expand the bellows inside the respirator, which was marked to indicate liters of air drawn in with a single breath. The therapist explained that I would become well acquainted with this little toy after the operation, since one of the critical recovery procedures would be to get air moving in and out of my lungs again, and to get them to reexpand, following their partial collapse when the chest was opened. I managed a maximum lung expansion of about 2700 cubic centimeters after a couple of test runs.

Somewhat later in the afternoon, just before supper was served, a gentleman came to the door of the room, wheeled in an enormous machine, and announced that he was going to weigh me. Since I had already been weighed twice on two different stand-up scales since arriving at the hospital, this struck me as a trifle superfluous, but this procedure must have been dead serious because it evolved into the most total weighing I have ever experienced in my life. My dinner tray was held up and I was first asked to go into the john and empty my bladder, then disrobe completely. Thereupon the technician spread a wide canvas sheet on the bed for me to lie on and then gathered the edges on both sides onto a long metal arm connected to the large machine, which proved to be essentially a small derrick that lifted me, canvas and all, completely off the bed. I knew vaguely that all this had something to do with the fact that anesthetic medication and other medications would be calculated on a per-kilogram-of-body-weight basis, but I had never imagined that this measurement of kilogramage had to be accurate down to plus or minus 10 milligrams. The whole procedure took about fifteen minutes, and the technician seemed terribly worried that being hoisted off the bed in this fashion would somehow alarm me. I merely found it fascinating, in a grotesque sort of way. To add to the grotesquerie, the man came back just before I retired that evening to go through the whole procedure again, saying that they hadn't gotten it right—then, repeated it again first thing in the morning when I woke up.

After the weighing procedure was over, and following the dinner hour, a young Oriental gentleman came in, suggested rather obliquely that Ann should leave the room (which I seem to recall she elected not to do on the grounds that she had seen me without any clothes on before), and then proceeded to give me a preoperative shave of my entire torso and lower extremities, sparing only my head, beard, neck and arms. I could remember from my internship days some of the jagged scratchy shaves that I had administered to unfortunate patients, using dull or resharpened razors, and I marveled at how remarkably smooth this dry shave proved to be with the little razor the man used. Since I have not actually used a razor on myself in over fifteen years, long before the days of the supersharp blade and the disposable razor, I found this dry shaving job very slick indeed.

As it happened, Dick Anderson made his appearance during this procedure, at a point when I was stark naked, flat on my belly on the bed with my rear upended, but I guess he had encountered this situation before. He didn't seem to be in any hurry and just sat down and chatted until the razor-wielder wrapped up his work and left. He said that he was mostly checking to see that I had gotten there all right, that nothing terrible had happened since I had seen him that evening ten days before, and that I was as mentally at ease as it was reasonably possible to be. He was dressed in casual sport clothes and leaned back in the chair, stretching his long legs out in front of him. He encouraged any further questions that we might have—very few—and then told Ann what she should expect the next morning. He would want her to wait in the special waiting room outside the operating room. She should bring a book along if she wanted to but really should plan to go out shopping or something during the morning because she'd have a long time to wait. She would be informed when I went in to surgery, and, he said, he would come out and report directly to her when the surgery was over.

He must have stayed fifteen or twenty minutes before leaving, a leisurely and unhurried visit, and it was amazing to me how much that simple visit contributed to my sense of confidence, and Ann's, even though clinically speaking it really had no importance at all. It improved my estimation of this man's capability and humanity by a quantum jump. He conversed with us like a friend, not like a doctor, and spoke of his son, who had been an undergraduate in physics at Cal Tech, the same place that our son was now in graduate school in geology. He even spoke a little bit of total inconsequentiae, and I was suddenly struck with the incredible contrast presented here with so many other surgeons I had observed in the past making such preoperative visits, marching in with their retinues of residents, interns, and medical students, brisk and abrupt, with their brusque patter going on while they made their equally brusque examinations, never pausing for a moment, moving into the room and back out again, always moving, always hurried. Presently, Dr. Anderson *did* listen to my chest, more with the attitude that it was expected of him than in any sense that he was learning anything. He warned us that his chief resident, who would assist at the operation, would be in a bit later for *his* preoperative visit, and that I would also have a visit from the anesthesiologist. "He's going to give you a long song and dance," Dr. Anderson warned. "Don't worry about it too much. If he gets too graphic or grisly, just turn him off—it's the way they do things these days." Finally, as he turned to leave, he said, "Really, the best thing that you can do is not to worry and get a good night's rest. Things are going to go just fine."

"Best that they do," I said. "You realize, of course, that I write books about everything that happens to me."

For a moment he looked startled, then he grinned. "Yes, I've heard about you," he said. "I'll bear that in mind."

A little later the senior surgical resident, Dr. Gregory Marrujo, did a brief review of history, made a more careful and thorough physical examination, and checked to make sure that there were no sleeping medicines that I had any particular trouble with, pointing out that I had nitroglycerin ordered, as well as other pain medicine, and I was to call for it during the night if I had the slightest need. "You're going to be seeing a lot of me for a while," he said, "beginning bright and early tomorrow morning."

The anesthesiologist was the last to make an appearance, a young man named Shaner, who must have been doing something serious that Sunday afternoon since he came in dressed in scrub suit and scrub hat, with his mask hanging around his neck, the working uniform of the day. He indeed did have a long, grisly tale to tell, starting with a brief account of the history of anesthesia, pointing out the kinds of anesthesia that would be used and why, then going through a long clinical list of all the horrible things that might reasonably be expected to happen, leaving the overall impression that something dreadful was almost certain to come to pass and that I must, in any event, give informed consent on paper for whatever it might be, before it happened. All that I could do was shrug my shoulders helplessly at Ann and thank God that my sense of the ridiculous was alive and well, else I would have been terrified. But at least I didn't tease this man; I think a divine hand must have restrained me.*

With the long parade of visitors finally over, we turned on the television and Ann and I sat for an hour watching Angela Lansbury in an episode of "Murder, She Wrote," an absolutely and appropriately ridiculous TV murder mystery that had the one redeeming grace that it starred Van Johnson in a guest role, the first that I'd seen him on the screen in at least twenty years. At nine o'clock the show was over, the sleeping pill came, Ann kissed me good night, and I retired for that all-important "good night's rest."

— 14 —

Cynics might say that the parade of visitors on that preoperative afternoon was deliberately designed to wear the patient down to a stump so that a good night's sleep was inevitable from sheer ex-

---

* This is probably grossly unfair. The truth is that the anesthesiologist has just as tough a job on his hands as the surgeon during a bypass operation, and Ann's impression was that this young man was genuinely concerned and worried about me.

haustion. I did, indeed, sleep well, with no trouble from angina, and had to be awakened by the cheery voice of a nurse at six-thirty in the morning as the bright lights of the room were turned on. It was a day of bright lights and oblivion. The preoperative medication was started before I was fairly awake, and things happened—the transfer from bed onto the wheeled gurney; the trip down brightly lighted corridors, into and out of an elevator, into other brightly lighted rooms; the anesthesiologist greeting me like a long-lost buddy, eager to ply his wares; the briefest glimpse of Dr. Anderson in his green scrub suit and cap, staring down at me, thick half-glasses hanging on his nose, saying something vaguely cheering; various nurses or others working away, placing IV tubes in my arms. I was aware of these things in retrospect, but not aware just when in the midst of all this that I drifted off on cue into my long morning's sleep. Again, Ann had agreed to keep tabs on what went on. She brought her little hand tape recorder along, and the best account of what happened then, and how, comes from the dictated journal she kept of that and the following days.

Sunday, November 25, 1984. It seems longer than six days since Alan called Janice, Dr. Anderson's office nurse, and set the target date for the operation, but at least I'm glad he opted to get it over with as quickly as possible, so that we didn't have the tension of waiting any longer, and also because he was not feeling well. At least we had a week to prepare ourselves, so to speak, partly gloomy, partly optimistic. We took the opportunity to talk over some of our long-term plans that I was very concerned about, especially in terms of the kids. Both of us knew that we had to talk about some things in case Alan shouldn't make it through the surgery or if he had terrible problems afterward, and this is always a frightening and depressing sort of thing.

We agreed that the kids should be notified that he was going to have the surgery and told something about the risks involved, although without dwelling on them, and Alan had called all of them on Monday evening. We spent part of that evening, in addition, talking about what we wanted to do with our financial arrangements with the children in case something went wrong, and once again I urged Alan to make me at least a list of where financial documents and so forth were located—deeds, notes, stocks and bonds, his will, insurance papers and so on—something that he had promised faithfully to do for months and months but had never actually done, and I had not felt right about pushing it. (He did produce the list, finally—on Sunday morning, just before we left for the hospital!)

We had a nice, quiet Thanksgiving. Bill and Mo had planned to come over, and Alan did not tell them about the pending surgery until after they had arrived—he was afraid they wouldn't come if they knew. Becky, who came up from Washougal, seemed extremely subdued. She agreed to take our dog, Gypsy, home with her so that I wouldn't have to worry about the dog during the time of the surgery.

This Sunday morning we left Thorp about ten o'clock. It was not bad weather that got us off to such an early start but concern that we might run into Thanksgiving holiday traffic, a hassle that I didn't need. We got to Seattle early, about lunchtime, so we went up to the Hunt Room at the Sorrento Hotel near the hospital, the elegant place we never could afford during internship days, and had a lovely lunch, but a pretty macabre conversation, since we both kept thinking of things that we hadn't discussed but really needed to. I'm afraid we rather distressed the elderly gentleman who was dining at a table nearby, since our conversation seemed preoccupied with death and dying. For instance, Alan remarked at one point that he supposed I already knew how he felt, but if he did die during surgery or the aftermath, he would want me to authorize an autopsy, since he felt that this was the absolute minimum one could do to advance knowledge of heart disease—which, of course, I knew perfectly well he believed, even though we had never specifically talked about it. He also expressed the feeling that if he came out of the surgery with such problems or complications that he would not be functional, I should pay attention carefully to what the doctors advised, but that he didn't want to prolong life pointlessly on machines—a feeling I was quite certain that we shared but he had never actually expressed. He pointed out that there was a vast difference between taking the necessary time on a respirator to aid normal recovery, or having oxygen support for a while in order to help the body heal and become capable of taking over for itself, on the one hand, as opposed to being tied to a machine forever. He also suggested that if I needed any advice about this or anything else that might transpire, I shouldn't hesitate to reach Fred Cleveland or David Hurlbut and ask either or both of them to guide me in any decisions I had to make. All this over fillet of sole meunière, broccoli au Hollandaise, and a bottle of Chablis.

After lunch, we walked over to the hospital. The admitting procedure didn't take too long. They had Alan's chart ready, a paramedic took us up to the room, and the parade started. This time, prior to going to the hospital, Alan had typed up a list of all the medications he was taking or had taken since his last admission there, together with doses and frequencies of doses (he called the list Form #28), then made twenty copies to take along, since the last time he'd been there everybody who had walked in the door wanted to know what medications he was taking and he had had to repeat it all until he was sick of it. This time, he just handed out the sheets like handbills, to anyone who walked in the door.

When Dr. Anderson came in, around five o'clock, he seemed particularly interested in Alan's legs. Alan had quite a bit of edema in the ankles at that time, but Dr. Anderson felt he had good veins and said that he might well take the saphenous veins from both legs in order to get as good material for grafts as possible, and that he intended to try to do as many grafts as he felt he could do to get a good job.

Later on, a Dr. Shaner came in, introducing himself as the chief resident in anesthesiology, who would be working directly with Alan tomorrow, although he said that a senior anesthesiologist would also be there. Dr. Shaner explained to Alan how he would be given some medicine first thing in the morning, to make him a little groggy, and then be taken on down to the operating room, where various connecting lines that would be necessary for support and monitoring what was going on would be installed. One thing he mentioned was a Swan-Ganz line, a catheter sort of thing that goes into the jugular vein in the neck, then is advanced down into the heart, one of the things that is used to monitor blood pressures, blood gases and other elements of heart activity. Dr. Shaner said that after the Swan-Ganz line was in, they would give Alan something by IV that would put him to sleep, and would then put in an endotracheal tube and start the anesthesia to get him ready to go about five minutes before eight, when the operation was scheduled to start.

I asked Dr. Shaner about the timing of the surgery, just to have some clue as to what would be going on. He said at eight o'clock Dr. Li, Dr. Anderson's operative partner, and Dr. Marrujo, the chief surgical resident, would begin opening the chest, and that meanwhile Dr. Anderson would be getting the veins from the legs. At about eight-thirty they would be putting Alan on the heart-lung machine and then would start doing the actual bypasses. The bypass surgery itself would probably take until ten or later, Dr. Shaner said. Once it was done, they would then begin the procedure of getting Alan off the heart-lung machine and getting his heart restarted and pumping on its own. He would be supported during this time on various other drugs and medications, and they would hope to be closing up the chest incision sometime before noon. Dr. Shaner indicated that it might well take longer, depending upon what they decided to do, and I remembered that Dr. Anderson had said that the operation might well go until one or two o'clock in the afternoon, although he was scheduling it for four and a half to five hours. Then, after the closure was completed, Alan would be taken directly to the Intensive Care Unit for support. The anesthesia people would breathe for him on the way, then hook him up to a respirator in the ICU. They anticipated keeping him deeply sedated, in order to let the heart rest and not have to work too hard, perhaps not letting him wake up until very late in the day, or even the next morning. Ordinarily, the respirator would be taken off the next morning, unless for some reason it was decided that he needed respiratory support for a bit longer.

About six-thirty that evening, I went out to get a little fast-food dinner to bring back to the room for me to have when Alan's tray came. When

I got back I found that he had another visitor, and I could tell that Alan was irritated. This was a young fellow in a business suit with a name tag on it who had apparently come in to ask Alan's permission for him to stand in and observe the surgery, and he wanted Alan to sign a special permission release for him. Alan had not understood who he was or where he came from, thought maybe he was a business administration student or something, and he couldn't see why he should have to sign permission to let just anybody who felt like it wander into the operating room. Finally, after much fumbling around, with Alan getting angrier and angrier, we managed to elicit that the young man was actually a student nurse from one of the local nursing schools and wanted to observe Alan's operation because he'd never seen one before. Alan finally reluctantly signed his permission form, but it seemed to me to be poor planning to spring something like this on a patient out of left field at the last minute.

About seven-thirty that evening, the admitting nurse came in and offered to take me down to the ICU to see what it was like. She said that many people visiting patients postoperatively were terrified by the machines, tubes, monitoring screens, and all that they encountered there the first few days postoperatively, and that it sometimes helped to see what it looked like in advance. The Intensive Care Unit happened to be very quiet at the time, but I did notice that it was in a different location than it had been previously when Alan had been here with his heart attack. I was also a little surprised that he was going to be going to the regular Intensive Care Unit, not the Coronary Unit. The ICU was a large space with a central nurses' station and rooms all around it, roughly about ten beds, some of them doubles, but mostly singles, each room equipped not only with a bed but a baffling array of machinery, wires, bedside stands, monitors, and other paraphernalia. I was introduced to the nurse in charge. She told me that the units were fully staffed twenty-four hours a day, and that once Alan was back from surgery, I would be allowed to come in whenever it was appropriate. She also said that they maintained full telephone contact so that if I was out of the hospital somewhere and wanted to come in, I could call in advance and make sure how things were going and whether I could visit at a given time.

After I got back to his room, Alan went in to take a shower with the Betadyne soap, an antiseptic soap that stained his skin a kind of yellow-brown. Then we watched a murder mystery on television for an hour before I left for the apartment to get some rest.

Monday, November 26, 1984. Since Alan was to be taken down to the operating room about a quarter of seven this morning, I decided to be there by six so that I'd be sure to see him before he went. Alan had just been wakened and given some kind of medicine before I arrived, and he seemed more asleep than awake. We talked about a couple of inconsequential things— getting to see the film *Amadeus* while we were there in Seattle, maybe doing some Christmas shopping, that sort of thing. He said he hoped maybe after the operation he could get off some of the medications he had been taking, and that this might make some difference in how he felt. A nurse came in and gave him two shots, one with morphine in it, the other some sort of antibiotic. I told him that I felt sure that things were going to go all right, which was not by any means true, and that I expected him to fight hard when the operation was over. By then Alan was becoming groggy from the morphine and kind of dozing off.

Right at 6:30, a man in surgical garb came with a cart to take him down to surgery. The attendant was pleasant, apparently knew that Alan had written *Intern*, and asked him a bit about what he was writing now. Alan's answers were brief; he really didn't seem to be tracking. I was allowed to go down with Alan to the entry to the surgical wing. I kissed him, and he said, "Take it easy, kid," and in he went.

At that point, I went down to the hospital cafeteria for some breakfast, then went back to the surgery waiting area, which was familiar because it was the same waiting area where I had waited during his heart caths. I had brought a lot of reading material with me, a couple of magazines, and our friend Robert Heinlein's new novel, *Job*, which I had started and hoped would keep me interested and not too agitated. The waiting area was well set up for families who had people in surgery. There was a volunteer who takes your name and lets you know as soon as they have any information from the operating room or recovery room. Dr. Anderson had said the evening before that he would come down as soon as the surgery was over and let me know how things were, but I didn't know whether to expect that to actually happen or not.

It turned out to be a very long wait. I suppose I should have taken Dr. Anderson's advice to go out shopping or something, since it was going to take so long, but I didn't want to be that far away. I stayed there and read, went to the john, drank a cup of coffee, tried to get interested in Heinlein's book. It was a good novel, too, but I found that Robert's most earnest efforts didn't seem to work too well at that time.

Along about eleven-thirty, a volunteer told me that there was going to be a service in the hospital's little Catholic chapel, so I went in. I was the only one there. The priest asked if I was Catholic and I said, no, I was Episcopalian, but that I was concerned about Alan, so he offered some prayers and administered Communion.

A little later, I went back to the waiting room and waited some more. At about a quarter of one Father Garlish came in, the Episcopal priest who has been the official chaplain at Virginia Mason Hospital for a number of years. He said that Nolan Redman, the priest at our church in Ellensburg, had called him about Alan, so he had come over.

Then, just as Father Garlish sat down, Dr. Anderson appeared. He was looking cheerful, almost elated, and he said that Alan was out of surgery and that everything had gone very well, from his point of view, in fact, much better than he had hoped. He said that when they had gotten into Alan's chest they had found the the situation with his coronary arteries had proved to be much more favorable than the angiograms had indicated. They had found another good pathway for a graft at the back of the heart that they had not anticipated at all, and they had been able to put in four grafts. He said he was especially pleased with this, because they were all good grafts. He said that about 25 percent of Alan's heart was not functioning, due to the old MI, but that the grafting should certainly help his angina problem. He said that Alan had gotten off the heart-lung machine without any trouble and begun to pump well on his own, so he would be going to the ICU very soon. Then, when Dr. Anderson left, Father Garlish said a couple of prayers with me and I decided to go get some lunch, since I would not be able to see Alan in the ICU for maybe half to three-quarters of an hour.

It was about ten minutes after one when I left the waiting area. I had lunch, came back to the ICU to see Alan at about a quarter to two, but they were still doing things with him, and said I could not go in for maybe another twenty minutes or so.

When I finally did go in, it was pretty much as I had expected. Alan was still unconscious, he had tubes coming from all orifices, and he was on the respirator. I saw that the Swan-Ganz line that Dr. Shaner had spoken of was itself hooked up to four or five different lines, and that nurses and doctors were busy adjusting things, taking readings, checking the connection of the respirator tube to the endotracheal tube. He also had some sort of nasogastric tube in place, had EKG leads on his chest, and there were two holes in his lower chest, or upper abdominal area, from which drains emerged connected to some kind of water trap on the floor. He also had some kind of wiring in his chest, I assumed something like a temporary pacemaker, which I was told was not being used—his heart was pacing itself all right—but they were there just in case they were needed, I suppose in case of an arrest. He had a unit of blood going into one arm and a unit of glucose going into the other, as well as a urinary catheter.

I remembered that somebody had once said that the number of tubes emerging from the patient immediately after a coronary bypass operation was highly significant; that if more than five tubes were in place, the patient wouldn't make it. Maybe that was true at one time, but I don't think that's the case anymore. Alan seemed to have seven or eight. The nurse said that his condition was stable, although he was, of course, considered critical, the standard status of any bypass patient immediately postop. When I talked with Dr. Anderson, I'd asked him then if I should let the kids know or if I should wait. He suggested that I wait until after four o'clock or so. When I asked the nurse in the ICU a little bit about how he was doing, she said that he was having some problems with cardiac output that they were trying to adjust with medications, but that there was nothing to be overly concerned about. I asked how long a patient was normally considered critical, and she said that she always heaved a sigh of relief after about twelve hours. I could see that Alan's color was good, but he was just lying there inert in the bed, I gather from the drugs he was on.

I only stayed a few minutes, then left because they had some more things to be done. That was at around 2:30 P.M.

At 3:30, I checked again briefly, but there was not much change. When I checked back again at 4:30, Dr. Anderson was just coming out of the room. He said that Alan had had some problems with cardiac output, but they were under control. "Don't expect too much too soon," he told me. "There won't be very much change for about six hours." I asked again about letting the kids know that he was okay, and he said he thought that this would be all right. When I went into the room, the nurse said that Alan had wakened a little when Dr. Anderson was in, that Dr. Anderson had talked to him, and that Alan had responded and moved all his extremities, and I knew enough to know that that was a good sign because it meant that he hadn't stroked out during the surgery.

I spent the next couple of hours at the apartment, tracking down the kids on the telephone, and also checking with Bill in Spokane. Back at the hospital, I had supper in the cafeteria and saw Alan again at about 6:30. I was glad I had come when I did, because he was a little bit awake then. I asked him if he recognized me, and he nodded. He didn't say very much, though—in fact, he didn't *say* anything at all because the endotracheal tube was still in place—and he dozed off again almost immediately. As I came out, the nurse told me that he was now on some different medication that seemed to be helping the cardiac output.

Back at about 8:30 P.M.; Alan was just barely arousing again, but not very much, and I only stayed a few minutes. Dr. Anderson came by in the hallway, saw me, and stopped in. He had on his raincoat, about to leave the hospital. He said things were going a little better now on the new medications and he felt that Alan was doing okay. Alan was still listed as critical, and things could happen, but Dr. Anderson felt confident that everything was under control and that the ICU team would be able to handle problems. A little later, Dr. Shaner, the anesthesiologist, stopped by. He seemed quite enthusiastic about how well Alan had done. At about ten I told the nurse that I would be going back to the apartment, to sleep, but that I would be back early in the morning, and I asked her to call me if there were any problems. She said that I could call to see how Alan was at any time and gave me a phone number.

Tuesday, November 27, 1984. I slept like a log that night, and when I woke up, as usual, at 5:15 A.M., the first thing I realized was that nobody had called *me* during the night, which had to be a good sign. I called the hospital and was told that Alan was doing okay and I could see him anytime

I wanted to come in. I got there at about 6:30, just as a nurse was coming out of his room. She said that I could go in, that Alan was awake; he was still having problems with cardiac output, which they were controlling by medication, but she didn't think that it was any major problem. She also said that blood gases were being run, and the doctors would be deciding whether to take him off the respirator this morning or not.

While I was in the room, Dr. Marrujo came in, apparently just prior to going into another surgery today. He said that Alan was doing very well, and I think he probably would have told me if it were otherwise. When I came back at about 8:30 to check again, Dr. Anderson had been in and they had taken the repirator off. Alan's bed was cranked up to a forty-five-degree sitting position, and he said hi to me in a very croaky voice. By ordinary standards, he looked like death warmed over, but by comparison to the day before he looked absolutely great to me. They had taken out the endotracheal tube and the nasogastric tube, and they had also discontinued the blood that had been running in all the previous day—he had had about four units in all. I asked him if he was comfortable, and he indicated that he was certainly more comfortable than with the endotracheal tube in. He said his chest only hurt when they made him cough, a procedure that involved moving him around so his legs were dangling, then placing a large fat pillow against his chest with his arms around it. Except for the coughing and deep-breathing exercise with the plastic air volume device, which apparently was extremely painful and distressing, he wasn't having any great pain—"but they keep me pretty well snowed, and I just tell them, 'Lasst mich schlafen' "—the dragon's famous line from Siegfried.* He said that they were still working on the stroke volume—I guess a reference to the output—and were trying to cut down the epinephrine they were using to stimulate heart activity. He asked about the kids, and I said I'd called them, talked to all of them, and had also talked to Carl Brandt, Bill, and others.

Back later at 10:30; things seemed to be going very smoothly—Alan's color looked good, and he was alert most of the time, although he kept dozing off. The place was like Grand Central Station, with different people coming in—the respiratory therapist who works with him on this coughing and breathing business, and a physical therapist, who said she was getting him started on his cardiac rehabilitation but was actually mostly seeing to it that he didn't just freeze up into an immobile lump. She carried him through a full range of motion of both arms and legs, tried to tell him how to practice tightening his leg muscles, using his biceps in the upper arms and pumping his forearms up and down. Since he was half-asleep through most of this, he seemed to have some difficulty understanding just what he was supposed to do, but at least it was a start toward physical activity.

* "Let me sleep."

I went out for lunch, then actually did go shopping for a while, returning toward evening. When I saw him then, I learned that the weaning him from the epinephrine was still going on but they were also reducing the dosage of dopamine, one of the drugs that helped maintain control of the heart activity. The nurse said that, after "checking the numbers," they had found that his blood pressure was a little high and, therefore, she didn't want to cut the dopamine off completely, so she had reduced it to a minimal dose. At eight o'clock the blood pressure was better. The nurse said they had been concerned about the "wedge pressure," or "wedge numbers," which I gather have something to do with internal blood pressures in the chambers of the heart and with stroke volume of the heart—how much blood was being put out with each heartbeat.

After a little supper in the cafeteria, I came back at around 9:30, told Alan good night, and went back to the apartment. In general, this day was one in which Alan was alert part of the time but doping off quite a bit; I'm not at all sure how much of it he's going to remember. Things have progressed sort of according to routine, and everyone seems very pleased with how much he had been able to do in getting rid of the various lines and tubes, starting on his deep-breathing exercises, and so on. I was struck that he was not very much with it half of the time and had difficulty understanding some directions, although he made responses that seemed to be appropriate.

Wednesday, November 28, 1984. When I got to the hospital at about 6:30 A.M. this morning, I found the doctors had already been there and had decided to pull even more of the various lines and tubes. They had taken out the Swan-Ganz line, removed the chest drain tubes, and also took out the urinary catheter. He still had some of the nasal oxygen going continuously, and one IV line was kept running. Shortly thereafter, the ward clerk came in and asked me about his belongings, since they planned, he said, to transfer Alan out of the ICU. This was the first clue I had that he was going to be transferred, and I considered this a sort of independent corroboration that the doctors must have thought he was doing very well.

At about 10:30 in the morning, the physical therapist came in to do exercises, and this time they were active exercises. He did well with the foot flexing and quad setting, once she reminded him about that. They did five to seven active hip and knee flexion exercises, hip abduction, and also some arm range-of-motion. During this time, Alan seemed sort of stupefied—he would follow the woman's directions for two or three exercises, then sort of doze off, and she would have to bring him back in order to do the rest. His right arm and shoulder were bothering him a great deal, apparently from an old bursitis he'd had for years. After all the exercises were done, the nurse got the therapist to transfer him to a wheelchair. Then she unhooked the oxygen and trundled him up to a room on the general surgical floor, fourth floor east. Once there, he took a couple of steps getting out of the chair and into the bed, with assistance. They hooked up the telemetry and restarted his oxygen, and he was back in a regular bed that he could control himself. Then—wonder of wonders—they mostly left him alone for much of the day. He didn't want much lunch when they brought it but did drink a couple of containers of milk. The respiratory therapist came up once or twice to make sure that he was doing his breathing business, which he really wasn't except when he was forced to. This is a problem because apparently it hurts a great deal to do the deep breathing and follow it with coughing. Ideally, they wanted him to go through this ritual for a couple of minutes at least every hour but had basically been settling for a few minutes every couple of hours.

Alan was still getting quite a bit of pain medication, so he was still quite dopey and would be alert for a while only to doze off again. Then, during the afternoon, he started developing a fever that went up to 103 degrees, probably a result of some atelectasis (still unexpanded lung area) that the deep breathing and coughing would help relieve. At about 5:30 in the afternoon, Dr. Anderson came in, indicating again that he was extremely pleased with Alan's progress. He said that his fluids were no longer restricted, and that getting more fluids into his system would help with the fever. He also said that Alan should certainly take the pain medication when he was uncomfortable, but that if he didn't need it, it would probably be a good idea not to have it because the medicine simply depressed respiration a little bit, and kept him groggy and not perfectly alert.

I asked Dr. Anderson what he had meant about being pleased to have been able to do four bypass grafts instead of the two he had originally anticipated. He said that the actual number of grafts wasn't as significant as the fact that he had been able to get a lot more blood to the myocardium, whereas he had been afraid that he would only be able to get a small amount more, judging from the angiographic findings. The fact that he had done four bypasses did not mean that Alan would take any longer to convalesce or that anything else would be different, except that he would have the benefit of as much blood getting to the myocardium as possible. Dr. Anderson pointed out that the first three or four days postoperative were pretty rocky for any bypass patient, but that then there should be a fairly good turnaround, that Alan would probably be agitating to go home before too many days passed.

Dr. Anderson also remarked that he had seen Dr. Jennings Borgen, Alan's former partner at the North Bend Clinic, in the surgeons' lounge on Monday morning. He said Jennings had not made any comment at the time, although he must have known that Alan was on the schedule, but that as soon as he saw Dr. Anderson in the hall on Monday afternoon, he instantly asked, "How did he do?" without even saying who he was asking about, and Dick knew it was Alan he meant. Jennings had commented that it was too bad Alan couldn't have some Irish whiskey in his IV lines, and Dick had said perhaps he'd rather have it straight a little bit later.

I think this kind of small, humorous touch did more for *me* during those first few days than maybe anything else. I had heard and read so often so many *bad* things about the Big Heart Surgeons—how hurried, abrupt, impersonal, and disinterested they often were—and I have to say that in all the times I have encountered Dick Anderson since the surgery, I have been more and more impressed with his patience and kindness. He never seems to be in a hurry, never seems to be trying to rush away or brush me off. He really seems to understand what the patient—and the patient's wife—is feeling and going through. I also get the impression that he knows exactly what's going on at any given minute with each patient that he has, whether he happens to be there at the moment or not.

That evening, at around eight o'clock, Robin Johnston came in, looking positively merry. He said that Alan's heart tracing from the telemetry looked good, in fact, looked better than prior to surgery. He asked Alan a few questions, listened to his chest, and so forth, but really didn't have a lot to add. Alan was still running some fever that evening, but nobody seemed very concerned about it.

Thursday, November 29, 1984. Alan apparently slept well during the night, and certainly on Thursday morning he was looking much better and brighter, still not much interested in eating, but relatively comfortable. He was getting pain medication, then, about every six hours instead of every four. He worked some on the deep breathing and coughing with me about three or four times, and was able to get the spirometer gadget up to 2600 cc, the highest he had made yet. Alan said the previous evening he had gotten up with assistance to go to the bathroom, and this morning they had put an extension cord on some of his wiring so he could get to the bathroom and back more freely on his own. This morning he was complaining about occasionally feeling a click or a "crunchy feeling" in his breastbone when he did his coughing or happened to move his torso the wrong way. Apparently, this wasn't painful, just uncomfortable, and a little unnerving, since it felt like something in there might be coming apart. Everyone he mentioned it to seemed to think it was a little movement of cartilage where it had been sewn back together again, and nothing to worry about. His fever had broken early in the morning, then seemed to go up a couple of degrees again in the afternoon, but this time it responded to a little Tylenol. This morning, Dr. Anderson came in with his chief resident, an intern, and a clinical nurse specialist, and he said he thought things seemed to be going along pretty routinely.

Dr. Anderson indicated that he wanted possibly to get rid of the nasal oxygen on Friday, and that they would take out the emergency pacing wires on Saturday, and think about possibly discharging Alan from the hospital as early as Tuesday or Wednesday of the next week. With that kind of scenario in mind I decided that I would plan to go home to Thorp on Sunday and see as many of my PT patients as I could on Monday—I'd just had a new part-time physical therapist to cover for me during my absence. Throughout this day Alan seemed to do well, but there was a little bit of drainage from his suture line, apparently a fairly common occurrence, and Alan continued to mention the click, or crunch, when he strained to get up out of bed or when he coughed. One of the nurses thought that it might be related to a tiny bit of movement of the wire sutures in the breastbone cartilage but said that there was no need to worry about anything coming apart—"They really anchor those things down."

The physical therapist took Alan through his exercises late in the afternoon, had him take a little walk with the extension cord, and he did very well. He was definitely more alert today when he was awake, but felt very tired, feeling that he was being pushed a lot, and wanting to sleep mostly, so we kept the door closed and he actually did get several hour-long stretches of uninterrupted rest. But Dick Anderson indicated that Alan *should* allow himself to be pushed now, because it was important that he get up and keep moving. His lungs sounded clear, not so much atelectasis (lung collapse) as before, but it was still important to keep working on the coughing so he wouldn't have so much fever problem.

Friday, November 30, 1984. Again, Alan slept very well. He seems to be able to get through until four or five in the morning before needing any pain medication. The fever had been up again during the evening, but was down again this morning. I helped Alan with his bath; he got up and sat in the chair for half an hour, brushed his teeth, ate a little bit of lunch. I went downtown to do a couple of hours of shopping, and when I came back, he said that Jennings Borgen had been by to say hello. By now he's pushing his little plastic respirator up to 2800 cc, coughing isn't hurting quite as much, and he's only requiring pain medication maybe twice during the day. Late in the afternoon they got a small portable oxygen tank on a cart, so that he could take it along with him, and he walked out and down the hall for a total of about three minutes, which everyone seemed to think was just fine. When Dick made rounds with his retinue that evening, they decided they would keep him on oxygen until tomorrow but probably discontinue it then. This made Alan happy because he is getting very sore in the nose. He keeps complaining of soreness in his mouth and throat as well—a common consequence, Dr. Marrujo said, of the length of time he had to have the endotracheal tube as a foreign body in his mouth and pressing against the back of his throat.

Late in the afternoon, Wilma Dlouhy called to see if she and Bob could come down, and they arrived in the early evening, stayed maybe twenty minutes, and had a nice visit. In all, Alan got up and sat in the chair three times today, for about an hour each time, did his three minutes of walking, plus several trips to the john by himself, and had a sponge bath and brushed his teeth. The doctor said there were still little moist sounds in the lower parts of his lungs, and he was still getting up a yellowish kind of phlegm, but the fever basically stayed down all day. The pacing wires are to be taken out tomorrow, and he will have to be on bed rest for a couple of hours after that. Later in the evening, Robin Johnston came by, as he has each of the last couple of mornings and evenings, keeping tabs on things and preparing to take over as cardiologist as soon as the surgeons spring Alan free. Robin didn't have much to say this evening, except to remark about how nice it was to have a thoroughly boring recovery.

After he had gone, the nurse came in to bring Alan the little paper with his second daily dose of Persantin and aspirin, the "anticlotting cocktail" that doctors think helps keep the bypass channels from plugging up again postoperatively. I saw Alan glance into the little paper cup as though startled, and then give me a very odd look as he took the pills with a little water. The funny look was still on his face when the nurse had left.

"What's the trouble?" I asked him.

"No particular trouble," he said, "but I just realized for the first time that they haven't been giving me any Inderal since I came back from surgery. They haven't been giving me any Procardia, either, or any Isordil, and even with all this jumping in and out of bed and walking up the hall and moving around, I haven't taken a single nitroglycerin tablet in five days. *There hasn't been any angina at all since I came back from surgery.*"

It was just as well that Ann kept a record of those confusing days, because I could never in the world have provided it. Any memories that I have at all of those first postop days are spotty, sporadic, and largely inconsequential. *Lasst mich schlafen*, indeed! The one thing they didn't do during that time was let me sleep. There were a million people wandering in to see that I didn't sleep—at least, not too much. I had never before undergone general anesthesia or a surgical operation in my life, but I am here to testify that all the nonsense one hears of weird dreams, fantasies, nightmares, and mental distortions during anesthesia are a lot of hooey. For me, it was as if someone had simply taken a chunk of time out of my life, like someone would clip a chunk out of a movie film and then splice the ends back together. I remembered being carted into a brightly lighted place the morning of the operation, after Dick Anderson had greeted me, and blinking out and then instantly blinking back in again, with a vague perception of Anderson's face very fuzzy above mine, and his voice telling me it was all over and things had gone fine, and the vague thought that this sure as hell wasn't heaven, so I must have survived. I have flash memories of nightmarish moments thereafter, of gagging and choking on the endotracheal tube, feeling as though I were being strangled and not being able to make a sound of protest no matter how hard I tried, the sort of thing I have occasionally experienced waking up from bad dreams. There were people making me grab a pillow and take deep breaths and cough, and flash memories of excruciating pain at those moments, and then dropping off almost instantly to oblivion again. What happened between the blinking out and blinking in again I cannot tell you from memory, but later I had the uncanny experience of reading my surgeon's formal operative report of my own bypass operation. For those with morbid curiosity, that entire report is reproduced on pages 258 to 260.

Later, I knew that Ann had been in many times, that the doctors had been in, that multitudes of nurses, interns, and orderlies had been in; and I was momentarily aware of some of those people from time to time, but with no coherent continuity whatever. It must have been Wednesday night, or Thursday, before I actually began to track, Friday by the time I was really conscious and aware all day long, getting out of bed, walking in the hall, going to the john, having a bath. Then, on Saturday morning, came the blinding realization that throughout all this, with the pain medication now reduced to a couple of Percodan tablets a day, I had had no antianginal medication of any kind since I came back from surgery and had not had a single twinge of angina pectoris.

Ann went home Sunday morning to Thorp, "to see if the place was still there," and pick up the mail, and she stayed over on Monday to see patients. Tuesday morning, Dick Anderson announced that as soon as Ann returned, I could be discharged to the Busbys' apartment, to stay there through the rest of the week, and then go home. Thus, on the evening of my eighth postop day, we left the hospital and went back to the apartment, and Buz and Elinor came over, and we did a rerun of an evening that had occurred four years before, pouring a small celebratory drink (not the Irish that Jennings had prescribed, but some moldy old Canadian that was sitting around the apartment)—the first booze I had had in ten days' time. Through the rest of that week I increased my activities, still flaking out for two or three hours' nap in the afternoon after lunch, still requiring some of the Percodan about twice a day to relieve the chest discomfort that was quite adequately relieved with Tylenol the rest of the time. Characteristically, there was a time about four in the afternoon that the pain began to wear me down, and again about four in the morning, but day by day the chest discomfort diminished.

As my activities increased, I kept waiting, and waiting, and waiting for a twinge of the angina, just a suggestion of the angina, each time that I pushed things a little bit further than the last time, waiting and expecting. But the angina did not come. My heart rate was much faster than it had ever been during the time I was taking the Inderal. It seemed to settle between 90 and 100 beats per minute most times. My color seemed better, at least as far as I could tell looking in the mirror, but I had a little bit of fever almost every afternoon. One other change that I noticed: Almost miraculously, even in that cold, wet early December in Seattle, in that cold little apartment, I felt more snuggly warm than I had felt in four years. It occurred to me that we might discover that I had a whole closet full of superfluous sweaters.

Back home at Thorp the following week, the main problem was an enormous lack of energy and a pair of extremely sore shoulders, a fierce flareup of the bursitis that I'd suffered years before, together with some continuing pain and stiffness in my chest, but that was all. No problem with the steps from the solarium up to our bedroom; no shortness of breath on waking up in the morning; no angina during activity, during the day, and no angina waking me at night— not one bit of angina, *none at all.*

The kids gathered for Christmas: Becky came up from her fish hatchery in Washougal, Ben from his work in San Francisco, Jon from his studies at Cal Tech. Only Chris wasn't there, since he had been sent once again back to New York to Coast Guard Radar School at Governor's Island, conveniently arranged to obliterate his holiday. Becky arrived a few days before Christmas and instantly demanded to see my scars, and I threw off the bathrobe I was wearing most of the time and displayed them in all their livid glory: a great purple stripe from my neck down to my abdomen in the front, and wobbly, slightly hacked away purple stripes down the inside of each lower leg. I was a bona fide member of the Zipper Club.

We had a great Christmas. I had some pain in the chest and could still sleep only on my back, and I pooped out after a couple of hours at a stretch on my feet, and I let other people do things, and I ate and drank in decided moderation, but I had no angina and no short- ness of breath—*none whatever.*

After Christmas I got back to work, after a fashion. Once again, I seemed to be limited to doing two beautiful things a day—writing two letters, reading two pages, stretching out work on the *Good Housekeeping* column over two weeks, playing as it lay and worrying not in the slightest. Carl Brandt wrote a cheerful note upon receipt of my first postop column, saying that he couldn't see any difference between it and any preop one, and the Ladies of the Club back at *Good Housekeeping* apparently agreed.

THE ELK HUNT

VIRGINIA MASON HOSPITAL
Seattle, Washington

OPERATIVE RECORD

21 51 39

Nourse, Alan E.
Date: 11-26-84

Preoperative diagnosis:
Coronary artery disease

Postoperative diagnosis:
Same

Operation:
Quadruple aortocoronary saphenous vein bypass graft to left
anterior descending, anterolateral, distal circumflex, and
right posterior descending coronary arteries with cardiopulmonary bypass.

Surgeon: Richard P. Anderson, M.D.
         Wei-i Li, M.D.
Assistants: Gregory Marrujo, M.D.
            Frederick Merchant, M.D.

Indications:
Dr. Nourse is a 56-year-old physician, writer, and former
Virginia Mason Hospital house officer who sustained a trans-
mural inferior wall myocardial infarction in 1980. Subsequently, he had angina, and in 1981 a heart catheterization
was performed demonstrating marked inferior wall akinesis
with a poor ejection fraction calculated at 45%. There were
two 40% stenoses in the proximal anterior descending coronary artery, the right dominant artery was totally occluded,
and the posterior descending branch filled on the left side at
injection. Circumflex appeared to be small and was nearly
totally occluded. A thallium treadmill test indicated a
fixed inferior wall defect with no adjacent ischemia. He was
treated with betablockers and nitrates, and remained about
functional class II for angina until 6 months ago when his
angina began to increase to functional class III levels. In
November, while hunting, he developed an episode of congestive heart failure and was hospitalized in Ellensburg in
pulmonary edema. Since that time, he has continued to notice
symptoms of congestive heart failure and his angina has progressed to functional class IV severity. Heart catheterization was performed by Dr. Robin Johnston on the 7th of November, 1984. This study demonstrated further deterioration in
left ventricular function with an ejection fraction calculated at a .35. The anterior descending artery showed a 70%

stenosis. The anterior descending artery proceeded downward on the anterior wall of the heart, and just distal to the stenosis a large anterolateral, and a separate diagonal branch arose. The circumflex artery was completely occluded and nothing could be seen of the distal circumflex circulation. The right coronary artery remained totally occluded and the posterior descending artery filled on a retrograde injection, but not as far as the distal right main coronary artery. Because of the marked progression in his symptoms and his functional class IV state despite the increasing risk occasioned by the poor left ventricular function, coronary bypass grafting was recommended to the patient and was accepted after a full discussion of the risks, benefits, and alternatives of the procedure.

Findings:
The heart was moderately enlarged with concentric left ventricular hypertrophy. The inferior wall was heavily scarred and thinned out, but not aneurysmal. There was diffuse coronary atherosclerosis in that portion of the arteries that could be visualized through the overlying fatty tissue and epicardium. The anterior decending coronary artery was grafted at its midportion where the lumen diameter was 2 mm. The graft inserted here carried a mean flow of 63 cc per minute. The anterolateral branch of the anterior descending was grafted in its proximal portion. Lumen diameter was 1.5 mm, and, aside from mild sclerosis of the wall, there were no occluding plaques. The graft flow through this diagonal branch was 63 cc per minute. A posterolateral descending branch was identified on the posterolateral aspect of the left ventricle. It was not possible to tell whether this was originally a component of the right system or, rather, represented the distal circumflex. The end of a double sequential graft was terminated in this vessel which was 1.5 mm in diameter. A natural Y branch was utilized to anastomose side to side to the posterior descending branch of the right coronary artery. This anastomosis was fashioned approximately 2 cm distal to the origin of the vessel from the right main, which was palpable as a heavily involved atheromatous cord. There was considerable atherosclerotic change in the right posterior descending artery, which was of the poorest quality of the 4 vessels grafted. Subsequently, mean flow of 32 cc per minute was measured through this double-sequential graft. Cardiopulmonary bypass was well tolerated and was terminated without need for vasopressor support of the circulation. Subsequently, however, an adrenaline infusion was utilized to enhance contractility and heartrate.

THE ELK HUNT

Procedure:

After induction of anesthesia, the skin of the anterior torso and both lower extremities was sterilely prepared and
drapes were applied. A median sternotomy incision was made
and pericardium was opened and sutured to the drapes. Meantime, the left greater saphenous vein was removed from ankle
to knee on both lower legs. It was prepared as an arterial
graft. The patient was heparinized, whereupon the right
atrium and ascending aorta were cannulated, and appropriate
attachments made to the pump oxygenator. Cardiopulmonary
bypass was instituted with cooling to 25° C. The left ventricle was vented by means of a catheter passed across the right
superior pulmonary vein. The aorta was cross-clamped and
cardioplegic solution was injected into the aortic root. The
pericardium was lavaged with iced Ringer's solution intermittently, and myocardial temperature maintained below 15°
C. throughout the duration of aortic cross-clamping, which
totalled 80 minutes. Each of the distal anastomoses was performed, in turn, using running 7-0 prolene technique. Sequence of grafting was anterior descending, anterolateral,
right posterior decending, and distal circumflex. Following
completion of the distal anastomoses, the proximal attachments of the grafts were made over a partially excluding aortic clamp, while the aorta remained cross-clamped. Running
5-0 prolene was used. Oval sections of aortic wall were removed with a punch. Following completion of these proximal
anastomoses, all air was evacuated from the excluded portion
of aorta, and grafts and occluding devices were released.
The aortic cross-clamp was released and rewarming was com-
menced. Various maneuvers were undertaken to be sure that
all air was evacuated from the left side of the heart. Following rewarming to normal body temperature, the left ventricular venting catheter was withdrawn and the vent site
secured by tying down over Teflon felt pledgets. Cardiopulmonary bypass was then slowly terminated as peripheral arterial pressure reached normal levels. Cardiac output was
satisfactory at this time. Cardiac rate was slow and a combination of adrenaline and atrial pacing was utilized. Cardiac
cannulae were withdrawn and the cannulation sites oversewn.
Protamine was administered to counteract heparin. Hemosta-
sis was secured in the mediastinal soft tissues. Temporary
pacing electrodes were applied to the surface of the heart
and brought out through the inferior aspect of the incision.
Pericardial space over the diaphragm and anterior medias-
tinum were drained by chest catheters brought out through
inferior stab wounds and attached to underwater seal. The
pericardium was closed over the aortic root, grafts, and
base of heart. The sternal edges were brought together with
multiple heavy Tevdeks and the soft tissues closed in layers. Dressings were applied and the patient returned to the
Intensive Care Unit with a nasotracheal tube in place.

RICHARD P. ANDERSON, M.D.

It took a couple of months for the energy level to begin to pick up enough to begin thinking of going back to the first draft of *The Elk Hunt* manuscript, which I had started just before the surgery—but there was no angina. In February, with deep snow all around, cabin fever set in, and Robin suggested a vacation trip to warmer country. We took his advice and went to Phoenix for a week. There was a medical meeting on headaches held at the Camelback Inn in Scottsdale, a beautiful and obscenely expensive resort, with accommodations for attendees at half rates—which were still obscenely expensive, but we decided, what the hell, archie, *toujours gai*, what else was life for? We had a splendid holiday, with much increased insight into why old folks like us, with bypasses, et cetera, are flocking to Arizona in the winter by the squadron.

Eight months ago, as I finished a first draft of this manuscript, I was very cautious about blowing the horn about how well I was doing. Six months after the surgery, almost to the day, I finished that first draft. At that time my energy and enthusiasm were back, far beyond what they had been anytime during the past four years; to that time there had been no angina, no recurrence of pulmonary edema, no more shortness of breath than one would ordinarily expect upon exertion. At that time I felt that the recovery period was essentially over, and, at least to that date, the reconstruction had been a stunning success. But I was very reluctant to proclaim any victories quite that soon. Six months is only six months. Anything could happen. What a disservice to readers to proclaim triumphant recovery, then drop dead the next day! What an ass I would seem to be. So I didn't say much in that first draft about how well I was doing.

At this final writing, it is now almost one year and seven months since my bypass operation, and I feel much more confident of what I can report. In late October, we had a fine 1985 deer season. I hunted, up hill and down dale, almost every day, from October 12 to October 30. I did not see a single buck deer, but I assure you I saw a million doe. The deer population in Washington State is alive and well.

During the past summer, I took on a number of "challenges" to see how well I really could do. In early August, Ben and Becky accompanied me on a backpack trip up Ingall's Creek to a fishing area I knew, some seven miles in from the road. I carried a thirty-pound backpack, and, somewhat to my surprise, had no problem at all. No angina. Shortness of breath only on the steeper pitches. No nighttime angina. Nothing.

Later, in early September, Ann and I tried a more extensive excursion, backpacking five miles in to Pete Lake from the Cooper Lake trailhead in the Salmon LeSac area, making camp in the rain, and then, next day, hiking four and a half miles, without packs, up to Spectacle Lake and back in one day. No trouble for me, and a tremendous sense of exhilaration that, maybe, possibly, the trials of angina were really over.

In October of 1985, I went to New York for two weeks to discuss the first draft of *The Elk Hunt* with Edward Chase, my editor at Macmillan, to see other editors, and to see my agent, Carl Brandt. During my visit, I spent a weekend with Carl at his home near Rhinebeck, New York, and he enlisted me on a Sunday hike in the Catskills. In one day he led me five and a half miles up a Catskill mountain and five and a half back down again. If I had realized the day's endeavor he had had in mind, I don't think I would have gone, but there were no ill effects. A little soreness of the legs, a little shortness of breath on steep pitches, nothing more.

What can I say now, today, nineteen months after my surgery? That I think I'm going to live forever? No way. I've had a good year—a *very* good year—better than any one in the last five. I am feeling better and working better than at any time since the night of my heart attack in late October 1980. How long is it going to last? Who can say? What does it matter? If I were to drop dead tomorrow—and maybe I will—the surgery would have been worth it for those nineteen fine months.

Probably I'm *not* going to drop dead tomorrow. It may be another year, or two, or seven, or ten before I have further trouble. *Sufficient unto the day is the evil thereof.* But when the time comes, I am now confident that there may be alternatives that never existed before. Because the cutting edge of new alternative treatments for coronary artery disease is moving forward very swiftly.

— 15 —

Where do we go from here?

It's a good question, in a way a fascinating question to ask during this early June of 1986. My personal history is unique, and yet today its pattern is becoming universal. Just nine and a half months before this date of writing I celebrated my fifty-seventh birthday, if "celebrated" is precisely the term you want to use. If I'm no longer a young man, I am by no means an old man, either, and despite the urgent mail entreaties I receive to join the American Association of Retired Persons, and the increasingly common inquiries on the part of merchants as to whether I am a senior citizen, I do not feel any older than the fifty-seven-odd years that I have achieved so far. Age and the appearance of age are relative; but as I proceed through my fifty-eighth year, the fact is that one may fairly say that I am a man in my prime, but a man with an old, bedraggled, beaten-up heart.

Six years ago, in 1980, I was a somewhat younger man in his prime who, without any knowledge, had already suffered severe progressive damage to his coronary arteries. During that year, 1980, I suffered a major heart attack. I believe that had I been fifty-two years old twenty years earlier, and this catastrophe had happened then, this book would never have been written, because I would not have survived that heart attack by as much as six years. But in the course of the last twenty years, medical understanding of coronary artery disease—and the approach to treatment of this disease—have undergone a staggering revolution.

This revolution has been very real. In large part it has been a technical revolution, one might almost say a mechanical revolution, involving new and immensely valuable tools and techniques for discovering exactly what is going on with a CAD patient's heart and coronary circulation; with new devices for monitoring progress and assessing damage; with new and very powerful medications that clearly act as powerful interventions to prolong life, reduce risk of death, control heart function, and minimize disability; and with new techniques of surgery and other forms of physical manipulation that can offer multitudes of patients real options and alternatives, very real new hope in place of the almost uniform gray hopelessness with which coronary artery disease was viewed twenty-five years ago. Precisely where *I* go from here will be a highly individual matter, a matter of the unique circumstances and chain of events that shape us as individuals, because I am different from anyone else and my CAD is different from anyone else's. Yet there are multitudes of people who have followed the same general pattern and pathway of illness and treatment that I have, and there will be many more, and it is at least possible to foresee *in general* where the path being followed by these people may ultimately lead.

One exciting truth stands out beyond any other: All of us who are or ever have been vulnerable to coronary artery disease—and there are literally millions—are living at the cutting edge of a fantastic medical and technological revolution. Things are becoming possible today that were not even remotely possible five years ago. New ideas and new approaches, which may provide quite new alternatives and options for multitudes of people, are being conceived and explored very rapidly, even as this book is being written. This is leading toward an exciting goal: less coronary artery disease and *less severe* disease for multitudes in the future, thanks to simple preventive measures; fewer unexpected catastrophes; more alternatives and options for treatment; more prolonged survival for those who are stricken; and a far higher quality of life for those who are enjoying that prolonged survival.

Of all the cutting-edge advancements that have appeared and are appearing, coronary artery bypass graft surgery has captured the imagination of the public most strongly because it seems to be the most immediate, most widely accessible, and most dramatic positive intervention in the progress of coronary artery disease ever to appear. CABG surgery *does* something to the patient upon which it is performed. In the right cases, it can alter the pattern and prognosis of that patient's disease. For the most part, we have dwelt upon the beneficial things that this surgery can do. In selected patients, it can completely eliminate or vastly relieve an agonizing and crippling pain syndrome—angina pectoris—that, in many cases, has previously made life intolerable. And although it has not yet been proved, there is good reason to suspect that this result of bypass surgery may have more basic significance than just relief of pain. It may also help prevent further deterioration of damaged heart muscle, thus shoring up the heart muscle's ability to continue functioning as a pump, and slowing down the tendency of that injured muscle to slowly die and fall into heart failure.

At the same time, a bypass graft provides new, open channels for the flow of blood across areas of coronary artery that have become badly diseased and obstructed, so that as long as the graft channels remain healthy and functioning, the atherosclerotic obstruction of the coronary vessels doesn't matter so much. We now know that in selected patients, bypassing such obstructive lesions may reduce the likelihood of a sudden catastrophic event, such as a myocardial infarction, simply by preempting and controlling the flow of blood across danger areas in advance of such a catastrophe—sort of analogous to removing all the bullets from a hijacker's gun before the hijack occurs—with the result of less risk of a disastrous infarction and potential prolongation of life in a patient who is walking around with a major infarction all ready to be triggered, just waiting for the right time to happen.

It is certainly true that all these benefits do not apply to every patient who has a bypass operation. What's more, in terms of what comes next, there are some very definite long-term disadvantages that a person must accept as part of the coronary bypass package. Obviously, for the patient to stay alive, adequate amounts of oxygenated blood must be transported, *somehow*, between the aorta and the myocardial muscle cells in order to keep the heart functioning and beating. When the graft is emplaced so that much of the blood to the myocardium is going through the graft channels, changes begin to take place both in the natural artery that has been bypassed and in the graft channel itself. Studies have shown that when a partially obstructed left main coronary artery, for example, has been bypassed by a graft, the blood flow through the natural vessel, which may have been going along fairly well past a partial obstruction, is greatly reduced. Although there is no certainty that atherosclerotic changes progress any more rapidly in those natural arteries that have been bypassed than without bypass, there is definite evidence that a bypassed natural artery soon begins to behave like an unused blood vessel that is tied off or isolated somewhere else in the body. The walls of the vessel begin to develop fibrous tissue, to scar, and gradually to close, essentially from disuse.

This means that the patient, after bypass, can't go back again to using that natural vessel later as effectively as before, or, maybe, even at all after a certain time, and he must depend upon the graft channel as the *only* channel through which blood can flow. In saphenous vein grafts, however, changes also go on. These thin-walled vessels are not thick-walled arteries. Inevitably, they undergo a certain amount of damage in the process of being taken out of the leg, of being held ready for use, and then being engrafted in place. These vessels are vulnerable to the collection of aggregations of sticky blood platelets and little bits of fibrin from the blood, and, thus, to a process of slowly plugging up almost as soon as they are implanted.

Studies done on early bypass graft patients reveal that grafts in some plugged up almost completely in as little as a month, while others remained open without discernible plugging for as long as seven years or more. But there is no absolute way of predicting how long a given graft will stay usefully open in any given patient. There is the strong probability that with every bypass, sooner or later each implanted graft will deteriorate to the point that it can't work anymore.

So then what?

So far, nobody knows the answer to that question, but there are three possible ones that are all being actively explored today on this cutting edge of a new surgical technology. Some surgeons felt that the fault lay in the choice of graft material, the use of a thin-walled vein to bypass a thick-walled artery. They believed that use of such a vessel for a graft subjects the thin-walled vessel to a strain it was never intended to carry, and that damage and deterioration, even atherosclerotic change in that vessel is inevitable, sooner or later. These surgeons began exploring the use of a different kind of vessel—the internal mammary artery—as the bypass graft channel.

This approach may, in fact, pay off well. Early in 1986, a study reported in the prestigious *New England Journal of Medicine* indicated that internal mammary artery grafts did not tend to plug up in the same way that saphenous vein grafts do—that the mammary grafts, indeed, seemed to enlarge somewhat after emplacement and seemed to be resistant to atherosclerotic change. There is the possibility that the patient with internal mammary grafts may have, on the average, a longer trouble-free postoperative period than those who have saphenous vein grafts. On the negative side, internal mammary grafts are technically more difficult for the surgeon to perform; the vessel (which remains attached at one end) may not reach parts of the heart where grafts are necessary; the time necessary for the operation is prolonged and the operative risk is somewhat greater. Many surgeons, at least today, feel that the problems may outweigh the advantages, especially with the long experience they have had using saphenous vein grafts successfully, and that it perhaps is wisest to keep the internal mammary arteries intact, holding them in reserve so that, when and if a patient's saphenous vein grafts plug up and he's again in trouble, there is an alternative, natural graft material to use to redo the bypass operation.

Of course, with either of these two answers, there is a clear recognition that the graft channel will not last forever. Bypass surgery in selected patients may indeed prove to set back the progress of coronary artery disease by ten years, as Robin Johnston suggested from his experience at the Mason Clinic and the Virginia Mason Hospital. Current figures from the University of Washington coronary artery disease group indicate seven years rather than ten. But either way, this implies that if the patients who have these grafts do not expire from other causes in the meantime, many of them may be faced with repeat bypass surgery sometime in the future, as an absolute lifesaving necessity.

Obviously, using natural graft materials, whether saphenous veins or internal mammary arteries, while feasible and workable, is not ideal, because these vessels, made of living tissue, can deteriorate in either case and ultimately become useless. This realization has led to a third possible answer now being explored by cardiovascular surgeons at such centers as the Bob Hope International Heart Research Institute, at Providence Hospital in Seattle: a search for a strong, durable, workable *artificial* graft material that might be used to form the bypass channels—a material that would not suffer the ravages of natural tissue, would not be damaged by atherosclerosis, would not cause clotting of blood, and might last and remain functional for as many years as the patient lives.

At present, the testing of such artificial graft materials is being done on laboratory animals. Nobody knows whether this search will eventually pay off. We do know that artificial vascular materials, such as Dacron fabric artery grafts and Teflon-coated artificial heart valves, have been used in reparative cardiovascular surgery for many decades. But none of these artificial materials has proved entirely free from problems. The fact that, today, in 1985, there are well over a dozen different types and styles of artificial heart valves in active use by various surgeons and medical centers throughout the world, with dozens more being tested experimentally, tells us rather clearly that no one artificial heart valve yet devised has been entirely ideal.

One major problem of all such artificial materials in the cardiovascular system is their tendency to induce blood clotting, certainly a major threat with any new artificial graft material. But the clotting problem can be minimized with the use of anticoagulant drugs, for example, so there is a good possibility that artificial bypass graft materials will find a place in coronary artery bypass surgery sometime in the future, perhaps very soon. And this would mean new alternatives, new options, an ever-expanding ability to tailor feasible and successful avenues of treatment to the specific needs of individual patients.

When CABG operations were first pioneered in the 1960s, there was a strongly fatalistic feeling that one bypass operation was essentially the end of the line for the patient who had it performed; he or she would survive as long as the graft did, and probably not much longer. Today, of course, that concept has changed. Reoperation, when necessary, is not only feasible but state of the art enough that surgeons more or less plan on it and try to hold natural graft material in reserve in case needed. Five years from now, it may be just as realistic and feasible to take artificial graft material off the shelf and implant it for the bypass channels, leaving the patient's saphenous veins or internal mammary arteries alone.

The Cutting Edge of Angioplasty

In the early 1980s, there was, and still is, one absolutely enormous and obvious disadvantage to CABG surgery as a major attack on obstructive coronary artery disease—a disadvantage nobody liked to talk about very much but that everyone was aware of, because it was sort of like an elephant in your bathroom: You couldn't ignore it. This was the simple fact that bypass surgery was a dangerous major operation, an operation involving extremely high morbidity and mortality rates for an elective procedure. It was also an operation that required a small army of people to make it float, all of whom had to be paid, and a staggering amount of major medical center and hospital resources, which also had to be paid for.

One of the main complaints about CABG surgery in the mid- and late 1970s was that its growing, widespread utilization was consuming far, far too much of the total medical resources of the country. Indeed, it evolved as a procedure feasible enough for widespread use for two reasons only—the risk and the cost of not doing the surgery were far greater, for many CAD patients, than the risk and cost of doing it; and, in terms of tackling coronary artery disease directly, bypass surgery was the only game in town. There weren't any alternatives. For any individual patient it meant that the surgery had to be done at a major medical center. It meant that somebody had to pay total costs that could range anywhere from fifteen to forty thousand dollars *per case*. Very clearly, the procedure was not "cost effective," as the medical economists like to express it; but there were a great many individuals, including myself, who were not terribly concerned about how cost effective it all might be for the rest of the world, since we chose to evaluate our own individual lives and futures perhaps more highly than the medical economists did.

It was during this time, in the late 1970s, that the cutting edge of technology led some cardiologists to explore another, much less costly and less traumatic alternative: tackling the lesions in coronary arteries directly.

By that time, it was often possible to identify people—by their symptoms, by treadmill testing, EKGs, and so forth—who had some degree of CAD that was surely going to give them trouble in the future. In those people it was also possible, by means of angiography, to identify precisely what lesions were located where in the coronary artery tree, and to determine what degree of obstruction there was in one vessel or another. In order to obtain this information, of course it was necessary to place a catheter in the patient's aortic bulb and poke the nose of the catheter into the orifices of coronary arteries, then squirt a contrast agent into the arteries in order to make X-ray pictures of the coronary artery pathways. These pictures could reveal areas of partial obstruction in individual coronary arteries—but what about the obstructive lesions themselves? What would happen, for example, if one used a very similar catheter to directly approach a partially obstructing lesion in such an artery and attempted to use the catheter to manipulate or alter the lesion?

The answer to such questions was the development of a very special kind of coronary artery catheter: thin, flexible, one that could be threaded directly into the mouth of a coronary artery, down the arterial channel to a partially obstructing lesion, then *on through* the area of obstruction. This special catheter was, in fact, a *double* catheter, with an outer layer near the tip that could act as a small, oval-shaped, inflatable balloon. In theory, such a catheter, delicately and skillfully maneuvered to place the balloon tip within the narrow channel of a partially obstructing coronary artery lesion, could then have the balloon inflated to actually expand the lumen—the interior channel—of the artery and squash the obstructing atherosclerotic lesion back against the artery wall. In Figure 10 (page 270) we can see how a coronary artery lesion might look before such a catheter is passed in, while it's in place and in use, and after it's withdrawn. This procedure was roughly analogous to dredging obstructing silt from the bottom of a river estuary in order to allow freer flow of river traffic up and down the waterway, except that, in this case, the obstructing material was not carried away but simply pressed back or compressed out of the way.

The idea was not entirely new. Such balloon catheters had been used quite successfully in dealing with atherosclerotic lesions in other blood vessels—in lesions involving the iliac arteries, for example, or the femoral arteries, or even the carotid artery. The technique was called *angioplasty*—literally, reconstructing a blood vessel—and, when applied to a lesion in a coronary artery, it became known as *percutaneous translumenal coronary angioplasty*, or PTCA, meaning the repair or reconstruction of a coronary artery lesion by approaching the lesion by means of a catheter through the lumen, or interior channel, of the coronary vessel itself.

This procedure was first tried on human patients in 1977 and

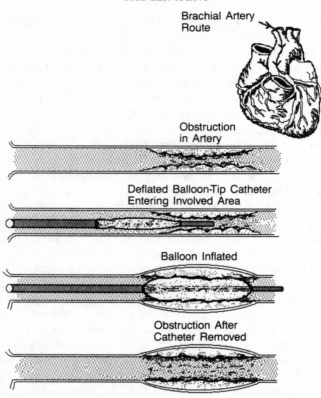

Figure 10   Percutaneous transluminal coronary angioplasty (PTCA). A balloon-tipped catheter, deflated, is passed into the narrowed segment of the coronary artery, then inflated to stretch the vessel open.

found to be successful in many cases. The patient suffering from severe angina as a result of an obstruction in a coronary artery branch could be taken not to an operating room, but to the cath lab, catheterized, have an angiography performed, and the partially obstructed channel reopened with a balloon catheter, right on the spot. That same patient could be returned to his hospital bed within an hour or so, relieved of his angina. The risk of major surgery, the trauma of major surgery, and the cost of major surgery could all be avoided in a carefully selected group of patients. The procedure was still confined to major medical centers: it required about $1,000,000 worth of radiology equipment and could only be performed safely with a cardiac surgery team on standby, to do an immediate CABG operation on the 4 percent of patients who ended up with complete obstruction of the artery. But angioplasty did not require a surgeon to perform it; today, coronary angioplasties are usually performed by the cardiologists who are already adept at and experienced in doing cardiac catheterization and coronary angiography. The procedure is nothing more than a simple and obvious extension of what such a physician is already doing.

Today, coronary angioplasty is performed on selected patients quite widely in a great many centers for the care of heart disease. It is still too early to assess clearly precisely how valuable this particular procedure is going to prove to be. Clearly, the patients have to be selected very carefully, because only certain kinds of coronary artery lesions lend themselves to angioplasty repair. Others, even with growing experience, remain clinically untouchable. There is also a great question today as to how permanent this procedure may be. Some studies indicate that the compressed atherosclerotic plaques often tend to reexpand and reobstruct within a matter of a few months in some patients—sometimes, almost immediately. Sometimes, this problem can be resolved by repeat angioplasty, sometimes not. Only the passage of time and the accumulation of a great deal of experience will tell us what real long-term usefulness there may be.

Despite these problems, there are certainly some patients for whom this kind of procedure can serve as a means of buying time: for example, easing a critical situation with obstructive coronary artery disease long enough to allow a patient to get into better shape for later bypass surgery. Once again, the development of percutaneous translumenal coronary angioplasty has opened up another alternative, another option for effective treatment for at least some patients with coronary artery disease. It will be interesting to see if the technique can also be used to deal with plugging and obstruction of bypass channels as well as natural coronary arteries. The possibilities are dazzling; it would certainly be splendid if a patient, seven or eight years after an initial bypass surgery, needed only to go into the hospital for an overnight admission to have relatively inexpensive angioplasty to open partially closed bypass channels, instead of having to repeat a complete CABG operation.

The Cutting Edge of Translumenal Coronary Thrombolysis

Exploratory procedures like translumenal angioplasty—and even coronary artery bypass surgery itself—are most applicable to people who have known atherosclerotic lesions threatening their lives. In particular, such procedures offer hope of preventing the catastrophe of myocardial infarction before it happens, or, by bridging obstructions and bringing fresh blood to myocardium injured by infarction, hope of providing relief from angina after a catastrophe has occurred. But these procedures obviously left one gaping hole in the armamentarium of alternatives and options. What about the patient who learned that he had advanced coronary artery disease for the first time when catastrophe struck? Some 40 percent of all first heart attack victims die within a few minutes or hours of the beginning of a heart attack—a staggering, appalling mortality rate. What option might there be for dealing with an MI *while it was actually going on*, and, perhaps, salvaging some of these lives?

Within the last five years, one such option has appeared on the scene, with truly exciting implications. Much has been learned in the last twenty years about the physiology of an acute myocardial infarction—what actually happens to cause it. Earlier I described, roughly, the chain of events that most cardiologists believe occurs when a myocardial infarction begins. Doctors have come to realize that by far the vast majority of MIs are related in some way to the formation of a blood clot in a damaged and partially obstructed coronary artery. In most MIs, it is a clot forming in the damaged interior of the artery that first causes the last vestige of blood flow through that branch of the artery to stop. Sometime *after* that clot has plugged up the vessel, edema and inflammation of the vessel wall completes the job. In theory, at least, it seemed to cardiologists that there might be a period of time after the onset of an acute MI when extensive myocardial damage and myocardial death or infarction might be prevented if there was some way to dissolve the clot, then and there, right away, where it had lodged itself in the coronary artery.

How could this be done? With cardiac catheterization, it seemed possible that one could deliver some clot-dissolving medicine or chemical, in concentrated form, directly to the place where the clot had lodged, if one could get to the patient soon enough. One problem was that there weren't very many such medicines known. A drug like heparin introduced into the circulation prevents clotting of blood very effectively by interfering with the clotting process before the event. But heparin has no effect whatever on a clot that has already formed. It can't make a clot *dissolve*. Medicines like warfarin or dicumerol presented the same problem—they interfered with the liver's production of prothrombin, one of the chemicals necessary in the stepwise chain of chemical events that leads to the formation of blood clots, so warfarin could also prevent formation of clots but couldn't dissolve a clot that was there already. In addition, both those drugs, once administered, made the patient vulnerable to bleeding from capillaries in various parts of the body, and, in the case of a fresh myocardial infarction, perhaps bleeding into the infarcted area, causing more damage rather than less.

Another kind of chemical suggested itself to cardiologists who were studying the possibility of thrombolysis (clot dissolving) as a way to tackle acute myocardial infarctions. This substance was an enzyme know as *streptokinase,* so called because it had first been isolated as a by-product of certain streptococcal bacteria. Streptokinase was essentially a protein-dissolving enzyme that had sometimes been used successfully in the past to dissolve hematomas (collections of clotted blood that occur in soft tissue, often as a result of some trauma or injury). Streptokinase tended to soften and break up the fibrin that formed the soft, gelatinous matrix of a blood clot, thus enabling a recently formed clot to dissolve without any particular ill effect on healthy living tissue in the surrounding area.

Once again, animal experimentation led the way. Researchers found that streptokinase injected into an injured coronary artery in laboratory animals could, indeed, dissolve fresh clots that formed there. Once its relative safety and efficacy was established in the laboratory, the drug was tried on humans, administered by the so-called translumenal route (through the artery itself). A catheter was placed in a coronary artery just above the point at which a clot associated with a myocardial infarction had formed, and a certain amount of streptokinase was infused directly at the clot site.

As was hoped, this type of treatment proved to be successful with certain cases. In early studies, it was found capable of dissolving an already-formed coronary artery clot and allowing the obstructed circulation through the coronary artery to be resumed. If done soon enough after the first symptoms of a heart attack occurred—like, within the first hour or two of onset—it could often prevent the ischemic death of myocardial cells, leading to a full-blown myocardial infarction, before this tragedy could occur. The procedure could be done in any cardiac cath laboratory and required the infusion of relatively large amounts of streptokinase over a period of time ranging from several minutes to half an hour or longer. It was found that if clot dissolution was going to occur, it would occur quite rapidly, and in many cases so treated, the EKG current of injury indicating myocardial damage would promptly disappear, the pain stop, the perfusion of oxygenated blood into the threatened area of the heart was immediately resumed, and, in effect, the catastrophe of a myocardial infarction prevented—literally—in midstream. And, indeed, when done on properly selected patients under ideal timing conditions, this procedure of translumenal intracoronary thrombolysis with streptokinase proved successful with a high percentage of patients and almost certainly saved lives in many cases.

The potential value of this procedure was obvious, but, as always, there were problems involved. You never seem to get home free. The large amounts of streptokinase required during treatment remained in the circulation for several hours before the kidneys could get rid of it, and during that time it could sometimes cause extensive bleeding elsewhere in the body, which was clearly not desirable. In addition, streptokinase, a foreign protein substance, is a powerful allergen, and a small number of people upon whom it was used had allergic reactions to it, sometimes quite severe. What's more, there was a certain amount of risk involved just manipulating a catheter in an area of the heart that that was under deadly attack already—the risk with a certain small number of patients, for example, of making the heart attack worse rather than better just by poking a catheter around.

Of course, one might live with problems like these in the interest of possibly saving a person's life in the midst of a myocardial infarction. But another problem was far more difficult to get around. It soon became apparent that the timing of this kind of streptokinase intervention was absolutely critical. The drug would dissolve only a fresh, newly formed clot in a coronary artery. It had to be used *fast*, before a great deal of myocardial damage was already done due to ischemia. This meant that it was most successful if used within a few minutes of the first onset of symptoms of a heart attack. The best results were obtained when the treatment was rendered within the first hour. Some help could be obtained, sometimes, as late as three or four hours after the beginning of symptoms, but experience showed that the success rate fell off sharply after that. Within five or six hours from the beginning of symptoms, this treatment was virtually useless—things had progressed too far by then for the procedure to work.

This kind of timing was just fine for the patient who had his heart attack while he was already in a hospital equipped with a functional cath lab, or for a victim lucky enough to live across the street from a major medical center. But most heart attack victims don't live that close to immediate help. For vast numbers, those precious first sixty minutes were often largely consumed just dithering around trying to decide whether something was wrong or not; still more time was consumed getting the patient to a medical center where the procedure might be done. There was no way that an outlying suburban hospital, emergency room, or a rural medical center without sophisticated equipment could make this treatment available at all. Thus, potentially promising as it seemed, translumenal coronary thrombolysis was terribly limited, and cardiologists began casting about to find ways somehow to increase its efficacy and application.

An obvious alternative approach was attempted. If too many patients lost too much time reaching a center where immediate cardiac catheterization could be done, to administer the streptokinase, maybe some benefit could be derived simply by injecting large amounts of the drug into a peripheral vein—a vein in the arm, for example— beginning as quickly after onset of symptoms as possible and continuing for a prolonged period, perhaps several hours. With such a procedure, the drug would be diluted in the bloodstream before it could reach a coronary artery, to be sure, but perhaps enough would reach the clot soon enough that way to begin the process of thrombolysis, and then a continued diluted dosage of the drug in the bloodstream, over a prolonged period of time, might allow the clot-dissolving to progress to completion. True, the large amounts of streptokinase and the prolonged period of administration would greatly increase the risk of unwanted bleeding in any given patient. But they were, after all, individuals who faced a very terrible risk of dropping dead of acute myocardial infarction if nothing were done, so it seemed that the added risk might well be worth taking. The really important thing was that this procedure, called *intravenous thrombolysis*, if it would work, could be started by virtually any doctor, anywhere, with any patient who seemed to be suffering an acute heart attack, thus getting the ball rolling fast. It could be started the moment the doctor saw the patient in some remote farmhouse bedroom, even if it was fifty miles away from any medical facility.

The procedure was duly tested—and didn't work very well. All the anticipated risks were there, all right, but the streptokinase administered in this way didn't seem to do much good in a large majority of patients. It helped some, but a smaller percentage compared to the 75 percent success rate of thrombolysis by the intracoronary delivery route, done within an hour or so of the attack. Clearly, some other clot-dissolving substance was needed besides streptokinase. And then in early 1983 and 1984, an alternative drug was identified and tested, and a wave of excitement spread through the world of medicine.

The new agent was an enzymatic substance known as *tissue plasminogen activator*, or Tpa, a chemical substance that is manufactured naturally in the human body, and, thus, does not cause allergic reactions. In concentrated doses delivered to a newly forming clot in a coronary artery by the translumenal catheter delivery route, the substance appeared even more effective than streptokinase in dissolving the clot. The same time limitations applied there as with streptokinase—the sooner the better, and not any later than five or six hours after the beginning of symptoms, if the drug was to be effective. And it did not seem to cause bleeding problems elsewhere in the body, so very large doses could be given without worrying about side effects.

Most exciting of all, however, was the discovery that the same drug, given intravenously, caused thrombolysis in a far greater percentage of cases than the streptokinase, intravenously. In fact, the studies that led to this discovery came to a most unusual end. The researchers testing Tpa had decided to try using this substance intravenously in a carefully controlled, randomized, double-blind study to compare the results with other patients receiving the streptokinase intravenously, and see which one worked better, if either. Patients who were candidates for intravenous thrombolysis treatment, after understanding the study fully and agreeing to participate in it, were assigned, at random, either to treatment with intravenous streptokinase or with intravenous Tpa, with assignment being made in such a way that neither patients nor doctors knew which patients were getting which drug. It was anticipated that the study would run for a period of a year or two as new patients were found who were suitable; at the end of that time, it was hoped there might be enough cases done with each drug that some statistical difference would appear showing one drug slightly more effective than the other.

That study was never finished, and for a remarkable reason: Very early on it became obvious to the physicians running the study that the drug being used in one group of patients was markedly more effective than the drug being used in the other group—so much more so, in fact, that the researchers could not ethically continue giving patients the less-effective drug. The study was abruptly terminated and the identification code broken to see which was the effective drug. As suspected, it was the tissue plasminogen activator that was so markedly more effective, even when delivered by the intravenous route. In early 1985, the preliminary results of this study were published in the *New England Journal of Medicine*, whose editors, as a matter of policy, practically never published preliminary reports of anything. They broke their own rules in this case because they considered these preliminary findings so important that the world of medicine should know about them immediately.

At the time of this writing, additional studies in the use of Tpa, both by intracoronary delivery and intravenous, are continuing. Only time will tell us if the intravenous approach with this drug will really prove effective enough to take its place as a major weapon in dealing with acute myocardial infarction. But some cardiologists, including Robin Johnston, are exceedingly sanguine about the efficacy of this form of treatment. When I talked to him, after the *New England Journal* article was published, he was clearly excited, envisioning revolutionary changes in the way acute myocardial infarctions might be dealt with in the future.

"Any doctor could carry this drug in his bag, with syringes and needles for intravenous administration," he said. "Any doctor or any emergency room, any dinky little rural hospital, could start administering this stuff just as soon as there was reasonable suspicion that the patient was having a myocardial infarction. Of course, it wouldn't be definitive treatment. It wouldn't fix the atherosclerotic lesion in a patient's coronary artery. But it could save his life, buy enough time to get him to a major medical center for a cardiac cath and angiogram, where angioplasty could be done, where bypass surgery could be done, according to what he needed. When you think of the lives that could be saved, the speed with which treatment could be started, the morbidity and disability that could be avoided— it really makes your head swim."

I suspect that, within a year or two, perhaps even before this book is published, we will have a much clearer idea of how much of this vision of the future may actually be in the cards. On this cutting edge of technology things are moving just that fast.

The Cutting Edge of Medical Treatment

Meanwhile, in very steady but less dramatic fashion, the search goes on for other solutions, other alternatives, other options, not only in the areas of surgery and advanced technology, but in the development of new medicines as well. The problem of medical treatment of angina pectoris remains with us today, and it's going to remain with us indefinitely. New drugs for dealing with angina are needed and are being studied and developed for future use. Among the finest drugs we have today to combat angina are the beta-blockers—Inderal and other drugs in that family—but when heart failure begins to emerge in a patient, these drugs tend to make the heart failure *worse* and may have to be withdrawn at just the time they are most desperately needed to control angina. Some hoped that the calcium slow-channel blockers might serve as alternatives, and, to some degree, they have, but these drugs also have a variety of drawbacks, not the least of which is the kind of erratic behavior that I experienced in using them. While they may help one patient a great deal, they may not help another at all, with no apparent reason why this should be so. Thus, new variations of calcium blockers are being investigated in the hope of identifying one or more that work more realiably and effectively than those used currently.

Digitalis is another old standby, used as a major weapon against congestive heart failure for over a hundred years. But even for this drug a good substitute is desperately needed. It does help combat congestive heart failure by acting on the cells of the myocardium to slow the pulse rate, increase the contractility of the myocardial cells, and, thus, improve the pumping efficiency of each heartbeat. The problem is that digitalis, or its purefied alkaloid digitoxin, is, as the name suggests, basically a myocardial poison. The margin between a *safe and effective* dose of digitoxin and a *toxic* dose is very narrow. In a patient who has suffered the terrible damage of a myocardial infarction, or the ongoing damage of myocardial ischemia, the heart-poisoning effect of the digitalis can become more and more ominous. People who have coronary artery disease badly need drugs available that have the beneficial heart-supporting effects of digitalis—the so-called *inotropic* effects—without the underlying toxic effects to contend with. A number of such drugs, very new and still highly experimental, are being studied intently by cardiologists, in hopes of finding some that offer real advantages in dealing with heart failure in myocardial infarction patients.

Finally, new drugs are also being investigated to combat cardiac arrythmias that can turn up in coronary artery disease and that may well be at the root of "cardiac sudden deaths." Here, already, technology—plain old bioengineering—has been lending a helping hand in recent years. It may be easy enough to determine that a patient has a cardiac arrhythmia—a disorder of the rate or rhythm of the heartbeat—but it can be difficult, even dangerous to treat an arrhythmia without first identifying what kind of arrhythmia it is; that is, where in the heart it originates, from what cause, whether or not it is likely to cause trouble, and whether it is even necessary to treat it at all. In most cases, the best way to "trap" an arrhythmia and identify its origin is to record it on an EKG and study the resulting tracing. This often can answer the basic question as to whether a given arrhythmia is dangerous and must be controlled at all costs, or if it is merely an annoyance that doesn't have any serious meaning in terms of health.

Unfortunately, arrhythmias often tend to come and go. They may not be so obliging as to occur when the patient is sitting in his or her doctor's office, where an EKG can be taken. But a couple of ingenious electronic devices have been invented to help get around this problem and make it possible to trap an arrhythmia on an electrocardiogram for identification, no matter when it occurs.

One of these gadgets is known as a Holter Monitor. Essentially, this is a highly miniaturized electrocardiograph machine that runs on batteries and can be connected by a single wire lead to the patient's chest, held in place with adhesive tape, and equipped with a twenty-four-hour supply of a special recording tape. The monitor is easily portable and not too inconvenient to carry, so the patient can hook it up at the beginning of a day, go about his business, go to bed at night, with the lead still in place and the machine still running, and wake up the next morning with a twenty-four-hour record of his heartbeat, including any episodes of arrhythmia that may have oc-cured.

Of course, there are some problems with this arrangement. The machine is very expensive, and rental costs, added on to the con-siderable cost of having the whole recording analyzed by a cardiol-ogist, makes a twenty-four-hour Holter Monitor record quite ex-pensive to obtain. In addition, the recorded tracing has to be transported physically to the doctor's office to have it analyzed, so there may be time delays in identifying the arrhythmia.

To meet these problems, another medical toy can be used as an alternative. Called a "memory cardiobeeper," this machine is an-other small, portable box that amounts to a miniaturized EKG ma-chine capable of recording several thirty-second EKG strips. When the patient is aware that a period of arrhythmia has started, he places the metal contact from this machine against his bare chest and turns on the machine. After recording a period of arrhythmia, the patient then can telephone the doctor's office, place the gadget's speaker in contact with the speaker on the telephone set, and rerun the recording of the arrhythmia. The machine converts the EKG into a sound signal, which is carried over the telephone line and picked up by a recording device on the doctor's telephone. This converts the tone directly into an electrocardiogram tracing. Thus, in a matter of min-utes, the doctor can have an actual physical EKG tracing of the arrhythmia that the patient, as soon as he became aware that it started, trapped. The machine is not as expensive as a Holter, and the only costs, other than rental, are those of the doctor's interpre-tation of a brief, ordinary EKG strip, so that the cardiobeeper can be used to identify the arrhythmia much more economically.

Once this has been done, there are a variety of medicines that can be used to quiet or "convert" it, depending on where it originates. Many of these, including the old-fashioned quinidine, or the Norpace that I used when my arrhythmia started, or lidocaine and other drugs, have been used for a number of years and can effectively control most arrhythmias. But all these drugs, like digitalis, are basically cardiotoxic, and doctors are reluctant to pile toxic effects on top of a sick, malfunctioning heart if there is any alternative. Currently, a wide variety of drugs are under investigation as better options for treating arrhythmias, with the emphasis not only on higher efficiency and efficacy, but on lower toxicity as well. A number of these drugs are likely to be available for general use in the near future.

Despite the number of drugs that are available now or under active investigation, however, some patients with severe, life-threatening arrhythmia problems just can't obtain reliable control of their disordered heart rhythms with the use of drugs. Many of these people have suffered irreparable damage to those portions of the heart through which the electrical conducting channels pass—as a result, for instance, of myocardial infarction—so the normal rhythm-establishing electrical patterns are broken and rhythm-disturbing feedback patterns occur, or responses to the natural pacemaker signals are interfered with. For many years now, some of these patients have been treated successfully with surgically implanted artificial pacemakers—electronic devices that are easily implanted under the skin of the chest and connected to the heart by just the sort of lead wires that I had implanted at the time of my by-pass surgery to be ready, "in case of emergency." These devices do not require really major surgery for implantation and need be disturbed only at infrequent intervals for battery recharging or replacement.

Certainly, artificial pacemakers have served an important purpose, but like everything else, there have been problems. Any mechanical device can break down unexpectedly, although these have an excellent history of prolonged, flawless function. Perhaps more important, most cardiac pacemaker devices have no way to adjust or accommodate to changing demands on the heart. They are preset to trigger so many heartbeats per minute, and that is the rate that is maintained. But of course, this, is not the way the heart ordinarily works. Under normal circumstances, when a person with a good, healthy heart engages in unusual physical exercise, the heart rate will increase to accommodate the body's increased need for oxygen. When that same person is relaxed or sleeping, the heart rate ordinarily will slow down, giving the heart a relative degree of rest. But these changes were not possible with the first artificial pacemakers, which were unable to adjust the heart rate according to the body's demand for oxygen.

Even this problem is being solved today. During 1985, doctors in various medical centers began implanting a new, "sophisticated" generation of cardiac pacemakers—"smart" pacemakers, so to speak. These new devices, in addition to delivering regular electrical impulses to trigger the heartbeat, also contain sensors capable of detecting increased or decreased physical activity on the part of the patient. Minicomputers can then cause an increase or decrease in the heart rate, triggered by the pacemaker, as demand waxes and wanes. For example, such a smart pacemaker might turn the pacemaking rate up to 90 or 95 during active physical exercise—brisk walking, jogging, or skiing—then, turn it down to 45 or 50 beats per minute while the patient is in deep sleep.

So far, these devices are used on an experimental basis only, and they have not been approved by the FDA for general application. No doubt glitches will be found in the function of these early models, but there is nothing in the concept that is beyond state-of-the-art electronic technology today. Probably such pacemakers, with appropriate modifications as experience is gained with their use, presently will replace the older variety, resulting in an overall net improvement in the alternatives available for dealing with problems of cardiac arrhythmia.

Reversing Cardiac Arrest

Even today, cardiac arrest—the sudden stoppage of effective heartbeat, without warning, usually due to sudden onset of ventricular fibrillation—remains a major and continuing threat to life for many victims of coronary artery disease, either before or after experiencing heart attacks. Cardiac arrest accounts for the vast majority of the thousands of "cardiac sudden deaths" that occur each year, and, once established, ventricular fibrillation won't correct itself spontaneously. Fortunately, in many cases cardiac arrest can be treated effectively and reversed if treatment can come quickly enough, and here another part of the cutting edge of modern heart technology is finding better ways to bring this about.

One way to deal with cardiac arrest, familiar to almost everyone by now, is the prompt performance of *cardiopulmonary resuscitation*, or CPR, on the victim. With some cases, nothing more than a sharp thump on the chest is required to restart an arrested heart; cardiologists argue about whether this is a good thing to do, but the conscensus seems to be that it's a very good thing if it works, and that it can't do anything much worse than is already happening if it doesn't. But in many cases, full CPR is necessary: using a formal resuscitation procedure to breathe for the patient while simultaneously compressing the chest over the breastbone, at approximately one-second intervals, to simulate heartbeat, and to help keep blood flowing to the brain and to other parts of the body, until the arrested heart can be jolted back to normal rhythm with an electroshocking device, or "shock box."

There has been quite enough publicity about the lifesaving benefits of CPR so that everybody knows what it is, at least vaguely, but there is a great difference between knowing what it is and knowing how to perform it. This book is not the place to try to teach CPR; learning to perform it requires not only instruction but guided, hands-on practice as well. Today, there are many places one can learn CPR, then follow up with periodical refresher courses. Virtually every hospital in the country provides CPR training to staff members, so most health workers at every level are trained. People staffing emergency rooms and Aid Cars are trained. Doctors and nurses are trained—but this isn't good enough. Ideally, *everyone* should be trained in CPR techniques, so that *anyone* could step in and perform it in an emergency. Certainly, somebody in every family should be trained. Local American Red Cross units provide courses regularly and usually announce them in local newspapers. Many local fire stations provide training courses. (Of course, all firefighters and police officers today are so trained.) Ask your doctor or someone at your local hospital where CPR training can be obtained—*and then obtain it*. Ordinarily, there is no charge for these training sessions; they are provided as public services. But if everyone took the very few hours necessary for CPR training, we could have an absolutely fantastic lifesaving public resource in this country without the expense of a single tax dollar.

CPR does not reverse cardiac arrest caused by ventricular fibrillation, but, in many cases, it can keep a patient alive long enough for an Aid Car, equipped with a shock box, to arrive for more definitive treatment. These electroshocking devices are kept on standby not only in Aid Cars and ambulances but in virtually every hospital, medical clinic, or doctor's office in the country. These devices, however, have always required technical knowledge and training to operate them. But recently in Seattle, Washington, an interesting experiment has been taking place to try to make shock boxes even more readily available to people who need them. A small, simplified version of a shock box unit has been invented—computerized and very portable—with stepwise digital readout instructions for use. Virtually anybody can use one by following built-in instructions, without any prior training.

In Seattle, these mini–shock boxes have been widely distributed on an experimental basis to local fire stations, doctors' offices, even to the homes of patients known to be at high risk for sudden cardiac arrest. The idea is that by having these simplified machines more readily available—and accessible for use—near more potential victims of cardiac arrest in the general population, the percentage of arrest victims who can be salvaged and kept alive may be greatly increased. Use of these devices is an ongoing experiment in Seattle at this time; only time will tell how successful it may prove to be.

The Ultimate Solutions

For all we can say about the rapid and remarkable progress in finding alternatives to use in dealing with coronary artery disease, the fact remains that many people still do, and will continue to, suffer catastrophic and massively damaging myocardial infarctions, or severe ischemia leading to crippling angina, and will proceed, inexorably, to develop congestive heart failure and die in spite of any alternatives for treatment that may be available. The heart is a living organ made of living tissue, and whereas one may help support it and help it to work more efficiently in the face of severe disease or injury, one cannot *make* it work when disease or injury ultimately overtakes it completely.

Everyone is aware of the two major "ultimate solutions" that have been explored in recent years as final avenues of escape, to preserve the lives of patients with irreversible terminal heart disease. Heart transplants—replacing a patient's diseased and dying heart with a healthy heart taken from a donor who has died from reasons having nothing to do with heart disease—have been explored since 1962, when they were first pioneered by Dr. Christiaan Barnard in South Africa. In the almost twenty-five years since the first heart transplant was attempted, hundreds of operations have been performed throughout the world, and, until recently, the record of success has been spotty indeed. In the earliest attempts, survival rates were very low, the total morbidity (overall gross illness) of the patient while surviving was extremely high, and the quality of life practically nil. For a number of years in the United States, only one medical center and one dedicated team of doctors continued to explore heart transplants as a means of treating selected terminally ill patients. The program, located at Stanford University in Palo Alto, California, was led by Dr. Norman Shumway and his associates. By carefully selecting only patients who had the most promising prospects possible for heart transplant, by developing and refining incredibly complex techniques of follow-up and support, by requiring truly dedicated effort on the part of the patients themselves, gradually the Stanford group has increased the rate of success with heart transplant patients, increasing the longevity of many while making possible at least a reasonable quality of life, despite the many elements of care that are necessary to help the patients survive.*

* The Stanford "careful selection" process was both arbitrary and intensely practical. No one over the age of fifty was considered; candidates could have no other illness except for absolutely terminal heart disease; and any candidate had to be able to provide an immense amount of money up front to cover at least part of the staggering cost of the operation and follow-up care. Thus there were very few people, relatively speaking, who could qualify as candidates.

Today, more and more major medical centers are resuming—or initiating—heart transplant programs. With the experience that has been acquired and shared with other doctors by the pioneers in this field, there is at least some reasonable hope that cardiac transplants may ultimately emerge as a plausible, feasible and widely available ultimate solution to terminal heart disease, at least for a select group of patients. According to the latest figures, approximately 50 percent of carefully selected patients given heart transplants can be expected to survive at least two years, and some have survived as long as ten.

But the problems with heart transplantation as a broad solution are legion. One enormous bottleneck has been the matter of acquiring enough healthy donor hearts to meet the growing demand. This problem, in the last twenty-five years, has forced medicine and society to completely reassess its definition of death, and even today there is still no good and reliable way to coordinate information about accidental death or other deaths, to ensure that a donor heart will be available when a dying patient needs one. At a recent meeting that I attended, one prominent cardiac surgeon, Dr. Denton Cooley of the University of Texas Medical Center in Houston, estimated that there might be as many as 33,000 eligible candidates for heart transplants in the United States in 1986—all of them people who will surely die without the opportunity of such surgery—but that only about 800 donor hearts can be expected to become available during that year, and not many more than perhaps 1,000 per year available by 1990. Obviously, this is not so much a medical problem as a terrible problem of logistics—simply identifying and acquiring enough suitable donor hearts. It will only be solved by widespread public education and such logistical solutions as an integrated, nationwide, before-death registry of potential heart donors. So far, no such registry is anywhere in sight.

The major *medical* problem with heart transplants is, of course, the problem of rejection—the continuing attempt of the recipient's immune system to reject or destroy the implanted donor heart as a threatening foreign body. This problem is far too complex to discuss here in any detail; let it suffice to say that, in order to enable a patient's body to accept and retain a transplanted heart, it is necessary to suppress or destroy many elements of that patient's natural immune protective system, so that if his or her body does retain the transplanted heart, it must be at the cost of leaving the patient vastly immunoincompetent, and thus highly vulnerable to attacks by bacteria, virus infections, various cancers, and so forth. At first, the very medications and drugs that were needed to suppress the patient's immune system were themselves so toxic that they could barely be tolerated. Today, one very special immunosuppressive drug, known as cyclosporin, has completely changed the picture for the better. It has proved highly effective in suppressing the immune system with far fewer toxic side effects than were caused by the drugs formerly used. As a result, the problem of rejection has become much easier to control in a great number of heart transplant patients, with significantly longer survival times.

There is reason to hope that ways may be found in the future to bridge these problems more and more effectively, but there are some other problems that may prove unbridgeable. The most obvious of these is the fact that any transplant patient, after surgery, must undergo intensive, continued, and prolonged medical and surgical follow-up for as long as he or she lives, and the overall gross cost of prolonging a single human life by means of heart transplantation is staggering. Few patients, indeed, can meet such costs from private resources; no one has yet found any equitable and feasible way to meet such costs with health insurance for any broad population of patients, and there is heated debate whether society, as a whole, even an affluent society such as ours, should have to assume the burden of such costs even for a relatively few selected individuals, to say nothing of tens of thousands of patients a year, at an aggregate cost of perhaps one-quarter of a million dollars or more per patient.

The other ultimate solution for dealing with terminal heart disease is a subject of even more controversy: the permanent implantation of completely artificial mechanical hearts as an alternative to implantation of natural donor hearts. This work was pioneered by Dr. William De Vries, a cardiac surgeon working first at the University of Utah, and later at the Humana Hospital in Lexington, Kentucky, utilizing an implantable mechanical heart designed by Dr. Robert Jarvik—the so-called Jarvik 7 heart. Later somewhat differently designed mechanical hearts have been utilized in Phoenix, Arizona, and Hershey, Pennsylvania, in human patients. At this time of writing such hearts have been used only in a handful of patients, and the procedure simply cannot yet be evaluated in any meaningful way. These operations have been undertaken only in patients who were so desperately and terminally ill as to be literally at death's doorstop before the surgery was done. The surgery is still on a completely experimental basis, and it has been performed regardless of the almost unbelievable expense; a number of these patients are still "in progress," with no way to guess to what degree these efforts may prove ultimately successful or even feasible. But the problems these efforts face are truly staggering. On the one hand, there is the problem of the emotional distress of a patient who must be tied to a pumping machine, perhaps to a single room, for as long as he or she may survive. This may not prove insurmountable. Polio victims have been known to live for decades in an iron lung, unable to move anything but their eyelids and cheek muscles, and have still led happy, productive lives. And surely, in time, the pumping apparatus will be miniaturized and made more portable.

Unfortunately, the medical and physiological problems of these early mechanical hearts are far more ominous. Those patients in whom they have been permanently installed have all suffered strokes or other cerebrovascular problems of one sort or another. The patients must be carried on anticoagulant drugs, and massive internal bleeding has been a recurrent problem. In addition, the mechanical hearts now in use all seem to destroy red blood cells prematurely, so the patient must have repeated transfusions. And other organ systems in the body, particularly the kidneys, may prove vulnerable to damage as a result of the mechanical heart's action.

Nobody yet knows why these medical problems occur in these patients. Some may arise simply because of unforeseen faults in design of the artificial hearts in their present form. But possibly the real problem lies much deeper than that. The artificial heart surgeons are attempting to install a rigid, inflexible pumping system into a living body made of soft tissue, flexible arteries and veins, and pliable organs and tissues that remain functional on the basis of biochemical reactions rather than electrical impulses or mechanical pounding. Many of the problems suffered by the early artificial heart patients— strokes, kidney failure, lung problems, blood cell destruction, and so forth—seem very much akin to the kinds of problems suffered by patients who have had to remain on the heart-lung machine too long. In a sense, the artificial heart, as it is presently designed, is a water-hammer, and a water-hammer will knock down anything if you give it long enough. It may well be that a rigid, inflexible artificial heart will sooner or later beat any patient's blood vascular system, kidneys, and lungs to death, so that the whole concept of the permanently implanted artificial heart as we understand it today may simply have to be discarded.

But it is far too soon to come to any such conclusion on the basis of what we know today. On October 25, 1985, an extraordinary conference took place in Washington, D.C.—a day-long dialogue between a panel of internationally recognized cardiac surgeons and representatives of the nation's newspaper, magazine, and broadcasting media. Among the doctors in attendance were Dr. William De Vries, who implanted the first permanent artificial heart in a patient (Dr. Barney Clark) at the University of Utah; Dr. Christiaan Barnard, who performed the first donor heart transplant; Dr. Denton Cooley of the University of Texas at Houston, the first surgeon to use an artificial heart in a patient temporarily while awaiting a donor heart for transplant; Dr. Jack Copeland of the University of Arizona in Tucson, who also implanted a permanent artificial heart in a patient; Dr. Robert Jarvik, designer of the Jarvik 7 artificial heart; Dr. Bjarne Semb, a cardiac surgeon from the Karolinska Institute in Stockholm, who has also implanted an artificial heart in a patient; and others. The purpose of the meeting was to review the state of the art of heart replacement surgery as of late 1985, and to discuss some of the ethical problems involved in reporting this work to the general public.

All the surgeons present were unanimous in their agreement that experimental work with artificial hearts must go on, and must continue to be done with human patients. But there was sharp disagreement as to what role the artificial heart would or should ultimately play in heart replacement surgery. Drs. Cooley and Barnard, for example, argued that there were far too many bugs in the artificial hearts currently available to use them as permanent heart replacements. At least in the short term—perhaps the next ten years— they felt that the highest, best, and safest use of the artificial heart should be as a temporary bridge to be used in a dying heart patient to keep him or her alive just long enough for a suitable donor heart to be obtained and implanted as a heart transplant. A second potential use—really a corollary of the first—would be to use the artificial heart as a lifesaving backup, ready for use in a case in which a transplanted donor heart went into failure within a few hours or days after transplantation (as some donor hearts do). Drs. De Vries and Semb, on the other hand, were much more optimistic that the artificial heart "bugs" could be resolved relatively quickly, so that a modified and improved artificial heart might soon offer the best hope for permanent heart replacement.

Certainly, that time is not yet. And in the meantime, ironing out the bugs must inevitably mean making hard choices and sacrifices. In a very real sense, the handful of patients so far receiving permanent artificial hearts have been sacrificial lambs, and continued work in this area will mean that more of them will be necessary. Dr. Robert Jarvik pointed out that he already had half a dozen or more possible improvements or modifications planned for his Jarvik hearts—but he wanted, ideally, to make those improvements just one at a time, not two or three simultaneously, in order to be able to learn which improvement helped and which didn't. Scientifically, this makes sense. But such a stepwise development program would require two, three, or more sacrificial lambs for each step along the way.

Some of the doctors speculated that a totally new and different approach to artificial heart design might be needed. Perhaps the water-hammer effect of a flexible diaphragm, to drive blood through the heart in a "normal" pulsating manner, might be avoided by devising a continuous flow pump, essentially producing blood circulation without a pulse! No one can guess how the body would deal with *that*. But it was pointed out that men spent centuries trying to fly by imitating nature—the flapping of birds' wings—and failed miserably in every attempt. It was not until the "unnatural" design of fixed-wing aircraft was devised that human flight became possible.

Thus, it may well be twenty-five years, fifty, or a hundred before we have final answers as to whether any permanently implanted artificial heart can ever be an ultimate solution to terminal heart disease. In the meantime there are some halfway measures that will surely be explored in the near future, not in terms of total heart transplants or total permanent artificial hearts, but in the development of various heart-assist devices, mechanical devices that can be used temporarily or permanently to relieve an ailing heart of much of the work that it has to do, and, thus, it is hoped, prolong survival should heart disease develop. The aortic-assist pump that I discussed earlier, used in some cases in the immediate postoperative care of coronary artery bypass graft patients, for example, is one of the simplest of such heart-assist devices—easy to install at the moment of need, by means of a catheter, and intended only for brief temporary use, over a period of a few hours or days, to help a recovering heart get over a temporary crisis. It could not be used for long-term assistance—but there are devices now existing that can be used for longer-term help, and a great deal of developmental work is being done on a variety of alternative devices of this sort. It is almost certain that such devices will, within a few years, become part of the regular armamentarium of treatment for extensive and severe coronary artery disease.

— 16 —

Forewarned is forearmed: You can't defend yourself against an enemy you don't understand. Twenty years ago, one of the most terrible things about coronary artery disease was that practically none of its victims knew anything much about it—where it came from, what caused it, how it might progress, how it might be treated, what might conceivably be done to protect against it, or, maybe, even prevent it altogether. It was a shadowy, devastating killer that struck out of the blue like an act of God, slaughtering many of its victims, crippling and shortening the lives of others. When it struck, it struck, and that was that; even for those who survived, nothing would ever be the same.

Today, we know that there is no need for that kind of ignorance anymore. This disease—still a killer, still a crippler—today is a perfectly comprehensible disease process, simple and straightforward in its nature. Everything about it makes sense. Anyone can understand a few basic, underlying facts about this killer. You don't have to be a physician or have a medical education, or even a great deal of medical sophistication, to grasp those basic facts and understand what coronary artery disease is all about.

The whole purpose of *The Elk Hunt* has been to provide a fairly simple information base, to explain in terms that any person can understand what the disease is, what it can do to you and how, what can be done about it today, and how it can be blocked or prevented. My personal experience, as I have related it here, has been unique, not universal, since every single individual's coronary artery disease is unique, but it has provided a springboard for explaining and clarifying a great many things about this devastating disease process.

One thing is blindingly clear: Prevention is the keystone to conquering coronary artery disease. We know a great deal more today about underlying *preventable* causes and risk factors connected with this disease than ever before. We have seen how each individual can assess his or her own individual risk and can actively work to protect him- or herself against coronary artery disease, not by massive and convulsive alterations in living patterns but through simple, livable, achievable modifications.

I have not dwelt heavily on specific detailed rules and guidelines for prevention in this book; there are many, far better sources for this information than any that I can provide. There are whole books, authoritative books, detailing the kind of dietary modifications that can and will help as powerful preventive measures. There are good books dealing with improving physical fitness and establishing exercise habits, which can contribute greatly not only to maintaining cardiovascular health but to maintaining a more active and interesting life. There are others detailing specific ways that you can help yourself eliminate your addictions to caffeine, alcohol, and, most especially, to cigarette smoking and the use of tobacco, which is such a major and completely eliminatable risk factor for the development of this disease. Still other books provide insight into dealing with the kinds of social, emotional, interpersonal, or business tensions that surely contribute equally, but less directly, to the progress and severity of this disease.

The Elk Hunt cannot provide detail in all these areas, but I have tried to provide an underlying baseline of knowledge, both for those of you who are so far free of coronary artery disease, at least as far as you know, and for those who have already had its presence demonstrated, whether spectacularly or not. I believe that we are entering a new era of understanding, prevention, and effective treatment of this killer disease, an era that will be marked by a sharp decrease in the incidence of acute, catastrophic coronary heart attacks, as well as a sharp decrease in coronary death rates, and with a great bursting forth of new alternatives and options in dealing with this disease when it appears. And in such an era, having the basic facts to know and recognize the enemy can make all the difference between life and death.

Toward the end of one sunny afternoon in late October of last year, almost five years to the day since my heart attack and approaching the first anniversary of my bypass operation, Ann and I drove our four-wheel-drive rig up the Taneum Canyon road, past the creekside campgrounds and logging spurs, then up an old road high into the mountain foothills—a ragged, rocky road climbing up out of the Shadow Creek Gully to the high wooded plateau above that we loved to hunt so much. The days had been dry and hot, but the nights chilly, so that the cottonwoods and tamaracks were in the full change of their fall colors.

At the top of the plateau we had a variety of choices. A road to the left went up to a hunter's camp area of steep wooded hills and gullies. Another road went out to a steep ridge that dropped off straight down to Shadow Creek, a favorite escapeway for elk on the move. To the right was a little road that dropped down to cross a creek bed and then wandered through an old forest area. The logging companies had spent the summer in this area, taking out forest in pieces and patches, disrupting great chunks of a beautiful wooded wilderness that we had hunted year after year. Now, with the year's elk hunt fast approaching, we were simply scouting to see what we could see.

We found that a new logging road had been cut through the area, built of crushed rock and soft dirt mixed with clay, still boggy from rain earlier in the fall, with mud holes and ruts. We were driving slowly up the road, bemoaning the ugliness of the logging operation, when the bull elk stood up from his bed, just below the road some twenty-five yards ahead of us.

We stopped the car and watched. He stepped up in front of us, crossing the road and going up the steep bank on the right with absolute effortlessness. Then he stopped to look back at us. He was sleek and handsome, in full fall color, his head, neck, and legs black, his body tawny, his rump white as snow. He had fine, high-spreading antlers, with three points on each side, and he flicked flies away with his ears as he stood there watching us for long seconds, completely unhurried. Then, as though dismissing us completely, he turned his head away, lifted his chin, lay his antlers back on his shoulders, and cantered on up to disappear into the thickets of tamarack and fir.

Something stirred in my mind then. Suddenly, it seemed to me that I had seen that same elk in that same place in that same way some time before. I thought to myself, stick around, my friend, I'll be back here just a few days from now, and maybe we'll meet again. I thought, maybe this year when the elk season opens, I can come up here and hunt, really *hunt*, again. But, then again, maybe not. Because, after all, I thought, like everybody else, both that elk and I are living on borrowed time.

— AFTERWORD —

In my final review of the manuscript of this book, it strikes me that I have been exceptionally hard on one group of people who deserve far better from me: the nurses who are engaged in all aspects of the care of people with coronary artery disease. Perhaps this is natural. Like many obsessive-compulsive people, I resent being ill and resent hospitalization as a totally unwelcome intrusion on my life. And, as a corollary, I tend to resent and reject nurses as part and parcel of illness and hospitalization. This is not only irrational, it's grossly unfair to nurses as well.

Dr. Richard Anderson, who did my bypass operation, presented a different view: "I view nurses as indispensable, compassionate, comforting presences who are the guardians of the patient's moment-to-moment well-being during dangerous times, and who, too often, are caught in the middle of a no-win sitaution between some physician's oversight and a system which impedes their independent initiative."

I can only say amen to that. I have not changed the manuscript, because I think the personal parts are only valid insofar as they reflect *how it was*, from my perception, not how it ought to have been. But I am clearly aware of how much I owe those nurses—far more than I have given them credit for—and I guarantee that I will give them a better (and more realistic) press in the future.

—A.E.N.

— INDEX —

A

Acute anterior marginal branch, 129, 130, 134
Adipose tissue, 21
Adrenal glands, 20, 84, 164
Adrenaline, 84; as risk factor for coronary artery disease, 67–68, 71, 84, 179
Adrenergic hormones, 84, 179
Adult onset diabetes, 166–67
Adventitia, 16, 17
Age, 28; as risk factor for coronary artery disease, 175–76, 180
Aid Cars, 282
Alcohol, 28, 45, 99, 164; as risk factor for coronary artery disease, 174–75, 180
Ambulances, 42–43
American Heart Association, 181n
American Red Cross, 282
Anatomy of heart and coronary arteries, 16–20, 127–34
Androgens, 20
Anesthesia, in bypass surgery, 225–26, 232, 242 and n, 255
Aneurysm, 147

Anger, as risk factor for coronary heart disease, 67–68, 84, 87, 178–79
Angina pectoris, 23–25, 59, 61–87, 91, 108–109, 201–202, 218; anger as trigger for, 67–68, 84, 87; bypass surgery relief of, 218–20, 230, 231, 255, 256–57, 261, 264; effect on sexual intercourse, 68, 156 and n, 192–93; EKG testing of, 73–76; exertional, 61–62, 63, 66–71, 79–80, 138, 139, 156, 189, 191; medication for, 63, 81–87, 148, 155–56, 186–92, 215, 277; nature and distribution of pain, 23–24, 69–70; at rest, 62–63, 67, 71–72, 87, 112–13, 138, 139, 156, 187–88, 191, 200, 215; treadmill testing of, 76–81; waxing and waning of, 214–15
Angiograms. *See* Coronary angiograms
Angioplasty, 268–71
Ankle edema, 193, 194
Annual physical exams, 30
Anticoagulant drugs, 267

Aorta, 18, 19, 127, 128; in bypass surgery, 222
Aortic arch, 19
Aortic assist pump, 234, 288
Arizona Heart Institute Cardiovascular Risk Factor Analysis, 181, 182
Arrhythmia, cardiac, 27–28, 31, 40, 90, 110–12, 155, 190; medication for, 278–80
Arteries, 15–16, 128; atheroma development in, 21–23; basic structure and function of, 16–20. *See also specific arteries*
Arterioles, 16
Artificial graft materials, 221, 267
Artificial heart valves, 267
Artificial mechanical hearts, 285–88
Artificial pacemakers, 280–81
Atelectasis, 252, 254
Atheromata, 25; development of, 20–23
Atherosclerosis, 70, 71, 76, 132; development of, 20–23; risk factors for, 160–83
Atherosclerotic heart disease (ASHD), 13, 21

B

Balloon catheters, 269–70
Balloon pump, 227
Barnard, Christiaan, 283, 286, 287
Beck, Claude, 29
Bernard, Claude, 118
Beta-blockers, 59, 84–85, 86, 148, 190 and *n*, 191–92, 207, 277; effect on sex drive, 156 and *n*, 193
Blacks, coronary artery disease as threat to, 165
Blood clots, 25–26, 138, 233, 272; induced by artificial graft materials, 267; and thrombolysis, 272–77
Blood flow, oxygenated, 15, 18–20, 127, 214; blockages of, 23–28, 64–72, 133, 136–38, 214–15; cigarette smoking effect on, 173; collateral sources of, 133–34, 219
Blood platelets, 25
Blood pressure, 27, 40, 84*n*; high, as risk factor for coronary artery disease, 165–66, 180
Blood vessels, 15–20
Bradycardia, 110
Brain, 128; blood flow to, 18, 23; damage, 28, 222
Breakfast meats, 176
Butter, 177, 178
Bypass surgery, 42, 110, 122, 130, 132, 148, 201–202, 217–62; anesthesia for, 225–26, 232, 242 and *n*, 255; angina relieved by, 218–20, 230, 231, 255, 256–57, 261, 264; angiogram analysis for, 217–19, 233, 269; benefits of, 264–65; cardiac conferences used in, 121–22, 147, 228; CASS study on, 229–30; costs of, 227, 228, 268; disadvantages of, 265–66, 268; double, 223; graft materials for, 220–22, 231, 265–67; and heart failure, 219–20, 226–27, 234; history of, 227–30; life extension statistics, 220, 266–67; medical staff and equipment for, 225; mortality in, 226, 228, 230, 232, 234, 236, 268; number of grafts, 224; operative record of, 258–60; overuse and abuse of, 227–28; postop appearance of patient, 248, 250, 251; postop compli-

cations, 232–34, 249, 254; procedure, 220–27, 260; recovery from, 248–62; reoperation, 230–31, 267–68; respiratory and physical therapy after, 233, 250–54; risks of, 222–23, 225–26, 228; triple, 223

C

Calan, 85, 187
Calcium, 22, 187
Calcium slow-channel blockers, 85, 148, 186–88, 277
Capillaries, 15; basic structure of, 16–20
Carbohydrates, 20–21, 171, 175
Carbon monoxide, 173
Cardiac arrest, 28, 31; reversing, 281–82
Cardiac attack, defined, 12–13
Cardiac catherization, 42, 91–92, 272; history of, 117–26; hospital procedure, 140–42
Cardiac conferences, 121–22, 147, 201, 228
Cardiac output, 80, 118, 249, 250
Cardiac surgery, history of, 117–18, 120–25. *See also* Bypass surgery
Cardiopulmonary resuscitation (CPR), 281–82
Cardiovascular system, basic structure and function of, 15–20
Cardizem, 85
Carotid arteries, 18, 23, 128
Cereal, 177
Cheeses, 176, 177
Chest pain. *See* Angina pectoris
Cheyne-Stokes breathing, 193
Cholesterol, 20, 57, 98 and *n*, 163, 175; defined, 20; dietary reduction of, 99, 177; excess deposits of, 21–23, 171, 176–77

Cigarette smoking, 30, 44, 164; quitting, 99–100, 155, 174 and *n*, 289; as risk factor for coronary artery disease, 172–74, 180
Circulatory system, basic structure and function of, 16–20
Circumflex artery, 129, 130, 131, 137, 147; bypass surgery for, 223
Circumstances at time of heart attack, 28–30
Clark, Barney, 286
Code Blue, 42
Cold-pressor test, 146
Cold weather, sensitivity to, 68, 87, 156–57
Collateral arteries, 69, 133, 219
Collateral circulation, 133–34
Complete revascularization, 224
Congenital heart disease, history of treatment for, 117–26
Congestive heart failure, 31, 194–95, 200, 201, 215–16, 278
Contrast agents, 122, 123, 135, 142
Cooking oils, 176, 177
Cooley, Denton, 286, 287
Copeland, Jack, 287
Coronary, 12, 13
Coronary angiography, 42, 92, 126, 134–39, 217; history of, 122–25; hospital procedure, 140–42; interpretation of, 136–39, 147–48, 217–19, 233, 269; technique of, 135–36
Coronary arteries, 13, 18; anatomy and function of, 127–34; collateral circulation in, 133–34

Coronary artery bypass graft surgery (CABG). *See* Bypass surgery

Coronary artery catherization. *See* Cardiac catherization

Coronary artery disease (CAD), 13; angiogram interpretation of, 136–39, 147–48, 217–19, 233, 269; basic facts of, 13–14; EKG testing of, 73–76; 1960s–1980s improvements in treatment of, 88–89; prevention of, 88–89, 289–90; risk factors for, 160–83; and size and shape of arteries, 132; treadmill testing of, 76–81; warning signs of, 23–30; world distribution of, 161–62. *See also specific arteries and types of disease*

Coronary Artery Surgery Study (CASS), 220, 229–30

Coronary occlusion, 12, 13, 26–28

Coronary thrombosis, 12, 13, 26–28

Counand, André, 120

Cyclosporin, 285

D

Dacron fabric artery grafts, 267

Dairy products, 99, 176, 177

Defibrillator, 29

Demerol, 34

Descending aorta, 19

De Vries, William, 285, 286, 287

Diabetes, 164; as risk factor for coronary artery disease, 166–67, 180

Diagonal branches, 129, 130

Dicumerol, 272

Diet, 20–21, 30, 57, 114, 155, 165; and angina, 68, 87; control program, 98–99, 117–78; food

preparation, 99, 177; high-cholesterol, 176–77; low-cholesterol, 177; red meat reduced in, 99; as risk factor for coronary artery disease, 166, 176–78, 180

Digitalis, 227, 277–78

Digitoxin, 209, 278

Diltiazem, 85

Donor hearts, 284, 287

Dopamine, 251

Double bypass surgery, 223

Drugs. *See* Medications

Dyspnea, 193–94, 207, 217

E

Edema, 193, 194, 221, 272; pulmonary, 206–209, 215, 217

Eggs, 176, 177

Einthoven, Willem, 72–73

Ejection fraction, 144–45, 148

Electrical activity of heart, 27, 73–76

Electrical shock, 28

Electrocardiogram (EKG), 27, 67n, 72–76, 78–79, 111, 146, 201; invention of, 72–73; memory cardiobeeper, 279; normal, 74–75

Electrocardiograph monitor, 32

Emergency room, 10–12

Emotional conflict, as risk factor for coronary artery disease, 67–68, 178–79, 180

Endotracheal tube, 232–33, 250

Enzymes, 27, 208, 273

Epinephrine, 84, 250, 251

Estrogens, 21, 164

Europe, coronary artery disease in, 161

Exercise, 114; and angina, 66–72, 79–80, 189, 191; lack of, and risk of coronary artery disease, 169–72; post–heart attack, 100–106, 158–60; types of, 171–72

Exertional angina, 61–62, 63, 66–71, 79–80, 138, 139, 156, 189, 191; patterns of, 68–72

F

Familial hypercholesterolemia, 163
Familial hyperlipidemia, 163
Family history, 30, 162–63
Family of heart attack victim, 36; reactions of, 36–40. *See also* Spouse of heart attack victim
Fats, 20–21, 171; excess, 21–23, 171, 176–77
Fatty acids, 20
Fight-flight reaction, 84
Finland, coronary artery disease in, 161
First heart attack, 28–29
Fish, 177
Food and Drug Administration (FDA), 85, 187
Forssmann, Werner, 117–20
Functional aerobic capacity (FAC), 80
Functional impairment, 138

G

Gastrointestinal tract, 15
Gender, as risk factor for coronary artery disase, 163–65, 176, 180
Gout, 55, 56
Graft materials, for bypass surgery, 231, 265–67

H

Hallucinations, 47–53
Harvard Step Test, 78–79

Headaches, as nitroglycerin side effect, 83, 87
Heart: basic anatomy and function of, 16–20, 127–34; electrical activity of, 27, 73–76; four major coronary vessels of, 128–30; normal muscle contraction and relaxation, 73–74; size of, 127
Heart attack, defined, 12–13
Heartbeat, 27; arrhythmic, 27–28, 31, 40, 90, 110–12, 155, 190, 278–80; average, 19; electrical stimulation of, 73–76
Heart failure, 27, 58, 86, 116, 206, 209, 277; and bypass surgery, 219–20, 226–27, 234; congestive, 194–95, 200, 201, 215–16, 278; medication for, 277–78
Heart-lung bypass machine, 120, 125, 222–23, 226, 245, 286
Heart transplants, 283–85; costs of, 285; problems with, 284–85; rate of success, 283
Heparin, 272
Heredity, as risk factor for coronary artery disease, 162–63, 180
Holter Monitor, 278–79
Hormones, 164; adrenergic, 84, 179; and cholesterol, 20
Hospital, choice of, 40–42
Hunter, Sir John, 67–68
Hypertension: medication for, 166; as risk factor for coronary artery disease, 165–66, 180

I

Impotence, 156n, 166
Inderal, 85, 86, 87, 110, 112, 155–

Inderal (*continued*)
56, 159, 186, 190 and *n*, 191–
92, 207, 257, 277
Indolence, physical, as risk factor
for coronary artery disease,
169–72, 180
Inferior vena cava, 19
Informed-consent forms, 140
Inhalation oxygen, 85–86
Insurance, 41
Intensive Care Unit (ICU), 246–51
Internal mammary artery grafts,
231, 266
Interventricular septum, 127, 130
Intima, 16, 17, 21
Intravenous thrombolysis, 275–77
Ischemia, 24, 26, 64–72, 76, 81,
132, 138, 172, 226; defined,
64
Isoptin, 85, 187
Isordil, 63, 83, 86, 87, 112, 113,
155, 159
Isosorbide dinitrite, 63, 83, 86

J

Japan, coronary artery disease in,
161
Jarvik, Robert, 286, 287
Jarvik 7 heart, 285
Jogging, 159–60
Juvenile onset diabetes, 166–67

K

Kidneys, 21, 166, 286; bypass surgery damage to, 234

L

Left anterior descending artery
(LAD), 129, 130, 131, 134,
137, 147; bypass surgery for,
223

Left atrium, 18, 19, 128
Left coronary arteriogram, 123–24
Left main coronary artery, 128,
137; anatomy and function
of, 128–34; bypass surgery
for, 230, 265
Left ventricle, 18, 19, 31, 127,
128, 129; severity of disease
based on impairment of, 143,
147–48; treadmill testing of,
144–46
Left Ventricular Assist Device
(LVAD), 227
Left ventricular branch, 129, 130
Left ventricular ejection fraction,
144–45, 148
Leg vein grafts, 220–23, 231, 245,
265, 266
Lesions, coronary artery, 269; angiogram interpretation of,
137–39, 269; PCTA recon-
struction of, 269–71
Lidocaine, 279
Lipoproteins, 20, 171, 175
Lithium, 193
Liver, 15, 31, 272; bypass surgery
damage to, 234
Lumen, 22
Lungs, 15, 18, 19, 64, 120; and
bypass surgery, 224, 227; cig-
arette smoking damage to,
172–73

M

Margarine, 177, 178
Marital problems during convalescence, 107–109, 193
Media, 16
Medications, 34, 40, 46, 57, 59,
88, 277–81; for angina, 63,
81–87, 148, 155–56, 186–92,
215, 277; for arrhythmia,
278–80; for blood clotting,

272–77; costs of, 190, 192; effect on sex drive, 156 and *n*, 193; for heart failure, 277–78; for high blood pressure, 166; toxicity of, 278, 279. *See also specific medicines*
Memory cardiobeeper, 279
Menopause, 164, 176
Mental defense mechanisms, 47
Metabolism, 162, 168, 171
Microobservation, 102–106
Morphine, 34, 207, 217
Mortality, 27–28, 290; in bypass surgery, 226, 228, 230, 232, 234, 236, 268; and number of major vessels involved, 131–32; rate statistics, 13, 29, 88, 183, 272; sudden death, 28, 29, 278, 281
Muscle tissue, 16–17, 21; injury to, 40
Muscularis, 16
Myocardial infarction (MI), defined, 12, 13
Myocardial ischemia. *See* Ischemia

N

Nausea, 27
New England Journal of Medicine, 266, 276
Nicotine, 172
Nifedipine, 85, 187, 191
Nitrates, 82–84, 86
Nitroglycerin paste, 34, 60, 83–84, 87, 113
Nitroglycerin pills, 59, 63, 82–83, 86–87, 191, 215; side effects of, 83, 87; under-the-tongue, 82–83
Nitrospan, 83
Norepinephrine, 84
Normal sinus rhythm, 74

Norpace, 112, 155, 190, 279
Nurses, 48–49, 293

O

Obesity, 21, 44; as risk factor for coronary artery disease, 167–69, 180
Obsessive-compulsive behavior, 178–79
Obstruction, angiogram interpretation of, 137–39, 147–48, 217–19, 233, 269
Obtuse marginal branch, 129, 130
Occlusion, 12, 13, 26–28, 138
Operative record of bypass surgery, 258–60
Organ meats, 176
Oxygen, inhalation, 85–86
Oxygenated blood flow. *See* Blood flow, oxygenated
Oxygen starvation, 23–28, 64–72

P

Pacemakers, cardiac, 280–81
Pasta, 177
Percutaneous translumenal coronary angioplasty (PTCA), 269–71
Peritrate, 83
Physical exams, annual, 30
Physical indolence, as risk factor for coronary artery disease, 169–72, 180
Physical therapy, after bypass surgery, 233, 250–54
Polydipsia, 167
Polyphagia, 167
Polyuria, 167
Portable respiratory tank, 239
Posterior descending branch, 129, 130
Posterolateral branch, 129, 130

Poultry, 177
Prevention of coronary artery disease, 14, 88–89, 289–90
Prinzmetal, M., 71
Prinzmetal's angina. *See* Variant angina
Private hospital room, 54–55
Procardia, 85, 187–88, 190
Progestogens, 20, 164
Propranolol, 59, 85, 86
Proteins, 20–21
Prothrombin, 272
Pulmonary arteries, 18, 31
Pulmonary circulation, 18, 19
Pulmonary edema, 206–209, 215, 217
Pulmonary embolus, 234
Pulmonary emphysema, 173
Pulmonary veins, 18
Pulse rate, 27, 159

Q

QRS complex, 75
Quadruple-vessel disease, 131

R

Race, as risk factor for coronary artery disease, 165, 180
Radioactive tracer studies, 143, 145–46
Red meats, 176; dietary reduction of, 99, 177
Referred pain, 24, 70
Retrograde amnesia, 35
Richards, Dickenson Woodruff, 120
Right atrium, 18, 19, 73, 128; catherization of, 119
Right coronary artery, 31, 128, 129, 137; anatomy and function of, 128–34; bypass surgery for, 223

Right ventricle, 18, 19, 31, 127, 128, 129, 143
Right ventricular branch, 129, 130
Risk factors for coronary artery disease, 160–83; age, 175–76, 180; alcohol, 174–75, 180; assessment of, 180–82; cigarette smoking, 172–74, 180; dealing with, 181–83; diabetes, 166–67, 180; diet, 166, 176–78, 180; emotional conflicts, 67–68, 178–79, 180; gender, 163–65, 176, 180; heredity, 162–63, 180; hypertension, 165–66, 180; obesity, 167–69, 180; physical indolence, 169–72, 180; race, 165, 180; and world distribution, 161–62
RISKO, 181*n*

S

Salt, dietary, 57, 99; and high blood pressure, 166
Saphenous vein grafts, 220–23, 231, 245, 265, 266
Saturated fats, 176, 177
Scar tissue, 113
Semb, Bjarne, 287
Septal branches, 130
Septal defects, 122, 123
Septum, 18, 127, 129
Severity of heart attack, 29
Sexual intercourse, 156*n*, 189, 192–93; and angina, 68, 156 and *n*, 192–93; effects of medication on, 156 and *n*, 193
Shock, 27
Shock box, 29, 281, 282
Single-vessel disease, 130, 131
Sino-atrial (S-A) node, 73, 74
Sinus of Valsalva, 127
Smoke-Enders, 174 and *n*
Sones, Mason, 122–24

Splenic artery, use in bypass surgery, 221
Spouse of heart attack victim, 36; reactions of, during bypass surgery, 243–55; reactions of, during convalescence, 107–109, 193; reactions of, immediately following heart attack, 36–40
Stanford University heart transplant program, 283 and *n*
Streptokinase, 273–76
Stress, as risk factor for coronary artery disease, 67–68, 108, 178–79, 180
Stroke, 41, 166, 222, 286; during bypass surgery, 233
Subclavian arteries, 128
Sudden death, 28, 29, 278, 281
Superior vena cava, 19
Surgery, cardiac, history of, 117–18, 120–25. *See also* Bypass surgery
Swan-Ganz line, 245, 248
Swimming, 171
Systemic circulation, 18, 19

T

Temperature changes, sensitivity to, 68, 87, 156–57
Tennis, 171
Tension, as risk factor for coronary artery disease, 67–68, 178–79, 180
Terminal heart disease, solutions for, 283–88
Thalium, radioactive, 145–46
Thrombolysis, 273–77
Thrombosis, 12, 13, 26–28
Tissue plasminogen activator (Tpa), 275–77

Transdermal nitroglycerin patches, 83–84
Translumenal coronary thrombolysis, 271–77
Transplants, heart. *See* Heart transplants
Treadmill test, 63, 67*n*, 76–81, 91, 143–44; development of, 78–79; procedure, 145–46
Triglycerides, 20, 163, 175, 176–77
Triple bypass surgery, 223
Triple-vessel disease, 130, 131–32
Two-vessel disease, 130, 131
Type A personality, 178, 179
Type B personality, 178, 179

U

Ulceration, 25–26
Underdeveloped countries, coronary artery disease in, 161–62

V

Variant angina, 62–63, 67, 71–72, 87, 112–13, 138, 139, 156, 187–88, 191, 200, 215; causes of, 187
Vascular system, basic structure and function of, 15–20
Veins, 15; basic structure and function of, 16–20; saphenous, use in bypass surgery, 220–23, 231, 245, 265, 266
Venous stasis, 233
Venous thrombi, 233
Ventricular fibrillation, 27–28, 29, 31, 111, 281
Verapimil, 85, 187

W

Walking, 171, 172; as post–heart
  attack exercise, 100–106, 158–
  60, 184
Warfarin, 272
Warning signs of coronary artery
  disease, 23–30
Women, coronary artery disease

as threat to, 163–65,
  176

X

X-ray image intensifier, 135
X rays, 118, 119, 123, 135–36. *See
  also* Coronary angiography